# AI and Machine Learning Applications in Sports Analytics

Tanupriya Choudhury
*University of Petroleum and Energy Studies, Dehradun, India*

Pradeep Kumar Arya
*Symbiosis International University, India*

Ketan Kotecha
*Symbiosis Centre for Applied Artificial Intelligence, Symbiosis International University, India*

Ashutosh Sharma
*Henan University of Science and Technology, China*

Jung-Sup Um
*Kyungpook National University, South Korea*

IGI Global
Scientific Publishing
Publishing Tomorrow's Research Today

Vice President of Editorial — Melissa Wagner
Director of Acquisitions — Mikaela Felty
Director of Book Development — Jocelynn Hessler
Production Manager — Mike Brehm
Cover Design — Phillip Shickler

Published in the United States of America by
IGI Global Scientific Publishing
701 East Chocolate Avenue
Hershey, PA, 17033, USA
Tel: 717-533-8845
Fax: 717-533-7115
Website: https://www.igi-global.com E-mail: cust@igi-global.com



Library of Congress Cataloging-in-Publication Data

Names: Choudhury, Tanupriya, editor. | Arya, Pradeep Kumar, 1985- editor. | Kotecha, Ketan, editor. | Sharma, Ashutosh, 1992- editor. | Um, Jung-Sup, 1956- editor.
Title: AI and machine learning applications in sports analytics / Edited by Tanupriya Choudhury, Pradeep Arya, Ketan Kotecha, Ashutosh Sharma, Jung-Sup Um.
Other titles: Aritfical intelligence and machine learning applications in sports analytics
Description: Hershey, PA : Business Science Reference (an imprint of IGI Global), [2025] | Includes bibliographical references and index. | Summary: "This book is an insightful exploration into how artificial intelligence (AI) and machine learning (ML) are transforming sports analytics. The book serves as a primer on AI and ML, making it accessible to novices while delving into their applications across various facets of sports, such as player performance analysis, game strategy optimization, injury prediction, talent scouting, and fan engagement"-- Provided by publisher.
Identifiers: LCCN 2024037882 | ISBN 9798369353851 (hardcover) | ISBN 9798369353868 (paperback) | ISBN 9798369353875 (ebook)
Subjects: LCSH: Sports--Statistical methods. | Artificial intelligence--Statistical methods. | Sports--Technological innovations. | Machine learning.
Classification: LCC GV741 .A32 2024 | DDC 796.02/1--dc23/eng/20240917
LC record available at https://lccn.loc.gov/2024037882
British Cataloguing in Publication Data
A Cataloguing in Publication record for this book is available from the British Library.

# Table of Contents

# Detailed Table of Contents

environments. The goal at the end of the road for AI-based systems is optimal athletic performance, but all this should be done with the aim of supporting long-term health and well-being.



This chapter will review the key building blocks and best practices to assemble an effective sports analytics team in the contemporary sports landscape. It covers the key functions, competence needs, hiring and recruitment strategies, and the design and dynamics of teamwork. It also articulates the technological tool requirements and the infrastructures involving data collection and processing, where it strongly emphasizes the importance of instituting a decision-making culture with data. It is, therefore, an examination of some trends that might shape the future of sports organizations, like being introduced by artificial intelligence and video analytics, and also challenges associated with such analyses and enhancements. From this analysis, sports organizations stand to position themselves accordingly to enable analytics help improve performances, inform decision-making, and engage fans better.



This chapter explores the transformative role of artificial intelligence (AI) and machine learning in optimizing game strategy within sports. By analyzing historical game data, AI enhances tactical decision-making, player development, and real-time adjustments during competitions. The integration of predictive analytics allows teams to anticipate future performance trends and adapt strategies accordingly, while AI-powered tools foster personalized training regimens and injury prevention. Furthermore, the collaboration between AI and human insight encourages a dynamic partnership that enriches coaching and gameplay. Despite its benefits, ethical considerations regarding data privacy, fairness, and competitive integrity must be addressed to ensure responsible AI use. As these technologies become more accessible, they will democratize strategy optimization, empowering teams at all levels. This chapter ultimately highlights the potential of AI to reshape the landscape of sports, driving innovation and improving overall performance.

This chapter explores the use of artificial intelligence (AI) to forecast injuries and put preventative measures in place in a variety of industries, including sports, healthcare, and workplace safety. It talks about the machine learning and data analytics techniques used in injury prediction with AI systems. The chapter also looks at the importance of proactive injury prevention techniques made possible by AI, emphasizing how they may reduce hazards and improve general safety. It also examines the difficulties and restrictions posed by this methodology, highlighting the significance of ethical issues, data privacy protection, and the interpretation of insights produced by AI. In summary, this chapter addresses relevant issues and concerns while offering insights into the exciting developments in injury prediction and prevention made possible by AI technology.



This chapter explores the transformative role of artificial intelligence (AI) in enhancing fan engagement within the sports industry. By examining key applications such as predictive ticket pricing, personalized content delivery, and immersive experiences through augmented and virtual reality, the chapter highlights how AI technologies create deeper connections between fans and sports organizations. It discusses the practical, managerial, societal, and ethical implications of integrating AI, emphasizing the importance of data privacy and fairness in AI-driven initiatives. As sports organizations leverage data analytics and machine learning, they can deliver customized experiences that resonate with diverse fan bases while fostering community engagement. Ultimately, this chapter underscores the potential of AI to reshape the future of fan interactions, making sports more accessible and engaging for everyone.

This chapter explores the role of machine learning (ML) in injury prevention and rehabilitation for athletes. It examines how ML models can predict injuries by analysing diverse data sources, such as biomechanics, wearables, and medical records, and highlights the potential for personalized, data-driven injury prevention strategies. The chapter also addresses how AI-driven rehabilitation programs can adapt in real-time to optimize recovery and reduce the risk of re-injury. Key challenges, such as data privacy, model complexity, and the need for explainable AI, are discussed, along with future trends like the integration of wearable technology, federated learning, and virtual reality in rehabilitation. These innovations promise to transform sports medicine by making injury prevention more accurate and rehabilitation more efficient, ultimately enhancing athlete performance and longevity.



In cricket, choosing the best team (Playing-11) is crucial. Cricket, as a sport, has witnessed a notable shift towards data-driven decision-making in recent years. We look at past players performance to understand how teams can predict their ideal players. This survey explores various data sources, tools, and techniques used in cricket analytics, offering insights into the broader landscape of data-driven decision-making and also shows the concept how data science and machine learning are changing the game. Serving as a guide for players, coaches, and fans, this paper provides a user-friendly exploration of the ways in which data science is reshaping cricket strategies and enhancing the precision of team selection. It's like a playbook for understanding how technology is making cricket team decisions smarter.

Artificial Intelligence (AI) is revolutionizing sports organizations by enhancing talent scouting, player development, and operational efficiency. This chapter explores the transformative role of AI and machine learning in identifying and nurturing athletic talent. It delves into the evolution of talent scouting, the integration of AI technologies such as predictive analytics and wearable sensors, and the implications for player development. Key sections address AI-driven scouting methods, player performance optimization, and the ethical and legal considerations of using AI. The chapter also discusses practical and managerial challenges in implementing AI systems, including data privacy and bias mitigation. By examining future trends and innovations, it provides a comprehensive overview of how AI is reshaping sports management and offers insights into the ethical and practical considerations that organizations must navigate.



In professional sports, there is potential to leverage extensive and detailed datasets generated from various aspects of the sports industry. However, challenges arise from the limited time available for data analysis and the vast amount and diversity of the data to be evaluated. Artificial Intelligence (AI) techniques can significantly aid decision-makers in addressing these challenges. Over the past twenty years, AI has significantly impacted how we analyze and engage with sports. This perspective paper offers a comprehensive overview of the machine learning paradigm, highlighting its potential to improve sports performance and business analytics. It reviews relevant research on AI and ML applications within the sports industry and presents hypothetical scenarios demonstrating how these technologies might influence the future of sports.

Talent identification and scouting are essential in sports, enabling organizations to identify and nurture talented players destined for success. This chapter focuses on how artificial neural networks (ANNs) have transformed these processes. It covers ANNs' basics, data collection, and preprocessing ideas specific to sports analytics. It shows various neural network types, like feedforward, convolutional, and recurrent networks, useful for tasks like injury prediction, performance measurement, and future prediction. Additionally, it includes a discussion of training and optimization algorithms, case studies, and real-world applications in various sports. The chapter concludes by addressing challenges and future research, including data quality, interpretability, ethical issues, and ANNs' integration with other modern technologies. Utilizing ANNs' potential may significantly develop sports organizations by helping them identify and nurture talented players and gain a competitive edge in a data and technology-based future of sport.



The integration of artificial intelligence (AI) and machine learning (ML) in sports analytics offers significant advancements in performance enhancement, strategy development, and injury prevention. However, it also presents critical ethical challenges that require careful consideration. This paper explores these ethical issues through four case studies: player privacy and data security in the New England Patriots, bias in talent identification at FC Barcelona's La Masia academy, the impact on coaching and decision-making in the Los Angeles Lakers, and long-term health implications at Manchester City. The analysis highlights the importance of transparency, fairness, and the safeguarding of athletes' well-being. Practical, ethical, theoretical, managerial, and societal implications are discussed, alongside limitations and future research directions. This paper emphasizes the need for a balanced approach that integrates AI insights with human expertise to ensure ethical and effective use in sports.

# Preface

We are pleased to present *AI and Machine Learning Applications in Sports Analytics*, a pioneering reference book that captures the profound transformation artificial intelligence (AI) and machine learning (ML) are bringing to the world of sports. This volume is the result of a shared vision to bridge the gap between cutting-edge technological advancements and practical applications in the dynamic and high-impact domain of sports analytics.

As editors, we have curated contributions from leading experts and researchers who delve into the many ways AI and ML are redefining how we understand, play, manage, and experience sports. From optimizing game strategy to predicting injuries, from analyzing player performance to enhancing fan engagement, this book offers a multifaceted exploration of how data-driven methodologies are shaping the present and future of sports.

The rapid proliferation of data sources — from high-resolution video footage to wearable sensors and social media — has made traditional methods of analysis insufficient. AI and ML offer the computational power and intelligence to process and interpret this data with remarkable precision and depth. Through this book, readers will discover how deep learning, reinforcement learning, and other AI techniques are being applied in real-world sports scenarios, yielding insights that were once unimaginable.

For instance, in chapters focused on performance analysis, readers will learn how advanced models extract meaningful patterns from thousands of gameplay hours, helping coaches fine-tune strategies and individual training regimens. Similarly, injury prediction models showcased in this volume demonstrate how AI can anticipate physical setbacks by considering a complex web of physiological and environmental factors. These innovations are not theoretical — they are already being adopted by elite sports organizations globally.

In compiling this book, we were guided by the belief that this knowledge should be accessible not only to experienced data scientists and industry professionals but also to educators, students, and decision-makers in the sports ecosystem. Thus, we have ensured that the content is both technically sound and pedagogically valuable. Each chapter is structured to build understanding progressively, making the book suitable as a textbook for subjects such as *Artificial Intelligence in Sports*, *Sports Analytics*, *Game Strategy Optimization*, and *Technology and Policy Studies*, offered in a range of academic programs including Computer Science, Engineering, and Sports Management.

## CHAPTER OVERVIEWS

Chapter 1 introduces a pioneering computer vision system designed to deliver real-time sports analysis by tracking player movements and interpreting game situations. This system leverages state-of-the-art computer vision techniques to overcome the inherent challenges of player tracking, activity recognition, and pose estimation in dynamic sporting environments. By extracting and analyzing data in real time, the research opens new avenues for strategy implementation and performance evaluation, ultimately providing an efficient and automated framework for understanding player dynamics and team interactions during gameplay.

Chapter 2 delves into the application of AI for player fatigue and workload monitoring, focusing on optimizing athletic performance while safeguarding long-term health. Through machine learning models that analyze physiological, biomechanical, and psychological data, this chapter illustrates how coaches can enhance training and recovery plans. The use of wearable technology and real-time predictive analytics is discussed alongside challenges such as data accuracy, privacy concerns, and ethical implications. Future trends like cognitive tracking and immersive training environments are also considered, highlighting the need for holistic, responsible AI integration in sports performance management.

Chapter 3 discusses the strategic assembly of a sports analytics team. It outlines the foundational elements required to build an effective analytics department, including roles, skill sets, recruitment strategies, and team dynamics. Emphasis is placed on the integration of advanced technologies and data infrastructures that support evidence-based decision-making. The chapter also explores the cultural shift toward data-driven practices in sports organizations and reflects on emerging trends such as AI and video analytics that are poised to reshape team operations, fan engagement, and performance optimization.

Chapter 4 focuses on AI and machine learning as game-changers in sports strategy and tactical optimization. By analyzing historical and real-time game data, AI enables more precise decision-making and the personalization of training regimens. This chapter presents how predictive analytics support adaptive strategy development and injury prevention, fostering synergy between AI tools and human coaching expertise. Ethical challenges related to fairness, data privacy, and competitive integrity are also examined, reinforcing the importance of responsible AI adoption as these technologies become more widely accessible.

Chapter 5 examines the use of logistic regression and machine learning in injury prediction and prevention across sports and other domains. This chapter details how AI systems utilize data analytics to identify risk factors and implement preventive strategies aimed at enhancing athlete safety. It underscores the benefits of proactive risk management while addressing significant hurdles such as model transparency, data quality, and ethical concerns. The discussion offers a comprehensive look at how AI is redefining injury prevention through predictive insights and real-time monitoring.

Chapter 6 highlights the power of AI to transform fan engagement in sports. It presents use cases such as predictive ticket pricing, personalized content, and immersive experiences enabled by augmented and virtual reality. The chapter also considers managerial and societal implications, especially regarding data ethics and user privacy. By leveraging data analytics and machine learning, sports organizations can deepen connections with fans, cater to diverse audiences, and foster community interaction, ultimately making sports more inclusive and engaging.

Chapter 7 explores how machine learning is revolutionizing injury prevention and rehabilitation for athletes. It showcases the integration of diverse data sources—such as biomechanical assessments and wearable sensors—into personalized ML models for injury prediction. AI-powered rehabilitation programs that adapt in real time are also discussed, emphasizing efficiency and reduced risk of re-injury. Challenges like model complexity, explainability, and data privacy are addressed, along with forward-looking innovations such as federated learning and virtual reality, which promise to transform sports medicine.

Chapter 8 investigates machine learning's application in selecting the optimal Playing-11 in competitive cricket. This chapter surveys the data-driven evolution of team selection, demonstrating how historical performance data and predictive models inform smarter lineup decisions. It explains how data science is influencing coaching strategies and making decision-making more precise. Designed for coaches, players, and fans, this chapter provides a practical guide to leveraging analytics for competitive advantage in team composition.

Chapter 9 discusses the role of AI and machine learning in revolutionizing talent scouting and player development. It covers how predictive analytics and wearable technology are being used to identify potential in athletes and optimize performance trajectories. The chapter outlines AI-driven methods for scouting and coaching, while addressing legal, ethical, and practical challenges such as data privacy and algorithmic bias. It also examines the evolving landscape of AI in sports management and its implications for long-term athlete development.

Chapter 10 provides a broad overview of AI and machine learning in sports research. It underscores the increasing volume and complexity of data in professional sports and the need for advanced analytical tools to process this information efficiently. The chapter traces the evolution of AI over the past two decades and illustrates its applications in performance improvement, tactical decision-making, and business operations. Hypothetical scenarios and real-world examples demonstrate the potential for AI to shape the future of sports in both competitive and commercial contexts.

Chapter 11 focuses on the use of artificial neural networks (ANNs) in talent identification and scouting. After covering ANN fundamentals and the types of networks suitable for sports applications, the chapter explores how these models aid in injury prediction, performance analysis, and talent forecasting. It presents case studies and practical applications in various sports while highlighting issues of data quality, model interpretability, and ethical use. The discussion also considers future directions involving the integration of ANNs with emerging technologies to create more accurate and holistic scouting systems.

Chapter 12 addresses the ethical dimensions of AI and machine learning in sports analytics. Through four detailed case studies, the chapter explores topics such as data privacy, algorithmic bias, the human-AI decision-making balance, and the long-term health implications of data-driven performance management. Practical, societal, and managerial implications are discussed, emphasizing the need for transparency and athlete-centered AI implementation. The chapter calls for a balanced approach that harmonizes technological innovation with ethical responsibility.

Chapter 13 presents a series of case studies showcasing the real-world impact of sports analytics on performance, injury management, and fan engagement. The chapter discusses how data accuracy, organizational resistance, and privacy concerns shape the implementation of analytics. Future trends such as advanced AI, wearable sensors, and immersive fan experiences are highlighted as key drivers of competitive advantage. The case studies demonstrate the practical relevance and evolving influence of data-driven decision-making across the sports industry.

Our target audience includes researchers, academics, AIML professionals, government and regulatory authorities, technology enthusiasts, and postgraduate students. Whether you are looking to integrate AI into training regimes, improve athlete selection, enhance broadcast analysis, or deepen fan interaction, this book provides a foundation and a roadmap.

We are grateful to our contributors, whose expertise and dedication made this publication possible. Their work reflects the global nature of this field, incorporating diverse perspectives from both academia and industry. We also acknowledge the growing community of practitioners and scholars whose continuous innovation inspires us to explore new frontiers.

It is our hope that *AI and Machine Learning Applications in Sports Analytics* will serve not only as a source of knowledge but also as a catalyst — encouraging collaboration, sparking new ideas, and guiding real-world implementation of AI-driven sports analytics.

# Chapter 1
# Real-Time Sports Analysis:
## A Novel Computer Vision System for Player Movement and Game Situations

**Toufique Ahammad Gazi**
https://orcid.org/0000-0002-3681-8213
*Techno International New Town, India*

**Kaushik Paul**
https://orcid.org/0009-0009-6929-7651
*Brainware University, India*

**Ranjan Bannerjee**
https://orcid.org/0009-0003-1950-7530
*Brainware University, India*

**Debmalya Mukherjee**
https://orcid.org/0009-0006-9946-0964
*Brainware University, India*

## ABSTRACT

*Player movement analysis, along with reading game situations, is very important in sports, especially for strategy implementation and performance evaluation. Real-time analysis of these elements through computer vision is implemented in this paper. In dynamic sporting environments, to address the challenges of player tracking, activity recognition, and pose estimation, the system will leverage cutting-edge computer vision techniques. Real-time data extraction and analysis using computer vision*

DOI: 10.4018/979-8-3693-5385-1.ch001

*provides valuable insights for those who are associated with sports. The proposed research has the potential to revolutionize sports analysis in real time, including metrics on player speed, interaction, and positioning, by offering an automated, objective, and efficient method for understanding player and team performance during games.*

## INTRODUCTION

Sports world floated with data. From strategies for game complexity to the statistics of player, data analysts and other sports peoples are constantly seeking new methods to gain a competitive edge. Post-match review and manual observation is the key component for traditional analysis which can be time-consuming and subjective. However, advancements in computer vision (CV) offer a powerful alternative for real-time, objective analysis of player movement and game situations.

This research proposes the development of a novel CV system specifically designed for real-time sports analysis. By leveraging the benefits of CV methods, this system will be able to overcome the shortcomings of traditional methodologies. Through the automation of player tracking, posture assessment, and activity detection, the technology is anticipated to produce an abundance of objective data regarding player movement and interactions inside the game. These findings will be used by the coaches to develop game strategies, the broadcasters to boost fan connection, and the viewers to better understand what is happening on the field. Furthermore, the system's real-time processing powers will enable quick analysis and feedback, encouraging a more dynamic and data-driven viewpoint on sports.

We'll go into more depth about the benefits and drawbacks of employing CV for real-time sports analysis in the sections that follow. We'll examine the intricacies of the suggested system and present a handful of its possible uses in the sports industry. Lastly, we will talk about the technology issues and potential developments for this cutting-edge method of sports analytics.

Figure 1 provide statistics from research on a range of sports for use in a number of applications, including player and ball detection and tracking, trajectory prediction, categorization, and video summarization. They are published in several of prominent journals.

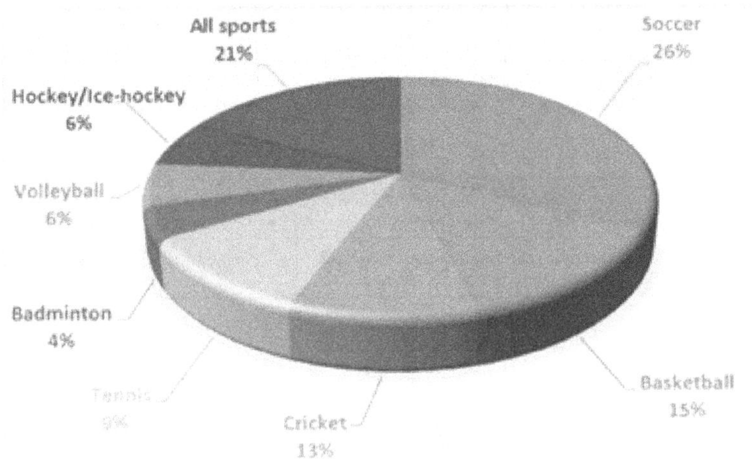


## LITERATURE REVIEW

Sports analysis using computer vision (CV) is a fast emerging discipline. The present state of gaming scenario analysis employing CV and real-time player mobility is the main topic of this study (Naik, Hashmi, & Bokde, 2022).

Player Monitoring: Colour tracking, backdrop reduction, and machine learning-based object recognition are some of the techniques used to identify and monitor participants in video streams. This data clarifies player location, gait patterns, and overall team strategy (Looser, Guntupalli, & Wheatley, 2012; Thomas et al., 2017; Huda et al., 2018).

Ball tracking: CV algorithms track the path of the ball during play, much as player tracking. This makes it possible to analyse shot placements, passing patterns, and the general flow of the game (Leo et al., 2008).

Player activities like as dribbling, passing, tackling, and shooting may be categorised using CV models. This makes it easier to identify tactical patterns and comprehend how players make decisions (Leo et al., 2008).

Formation Analysis: The technology is able to identify team formations and monitor changes made to them throughout a game by monitoring player placements. This provides information about team tactics and modifications (Khan & Shah, 2005).

*Table 1. Area of sports analysis using computer vision (CV)*

| Functionalities | Descriptions | Benefits |
|---|---|---|
| Player Tracking | Use machine learning to track players via color tracking, background removal, and object identification. | Gives information on the positioning of players, their gaits, and the team's general strategy. |
| Ball Tracking | Throughout the game, track the ball's trajectory with CV algorithms. | Makes it possible to analyses the game's general flow, shot placements, and passing patterns. |
| Action Recognition | Use CV models to categories player activities such as tackling, dribbling, passing, and shooting. | Helps recognize tactical patterns and comprehend how players make decisions. |
| Formation Analysis | Examine team lineups and how they alter throughout the match by examining player placements. | Provides information about team tactics and modifications. |

## Benefits

Real-time analysis: Coaches, commentators, and spectators may receive instant information from CV systems during live games.

Performance analysis: Coaches can create training programmes with the use of automatically generated player and team performance measurements.

The capacity of CV to detect important occurrences automatically, such goals or close plays, speeds up the compilation of highlights.

*Table 2. Comparison table on Real-time analysis, Performance analysis, and Highlight generation*

| Applications | Descriptions | Benefits | Challenges |
|---|---|---|---|
| Real-time analysis | During live games, CV systems instantly offer information on player positioning, ball movement, and game circumstances. | * Coaches making better decisions throughout games; * Viewers receiving richer commentary with real-time information. * Higher audience participation when data-driven visualizations are used. | * Video data processing latency can lead to information delivery delays; * System failures can interfere with real-time analysis. |
| Performance analysis | Measurements for team and player performance that are automatically created depending on formations, movements, and actions of the players. | * Makes it possible for coaches to pinpoint training programmers by identifying strengths and deficiencies. * Increases training efficiency by concentrating on areas that require improvement. * Offers objective data for player evaluation and selection. | * depends on how well CV's tracking and action recognition algorithms work. * Some characteristics of a player's success, such mental toughness and leadership, may not be fully captured by metrics. |
| Highlight generation | By automatically identifying crucial events like goals, close plays, and remarkable deeds, CV streamlines the process of creating highlights. | * Saves broadcasters and content producers time and money during post-production. * Guarantees that every important moment is recorded, even in action-packed games. Gives audiences a carefully chosen collection of the most thrilling plays. | CV might not include subjective highlights like outstanding saves or good sportsmanship. Depends on pre-established criteria for highlight identification, which might lead to the omission of noteworthy events. |

## Challenges:

Occlusion: If players obstruct one another's view, it might be difficult to follow.

Camera angles: Wide-angle views have the potential to misrepresent players' positions, hence calibration techniques are required.

Real-time processing: Accurate and timely processing is necessary for real-time analysis, and this requires strong hardware and efficient algorithms.

*Table 3. Challenges in Real-time Sports Analysis using Computer Vision*

| Challenge | Description | Impact |
|---|---|---|
| Occlusion | It is difficult for CV algorithms to properly track players since they can block each other from the camera's view. | Inaccurate player tracking data may lead to false conclusions about player movement, formations, and overall game analysis. |
| Camera Angles | Wide-angle camera views may alter player placements due to perspective changes. | Player position distortion can lead to mistakes in tracking data, formation analysis, and action detection. |
| Real-time Processing | Real-time analysis requires fast and precise processing of video data. This might have a significant computational cost. | Information distribution may lag as a result of delays in the processing of video data, which can impair the effectiveness of real-time analysis. |

Prospective Courses: To gain a deeper understanding of player movements and formations, 3D reconstruction integrates depth data.

Systems with several cameras: using many cameras to improve tracking accuracy and record a wider range of view.

Artificial Intelligence-driven game analysis: Applying AI to get a deeper comprehension of player behavior and game strategy.

Real-time sports analysis is being revolutionized by computer vision. For coaches, broadcasters, and spectators, CV offers useful information by monitoring players and the ball, as well as identifying movements and formations. We may anticipate much more in-depth research and insights into the sports industry as technology advances.

## EVALUATION OF EXISTING PLAYER TRACKING TECHNIQUES

It is crucial to evaluate player tracking techniques in computer vision (CV) for sports analysis to ascertain their benefits, drawbacks, and suitability for different situations. The following is a list of crucial considerations:

By far the most significant metric is accuracy. It evaluates how closely the tracker matches the actual positions of the players on the pitch. Common measures include: The Average Distance Error (ADE) is the mean difference between the observed and actual player locations. The Centre Point Error, or CPE, is the average difference between the players' true and monitored center points. False positive refers to the inaccurate identification of a non-player as a player, whereas false negative refers to the tracker's inability to detect a player.

Processing speed is essential for real-time applications. Frames per Second (FPS), or the number of frames processed in a second, is one of the measurements. The amount of time that passes between a video's capture and the monitored data's display. The ability to handle challenging circumstances like: Occlusion: when participants block one another's path changes in the angle of view (wide-angle distortion) and Variations in illumination (shadows, games at night).

Benchmark Datasets: Openly available datasets with player locations annotated are used for standardized evaluation. As illustrations, think about: Multiple Object Tracking Challenge (MOTChallenge) Ground Truth Data Monitored positions may be compared to baselines found in sports-specific datasets like UCF101 or Labelled Sports Dataset Player placements in video frames with human annotations. Highlight the inadequacies of the currently employed techniques and potential avenues for improvement (e.g., merging several camera viewpoints, using three-dimensional data).

The evaluation of player tracking techniques helps identify the optimal approach for a certain use case. Techniques that optimize performance for real-time sports analysis may be chosen or developed by researchers and developers by taking into account variables such as accuracy, speed, resilience, and processing needs.

*Table 4. Comparison of Player Tracking Techniques in Computer Vision (CV) for Sports Analysis*

| Criteria | Description | Importance | Example Techniques |
|---|---|---|---|
| Accuracy | Measures how well the tracker matches actual player positions. | High Importance | * Average Distance Error (ADE) * Center Point Error (CPE) * False Positives (FP) * False Negatives (FN) |
| Speed | Processing speed is crucial for real-time applications. | High Importance | * Frames Per Second (FPS) * Latency |
| Robustness | Ability to handle challenging scenarios. | Important | * Occlusion (player blocking) * Camera angle variations * Lighting changes |
| Computational Cost | Processing power required by the technique. | Important | * Color Tracking (Low) * Object Detection (Medium) * Deep Learning (High) |
| Evaluation Methods | Standardized methods for comparing techniques. | Important | * Benchmark Datasets (MOTChallenge) * Ground Truth Data |
| Limitations of Existing Techniques | Areas for improvement in current methods. | Informative | * Limited robustness * High computational cost |
| Future Directions | Potential advancements in player tracking. | Informative | * Multi-camera integration * 3D information utilization |

## BENEFITS OF INTERPRETABLE AI IN SPORTS ANALYSIS

The use of AI in sports analysis is growing in popularity, which has prompted the creation of efficient techniques for evaluating both individual and team performance. However, the incomprehensibility of many AI models—often referred to as "black box" models—is a serious disadvantage. This is where interpretable AI (IAI) comes in, offering a number of noteworthy benefits for sports analysis that are discussed in the table below:

*Table 5. Interpretable AI (IAI) in Sports Analysis*

| Benefit | Description | Impact on Sports Analysis |
|---|---|---|
| Enhanced Transparency and Trust | Conventional AI models are "black boxes," producing insights without disclosing their logic. On the other hand, IAI models are able to describe how they make decisions. | * Promotes trust between players, coaches, analysts, and spectators. Because users can comprehend the reasoning behind the AI's suggestions, more people will embrace and use analysis driven by AI. |
| Practical Takeaways | Performance measures are influenced by player actions, formations, and other factors, which are explained by IAI models. | * gives instructors useful information to create specialized training plans. Gives analysts the ability to maximize game plans by using their knowledge of the causal linkages between player behavior and performance results. |
| Analysis of Debasing | Biases found in the training set of data can be reinforced by traditional AI models. IAI models enable analysts to recognized and correct any biases by disclosing their decision-making processes. | Assists in reducing the possibility of biased decision-making based on past data trends. * Guarantees impartiality and fairness in AI-powered analysis. |
| In-the-Loop Human Analysis | IAI models provide human analysts more insight into the AI's conclusions, empowering them in the process. | * Allows for the model to be refined based on human feedback, boosting its accuracy over time; this enables analysts to take advantage of the AI's insights in addition to their own experience. * enables well-informed decision-making by fusing analysis produced by AI with human judgement. |
| Reasonable Forecasts | IAI models go beyond simple historical performance explanations to provide comprehensible forecasts of future events. | * Coaches and analysts are able to comprehend the rationale behind projected plays, opponents' advantages and disadvantages, and possible game situations. Enables proactive tactics depending on expected game circumstances. |
| Speaking and Narrating | By elucidating the "why" underlying the data, IAI models may be utilized to craft appealing narratives about individual and team success. | * Improves correspondence with players, coaches, and even supporters. * * Encourages a better comprehension of the game by giving concise justifications for performance indicators and patterns. Enables data-driven narrative to captivate audiences and inspire gamers. |

## PROPOSED SYSTEM

This proposed system is built on a powerful combination of computer vision techniques designed to extract real-time insights from live sports broadcasts. Deep learning models, such YOLO and Faster R-CNN, function as the system's eyes, efficiently identifying players and the ball in each video frame. Tracking algorithms such as Kalman Filters or DeepSORT are utilized to maintain identification even when players obstruct one other's view or when camera angles shift. By ensuring that participants are never lost in the shuffle, these algorithms create the foundation for future studies.

The system expands on this basis by analyzing player behavior and game conditions in greater detail. 3D Convolutional Neural Networks, or CNNs for short, are used to classify player activities like as dribbling, passing, and shooting. Based on their analysis of the temporal and geographical information included in video frames, these models are quite good at identifying activities. Large-scale tagged video datasets were used to train them. Furthermore, the system employs an intricate technique to identify significant occurrences like as goals, fouls, and offsides. In addition to the temporal information from player and ball trajectories, it takes into account the spatial interactions between players, the ball, and specified game zones. Instant alerts for important instant alerts for important notifications for important.

The raw data is processed and visualized by the system to generate actionable insights. Players' and teams' real-time performance metrics are produced using a combination of monitored data and action recognition results. Then, using interactive dashboards or on-screen visualizations, this data is displayed in an understandable and instructive way. These visualizations satisfy the specific needs of each user group, giving coaches data-driven strategy, broadcaster's additional content, and spectators a better understanding of the game.

### Proposed Pseudo code

This Pseudo code illustrates the role of Convolutional Neural Networks (CNNs) in real-time sports analysis.

```
def recognize_action(video_frame):

Should pre processing be enabled:

pre_process_frame(video_frame) = video_frame
```

```
Send cnn_input = video_frame to 2D CNN.reshape((1, channels,
width, height))

Convolutional Layers for Feature Extraction: features = cnn_
model(cnn_input)

Full Connected Layer Classification action_probabilities =
softmax(features)

Action Acknowledgment Predicted_action_id = np.argmax(ac-
tion_probabilities) is the output.

Predicted_action = action_labels[predicted_action_id]

predict_action in return

Assistance functions (substitute with real implementations)

pre_process_frame(frame) def pre:
```

Carry out normalisation, scaling, or other pre-processing actions pass

Use the softmax function to implement the probability distribution pass def softmax(x)

## System Implementation

Initialization of the System: The initial stage is loading a 2D Convolutional Neural Network model that has been pre-trained to identify player movements in sports footage. A sizable dataset of labelled video frames with a variety of activities (dribbling, passing, shooting, etc.) should be used to train this model. Make a list with names for every player activity that the system is capable of identifying, such as ["dribbling," "passing," "shooting," and "standing"]. The anticipated action ID from the CNN will be mapped to a label that can be read by humans using this list.

Loop for Video Processing: Capture Video Frame: Keep capturing frames from the live sports feed at all times. Use the pre_process_frame function to carry out tasks like normalization, scaling, or color space conversion if the recognize_action function allows pre-processing (based on your model's criteria). Provide the recorded (or previously processed) video frame to the recognize_action function. This function will: Run the frame through the CNN model that has been loaded, extracting features and classifying the data. Use np.argmax to determine which action has the highest probability score. Using the expected ID, look up the matching action label in the action_labels list. Depending on how the recognized action is applied, the system can handle it in a variety of ways. Show viewers the video feed and the identified action label on the screen. Record the action that was recognized, the timestamp, and the frame number for further analysis or performance statistic generation. Send out instant alerts or messages in response to important events (such as goals or fouls).

Monitoring and Enhancing the System: Keep an eye on the system's efficiency at all times, taking note of its accuracy and processing speed. Consider retraining the CNN model using a larger or more recent dataset if performance deteriorates over time in order to increase accuracy.

*Table 6. System implementation model*

| Step | Description |
|---|---|
| Initialization | |
| 1.1 | Load Pre-trained CNN Model |
| 1.2 | Define Action Labels |
| Video Processing Loop | |
| 2.1 | Capture Video Frame |
| 2.2 | Pre-process Video Frame (Optional) |
| 2.3 | Recognize Action |
| 2.3.1 | Call recognize_action function with the captured (or pre-processed) video frame. |
| 2.3.2 | The function processes the frame through the loaded CNN model, extracting features and performing classification. |
| 2.3.3 | Identify the action with the highest probability score using np.argmax. |
| 2.3.4 | Look up the corresponding action label from the action_labels list based on the predicted ID. |
| 2.4 | Output and Processing |

continued on following page

*Table 6. Continued*

| Step | Description |
|---|---|
| 2.4.1 | Real-time Visualization: Display the recognized action label on the screen along with the video feed for viewers. |
| 2.4.2 | Data Logging: Log the frame number, timestamp, and recognized action for further analysis or generating performance metrics. |
| 2.4.3 | Trigger Events (Optional): For critical actions (goal, foul), trigger real-time notifications or alerts. |
| Monitoring and Improvement | |
| 3.1 | Performance Monitoring |
| 3.2 | Model Retraining (Optional) |

## EVALUATION AND RESULTS

The article "Real-Time Sports Analysis: A Novel Computer Vision System for Player Movement and Game Situations" provides an in-depth analysis of computer vision methods used in sports video analysis for a range of purposes, such as player identification and classification, tracking of players or the ball, trajectory prediction, team strategy recognition, and event classification. The writers talk about the difficulties in deciphering sports footage, including player and ball zigzag motions, ball switching between players, and extreme ball occlusion. Additionally, they divide sports, after thorough examination, into two categories: ball-centered sports and player-centered sports.

The study focuses on how computer vision techniques might improve team performance in volleyball, badminton, hockey, and soccer, among other sports. It discusses the most recent developments in sports video analysis, focusing on the features of computer vision techniques used to complete specific jobs. The authors also provide publicly accessible datasets of several sports along with a roadmap of the selection and evaluation criteria used by various AI systems.

## APPLICATIONS AND FUTURE DIRECTIONS

Real-time sports analysis using a special computer vision system for player movement and game circumstances has several possible applications and methods. Sports computer vision technology has the power to fundamentally alter how competitions are seen, played, and rated. Here are some significant applications and potential future paths based on the provided sources:

Applications: Computer vision technology like Hawk-Eye are used in tennis and football to accurately track the trajectory of the ball, helping referees make accurate calls. Computer vision provides athletes with thorough insights into their performances by analyzing biomechanics and kinematics and providing customized feedback for training development. By using computer vision-based athlete tracking, coaches may better evaluate player performance, spot potential injuries, and boost team output. To track player performance, spot injury signs early, and lower health risks in professional sports, wearables and computer vision combine. Computer vision enhances fan engagement by bringing in greater audiences and creating unique viewing experiences by overlaying dynamic content on live sports broadcasts. Advanced computer vision technologies have the potential to provide precise insights into a player's worth, which may aid in player acquisition and team performance optimization.

Future Directions: Sports data may be efficiently visualized and analyzed to evaluate performance potential, reduce injury risks, and understand collective tactical behavior by merging artificial intelligence and big data analytics. Identifying the top prospects, projecting their future growth, and streamlining decision-making processes via the use of data-intensive methodologies. Machine learning, artificial intelligence, and data analytics are a few of these methods. Increasing revenue and providing sports leagues and organizations with valuable information by applying analytical techniques in critical commercial domains like CRM and ticket pricing systems.

## CONCLUSION

The integration of a cutting-edge computer vision system for real-time sports analysis, with a focus on player mobility and game circumstances, is a notable advance in the field of sports technology. This innovative method has several benefits, including increased player performance evaluation, precise game situation monitoring, and increased audience engagement.

By employing computer vision technology, sports companies may get valuable insights into player movements, tactical approaches, and performance metrics in real-time. This gives fans a more dynamic and engaging experience while also assisting athletes and coaches in improving their training regimens and strategies.

Additionally, the application of computer vision in sports analysis opens up new avenues for talent identification, injury prevention, and performance prediction. The ability to quickly and precisely measure and analyse player motions enables data-driven decision-making processes that have the power to fundamentally alter how sports are taught, played, and enjoyed.

In conclusion, the use of a special computer vision system for in-the-moment sports analysis has enormous potential to transform sports technology. These advancements are expected to lead to further innovations in player performance, game analysis, and fan involvement, ushering in a new era of excitement and innovation in the sports business.

## REFERENCES

Huda, N. U., Jensen, K., Gade, R., & Moeslund, T. B. (2018). Estimating the number of soccer players using simulation-based occlusion handling. *2018 IEEE/CVF Conference on Computer Vision and Pattern Recognition Workshops (CVPRW).* DOI: 10.1109/CVPRW.2018.00236

Khan, S. M., & Shah, M. (2005, November). Detecting group activities using rigidity of formation. In *Proceedings of the 13th annual ACM international conference on Multimedia* (pp. 403-406).

Leo, M., Mosca, N., Spagnolo, P., Mazzeo, P. L., D'Orazio, T., & Distante, A. (2008, July). Real-time multiview analysis of soccer matches for understanding interactions between ball and players. In *Proceedings of the 2008 international conference on Content-based image and video retrieval* (pp. 525-534).

Looser, C. E., Guntupalli, J. S., & Wheatley, T. (2013). Multivoxel patterns in face-sensitive temporal regions reveal an encoding schema based on detecting life in a face. *Social Cognitive and Affective Neuroscience*, *8*(7), 799–805.

Naik, B. T., Hashmi, M. F., & Bokde, N. D. (2022). A comprehensive review of computer vision in sports: Open issues, future trends and research directions. *Applied Sciences (Basel, Switzerland)*, *12*(9), 4429. DOI: 10.3390/app12094429

Thomas, G., Gade, R., Moeslund, T. B., Carr, P., & Hilton, A. (2017). Computer vision for sports: Current applications and research topics. *Computer Vision and Image Understanding*, *159*, 3–18. DOI: 10.1016/j.cviu.2017.04.011

# Chapter 2
# AI-Based Player Fatigue and Workload Monitoring Systems

**Shashank Mittal**
https://orcid.org/0000-0002-8666-5323
*O.P. Jindal Global University, India*

**Ajay Chandel**
https://orcid.org/0000-0002-4585-6406
*Lovely Professional University, India*

**Huy Hung Ta**
https://orcid.org/0009-0008-6835-3036
*International School, Vietnam National University, Hanoi, Vietnam*

## ABSTRACT

*The Present chapter examines AI-based player fatigue and workload monitoring systems in optimizing the performance of athletes while preventing them from burning out. These are harnessed from advanced models of machine learning, analyzing physiological, biomechanical, and mental health data to improve training and recovery strategies. Advances in wearable technologies will dramatically change the way coaches and athletes approach the world of performance management by harnessed real-time data and predictive analytics. This chapter also deals with some of the difficulties, including data accuracy, privacy and ethical issues, associated with athlete autonomy. Other possible future trends relate to cognitive metrics, multisport data sharing, and involvement of virtual or augmented reality in training environments. The goal at the end of the road for AI-based systems is optimal athletic performance, but all this should be done with the aim of supporting*

DOI: 10.4018/979-8-3693-5385-1.ch002

*long-term health and well-being.*

## INTRODUCTION

The demands placed on today's sport mean that management of player fatigue and workload needs to be better controlled. Athletes are asked to perform at elite levels, either through intense training or high-level competition, to the point of potential exhaustion, injury, or, in some cases, burnout if not monitored appropriately. Fatigue can also be physical or mental. It is one of the important factors that may actually have an impact on an athlete's performance in the activity and alter an athlete's career in the long run. Overtraining or undertraining could also negatively affect the health of the athletes and performances if the workload is not appropriately distributed (Akyıldız et al., 2022). Against this backdrop, new AI and ML technologies are opening up new avenues to achieving more accurate and efficient fatigue and workload monitoring systems.

AI and ML indeed revolutionized many industries and are quickly permeating the world of sports analytics. Monitoring athletes is becoming yet another area that is increasingly amenable to AI-based systems that track and analyze player data so as to provide coaches, sports scientists, and medical teams with valuable insights into the physical condition of an athlete (Biró, 2023). Such technology makes it possible to switch from a more traditional reactive approach to managing player fatigue and workload to one that is based on data. With AI, sports teams can then predict when a player is likely to experience overtraining or burnout, thus averting the latter and ensuring recovery (Clemente et al., 2021).

These innovations are rooted in machine learning models that analyze large amounts of data culled from different sources, including wearables, GPS trackers, and biometric sensors. All of these metrics-instant heart rate, distance covered, sleep pattern, and recovery time-were captured and then analyzed by AI algorithms in order to predict levels of fatigue and suggest training load adjustments. The potential of machine learning to make predictions is extremely valuable in this respect: instant, in-depth adjustments to the intensity of training and game decisions to avoid overwork and underprep of the athletes can be made. Such systems not only improve athletic performance but also extend the career span of an athlete as they limit the chance of long-term injuries associated with overreaching and burnout (Coutinho et al., 2018).

Moreover, AI-driven monitoring system of workload delivers specific information that is crucial for each athlete. Unlike traditionally applied measures taking a one-size-fits-all approach, AI models consider individual variations between athletes concerning their level of fitness, ability to recover, and psychological resilience as well. At this level, every player's workload is optimized based on his specific needs, leading to better performance and reduces the risk of getting injured. As these systems continue their trend, they also begin to absorb psychological and mental markers of fatigue, which provides a more holistic approach to athlete health.

Some challenges as well as ethical consideration have to be met in this arena of AI:. Of course, such concerns are still related to data privacy, overreliance on AI, and lack of human oversight. However, with technological advancements in AI and machine learning, the skills of these technologies in monitoring player fatigue and workloads will be expanded, providing potential paths for developing athletes who can achieve better performance while conserving long-term sound health. This chapter addresses the status of the current AI-based monitoring of fatigue and workload, their applications in a real-life perspective, and the challenges involved in implementing these systems in modern sports (Daly et al., 2022).

## UNDERSTANDING FATIGUE AND WORKLOAD IN SPORTS

Fatigue and workload are integral aspects of sports performance that determine an athlete's ability to perform at their peak and sustain health over the long term. Fatigue is generally regarded as a diminution in the level of physical or mental performance following prolonged exertion, and it may be either physical, mental, or emotional. At a physical level, it includes depletion of stored energy in the body, muscle damage, or reduced ability to maintain an effort. At a mental level, it results from cognitive overload that impairs decision-making and concentration. Emotional fatigue often is linked with the stresses, pressures, and demands from being in competition, all contributing to the effects of physical and mental fatigue. The two forms of fatigue are intertwined and can also be additive, hence it is an important factor in athlete performance and well-being research (Delecroix et al., 2018).

Workload is the term in use commonly in the training environment for describing the physical and mental load exerted on an athlete in the process of training or competition. The management of workload attempts to apportion intensity, frequency, and volume of activity in a manner that maximizes performance without overstraining the athlete. In sports, workload is divided into internal and external workload. Internal workload refers to a representation of physiological and psychological stress acquired through the athlete's heart rate, perceived exertion, and other bodily responses to activities (Mandorino, 2023). External workload represents objective quantification of physical workload such as distance run, number of sprint performed, or weight lifted during a training session. Appropriate management of both internal and external workloads is necessary to avert overtraining and undertraining that may have significant implications for performance and injury risk.

Then proper workload management should be taken so that when athletes start reaching beyond their ability to cope with a specific workload, they become susceptible to injury, exhaustion, and long-term burnout. An overtraining syndrome is an incident most often encountered in high-performance sport when athletes are stretched too far beyond recovery, leading to a halt in performance capabilities, chronic fatigue, and susceptibility to injury. This is particularly problematic in sports with high competition frequency or intense training regimes, such as football, basketball, and endurance sports. Conversely, undertraining can leave the athlete with a workload that is less than that expected to improve performance such that a state of detraining occurs, fitness levels are lowered, and, thus, performance during competition is suboptimal. Thus, proper balance in workload is vital for athletic success (Martinho, 2024).

The traditional ways of measuring fatigue and workload rely on subjective estimation of the degree of rating the exertion with self-reporting or through coach observation, which may present biases and errors. Despite these remaining powerful, they have no precision and live feedback that modern technology can provide. With recent progress in sports science, objective measures of fatigue and workload have now been more technologically advanced through the use of wearable technology, GPS tracking, heart rate monitors, and even advanced biomarkers to trace how an athlete's physiological responses behave following training and competitions. This allows for the capture of more precise real-time data that may be able to track athletes' responses to workload and predict levels of fatigue (Nobari et al., 2023).

Understanding the underlying mechanisms of fatigue and the effects of workload mismanagement is essential in implementing strategies to optimize performance and prevent injuries. There is an increasing body of evidence within sports science research that necessitates a data-driven approach towards tracking and adjusting workload based upon an athlete's specific needs and recovery capacities. This is where AI and machine learning models come into play, providing a much more dynamic and personal approach to fatigue prediction and workload management, further improving performance and athlete well-being.

## AI AND MACHINE LEARNING IN SPORTS ANALYTICS

Artificial intelligence, or AI, and machine learning, or ML, are revolutionizing sports analytics by delivering innovative capabilities to advance performance, prevent injuries, and optimize training regimens. Traditionally, sports analytics are based on post-game performance reviews, which are characterized by data that has been manually collected and analyzed with basic statistics. In contrast, with AI and ML, the scope of analytics has totally transformed into real-time data-driven decisions that can predict outcomes, provide insights regarding athlete health, and even personalize training programs (Selmi et al., 2022). This interaction of AI and ML in sports enables teams and athletes to change the paradigm from reactive to proactive strategies. All these factors have been empowered more than ever by increasing the capabilities in monitoring performance, managing fatigue, or keeping injuries at minimum risk.

The drivers behind AI and ML in sports are largely the analysis of large datasets collected through various technologies such as GPS trackers, wearable sensors, cameras, and even social media platforms. This contains perhaps the richest variables: player movement, physiological data from sensors (heart rate, oxygen levels), and environmental factors, like temperature and humidity. These are complex datasets that can be utilised in machine learning to analyze patterns and relationships that are less obvious for human observation. This will be useful in building models to predict performance, for example, in terms of a player's fatigue, chances of injury, or even peaks in performance, which can then be applied to amend training schedules or even the strategies during games (Starling et al., 2019).

In terms of monitoring fatigue and workload, AI-based systems have come in handy. Thus, there is a possibility to train machine learning models into the detection of patterns in player data that would indicate the onset of signs of fatigue before actual performance decline or injury might happen. This would be through continuous data streaming from wearable devices like heart rate monitors, accelerometers, and GPS trackers. On this basis, ML algorithms would take into account the elements of training load, recovery time, and physiological strain to predict when a player is at the brink of overexertion (Starling et al., 2020). It can be used by the coaches and sports scientists to determine whether it's the right time to reduce the workload for the athlete, allow more recovery time, or even modify the training intensity in a way that will prevent injury and optimize long-term performance.

Besides that, AI and ML have enabled the training and recovery plans of an athlete to be individualized. Variable responses to a sport may mean that an athlete demands more and, potentially, inefficient as well as more injury-prone one-size-fits-all training regimes. Player data can be analyzed and customized into training plans according to the needs and recovery capacity of each athlete. For example, some have a greater requirement for recovery compared to others after high-intensity sessions, while others can be returned more quickly to activity. This level of personalization is tough to achieve without AI and its learning to process massive, heterogeneous data sets that lead to the extremely fine-tuned personalization in training and recovery (Costa et al., 2019).

The injury prevention is another major application of AI in sports. A machine learning-based model in the workout data combination with biomechanical movements and past injury records can predict the risk of injury. This allows teams and coaches to be proactive, such as by adjusting workload, focusing on specific muscle groups, or contacting individual players to avoid overwork. For example, AI systems may monitor patterns of running and workload in soccer players relating soft-tissue injuries, for instance, hamstring strains that have a direct correlation with a high level of fatigue and incorrect workload management. This enables pre-intervention, thereby minimizing the period taken to injuries and prolonging an athlete's life span. Besides preventing a downfall due to fatigue and injury, AI and ML are further employed in the sectors of tactical analysis and performance optimization. Through the utilization of advanced algorithms in AI, game footage and real-time in-game data can be analyzed to derive insights on team strategy, opponent weaknesses, and optimal player positioning. This allows coaches to have an even stronger edge at coming up with game plans that are data-informed and attuned to certain situations. More importantly, real-time processing and analysis of data by AI still leave room for tactical changes at a game-by-game basis, thus keeping the competition on their feet as well in terms of responding to new situations on the playing field (Vasiljevas et al., 2023).

Even as AI and ML impose immediate benefits on sports analytics, there are still issues at hand. There's the problem of data privacy. Since most of the biometric information is going to be sensitive in nature, reliance on huge amounts of such data is a concern with regard to the privacy of such data. Over dependence on AI might lead to reliance on technology; how effective is human intuition and experience in sports?. However, AI and ML can remarkably complement the traditional methods so that decisions based on athletes shall improve much more holistically and accurately optimized athlete management and performance.

In sum, the AI and machine learning will open a new horizon in the world of sports analytics-through highly real-time, data-driven insights into training, performance, and recovery. Artificially intelligent prediction of fatigue, injury prevention, and personalization of athlete workloads are changing the landscape. This revolutionizes sports, making them safer and more efficient. Sports will indeed take more aspects of technological advancements while providing even more doors for innovation and better performance (Munoz-Macho et al., 2024).

## AI MODELS FOR FATIGUE PREDICTION

The AI models of fatigue prediction go along with the modern game. These ensure that teams and athletes can easily quantify and control their levels of fatigue. They make use of machine learning algorithms to undertake comprehensive analysis on physiological, biomechanical, and performance data to predict the onset of overexertion and current fatigue levels. In short, such AI systems help prevent injuries, optimal recovery, and performance by having an accurate fatigue forecast. This is the big leap in sports science where AI models predict early signs of fatigue that would appear before their decline in performance, indicating a proactive approach to workload management (Giorgi et al., 2023).

The various types of machine learning models that can be used are comprised to orient at different aspects of athlete tracking; for instance, supervised learning models, which will have already been trained on labelled data, containing all historical athlete performance, workload, and recovery times. These models will seek patterns within the data and predict fatigue based on input features like heart rate variability, distance covered, training intensity, and periods of recovery. As they learn with new data, they become successively closer to the ideal output and can provide the most accurate predictions. This is where the model comes in very handy in sports such as cycling or running marathons since knowing an athlete's limits could be very important for performance or prevention of injuries and generally for other endurance sports (Biró et al., 2024).

The kinds of unsupervised models are those that work based on pre-labeled data but seek hidden patterns within the data itself. These models would prove really effective in finding something so subtle regarding fatigue that might not have been easily identifiable through the typical model. For example, an unsupervised model might cluster the athletes with regard to the performance metrics and then figure out unique recovery patterns or trends associated with certain groups of athletes. Such insights could lead to more personalized approaches in managing fatigue, which coaches can incorporate into personalized training programs for each athlete.

The most advanced AI approach involves the application of deep learning techniques, such as RNNs and LSTMs, specifically designed to process time-series data. These models are particularly appropriate for the task as they can better capture temporal relationships in athlete data, thus being particularly well-suited for predicting fatigue. For instance, LSTM models can capture the natural fluctuations of an athlete's performance over time by considering not only the current state but also how previous workloads and recovery patterns explain those same states. Therefore, the model can better predict fatigue and related declines in performance as it understands how for instance, the pattern of fatigue accrual contributes to these changes over time and the impact of recovery on future performance (Silacci et al., 2020).

The quality of input data may affect the success of these AI models. The wearable devices include heart rate monitors, GPS trackers, and sleep monitors, which go on to produce continuous streams of data that feed into AI systems. These devices measure the most important physiological metrics and external metrics like distance traveled, speed, acceleration, and other factors like body temperature and oxygen saturation. The combination of all these data makes it possible for the AI models to see a more holistic view of the athlete's physical health status and identify early warning signs that may not be noticed by the human eye.

Some of the well-known AI models in the prediction of fatigue include HRV data. HRV is the established marker for an athlete's level of activity of his autonomic nervous system and very commonly used in assessing recovery and level of fatigue. Machine learning algorithms trained on HRV data can then identify deviations from baselines that would signal for real-time adjustments in training intensity (Nahavandi et al., 2022). Similarly, GPS monitoring the movement pattern will hint that the athlete is slowing down or moving for shorter distances with time passing; these are typical symptoms of fatigue.

There are many case studies that demonstrate that AI-driven models are very effective at predicting fatigue in most sports. For instance, soccer teams can use AI-driven models monitoring player fatigue, based on GPS and accelerometer data. These models can predict when a player might hit the level of fatigue, giving one ample time to replace that player with another or to reduce their workload in training. For endurance sports, such as cycling and distance running, AI models are used to fine-tune specific training regimens based on individually customized metrics for fatigue. It enhances performance while minimizing the risk of overtraining (Sandamal et al., 2024).

Continuous learning and adaptation of AI models make them a rare resource for sports teams. With the continuous generation of data analyzed, more refined models are resultant, thus doing a more precise and accurate fatigue prediction tailored to individual athletes. This precision enables transitions from generalised training programmes to very specific workload management strategies, thus ensuring that athletes train at their optimal capacity and do not exceed these physical limits (Akyıldız et al., 2022).

While AI models for the prediction of fatigue have taken off, they have problems in the first place: data quality and consistency, namely, the credibility of the inputted data is by what the actual prediction of fatigue is dependent. For example, wearable device inputs might be noisy or partially missing at times. Even if AI models can generate predictions by patterns of data, this requires human oversight in terms of interpretation of results or decisions over training adjustments or recovery protocols.

Overall, AI models for fatigue prediction are a giant step forward in athlete monitoring and performance optimization. These models analyze data of every range using the power of machine learning algorithms to give actionable insights into different actions helping athletes avoid overtraining, recover well, and perform at their peak. Technologies about AI continue to evolve. It is expected that their role in the management of fatigue shall be larger, along with offering even more sophisticated tools and techniques through which sports teams can improve the performances and welfare of athletes (Biró, 2023).

## WORKLOAD MONITORING SYSTEMS

Workload monitoring systems play a very crucial role in modern sports, as it allows constant monitoring of the physical and physiological load on an athlete. Both internal and external workloads can be monitored, which enables coaches, sports scientists, and medical teams to optimize training programs, avoid injuries, and, thus, improve performance in the long term. The advancement in high-tech technology such as wearable devices, GPS trackers, and complicated software platforms has really enhanced the precise and effective workload monitoring that has, in turn, given teams an opportunity to make decisions on training that best align with an athlete's individual needs and capacities (Clemente et al., 2021).

Workload in sports is usually categorized into two broad types: external workload. External workload encompasses the measurable outputs or the quantities, clearly visible metrics that determine to what extent an athlete has worked while at training or in competition. A few examples of the external workload include total distance covered during a session; numbers of sprints or high-intensity movements; weight lifted; and amount of time spent being active (Coutinho et al., 2018). These loads can be tracked with reasonable accuracy employing wearable technology, such as GPS systems or accelerometers that could continuously feed back real-time data pertaining to the movement and exertion of an athlete.

Internal workload refers to the athlete's physiological and psychological responses to the imposed external workload. These consist of heart rate, heart rate variability (HRV), oxygen consumption, perceived exertion, and biochemical markers such as lactate levels. It is essential to monitor the internal workload because two athletes with the same external workload will respond differently due to fitness levels, recovery status, or health status. For example, an athlete recovering from injury may indicate fatigue at a lower external workload than a fully fit athlete. Monitoring internal workload can explain how well a person is coping with the total demand placed upon him, therefore tailoring training adjustments more personally (Daly et al., 2022).

Wearable technologies form the key component of workload monitoring systems. GPS trackers, accelerometers, and heart rate monitors are often used to collect data on external and internal workloads. Such devices provide real-time data during training and competition, offering insights into an athlete's performance. For instance, GPS trackers can track metrics such as speed, distance, and acceleration, while heart rate monitors can assess the cardiovascular strain imposed by physical activity. Put together, such devices provide a very full view of how an athlete is performing and how their body is responding to the workload (Delecroix et al., 2018).

A very important advantage of workload monitoring systems is their ability to prevent injuries through training load management. Injuries have been found to occur more often when there is an abrupt increase in workload, such as when training becomes extremely intensive or prolonged without corresponding time for recovery. By applying workload monitoring systems, teams are enabled to monitor an athlete's Acute

Workload Ratio (ACWR): it calculates the acute workload in comparison to the chronic workload. Balanced ACWR values will show that an athlete maintains his workload consistent with what his body is used to, and if a higher value of ACWR comes up, he is most likely at risk of overtraining or injury. From this data, coaches can adjust training loads to enable athletes to stay in an optimal training zone and avoid developing overuse injuries (Mandorino, 2023).

Workload monitoring systems improve performance through information on when athletes are ready to produce peak performances. This is through continuous data collection, which shows periods of high readiness, whereby athletes have completely recovered and can withstand more intense training or competition. In periods whereby the data shows fatigue signals or poor recovery, training loads can be depleted to prevent over strain. This aids a periodized training plan that matches the physiological state of the athlete, thereby having him or her fit at the right time for major competitions (Martinho, 2024).

There is an increment use of AI and machine learning technologies in workload monitoring systems, which enables the analysis of much more sophisticated data and enables prediction capabilities. Scientists can analyze the past data; look for patterns and predict how the amount of workload that an athlete applies today will impact his or her performance in the future or risk of injuries by using machine learning algorithms (Nobari et al., 2023). For example, AI models can apply data from wearable devices to predict when an athlete is at the risk of soft tissue injuries such as hamstring strains. These types of injuries have been mostly associated with mismanagement of workload. In this aspect, such prediction models allow teams to pre manage the workload and calibrate training intensity in advance of when the injuries will actually strike instead of reacting once they do.

Other very significant part of the modern systems for workload monitoring is cloud-based. They centralize data from a number of wearable devices, allowing medical staff, coaches, and athletes to access performance metrics in real-time. Such platforms offer a holistic overview of athlete health and workload if integrated with data from several sources, such as GPS, heart rate monitors, and subjective wellness surveys. Cloud-based systems also improve the collaboration between various team members because these allow team members to make decisions about training, recovery, and injury management based on data (Selmi et al., 2022).

Workload monitoring is viewed as extremely useful for team sports in managing huge teams of athletes. This means that workload monitoring systems allow the coach to individualize the training program for each player considering the position, role, and playing time of different players. In soccer, for instance, if a midfielder runs more ground than a forward, or simply puts in more sprints, then the player would require more recovery time. This would enable the team to ensure that different squads of players are neither over-trained nor under-trained.

Workload monitoring systems have several merits, but they're not without problems. The main problem is data overflow from wearable devices, which would wash away without proper tools by giving into their rigidity to manage or analyze it. Variability in the way in which individual athletes respond to workloads and is quite difficult to standardize for the whole team makes things more complicated. The coaches and sports scientists also need not rely on data at an exclusion of the more human coaching skills about understanding the mental state of the athlete and his or her levels of motivation and resilience in the approach to workloads.

Workload monitoring systems are very significant in the new world of sports, providing data useful for optimizing performance, preventing injury, and personalizing training. They are advanced with AI, machine learning, and based on cloud platforms, making them more advanced and accurate, enabling teams to dynamically and in real-time manage workload. With the advancement of technology, tracking systems for workload will undoubtedly be an integral part of the future of sports performance and athlete management (Starling et al., 2020).

## PREVENTING BURNOUT WITH AI-BASED SYSTEMS

A very vast area in sports science and performance management has been prevention of burnout among athletes, as much importance has been granted because over-training leading to high workloads has been extremely linked with the initiation of fatigue, injuries, and poor performance. With respect to burnout issues, AI-based systems prove to be highly valuable tools by providing data-driven insights into the physical and mental state of an athlete in a personalized fashion. These help detect early on the risks associated with overtraining, enable real-time adjustment of workload to prevent burnout, and help athletes attain a balance between training intensity and recovery, thus reducing the likelihood of burnout.

## Understanding Burnout in Sports

Athlete burnout is primarily the result of a prolongation of physical and mental strain without adequate recovery. It occurs in numerous forms, such as chronic fatigue, lack of motivation, performing at poor levels, and an increased susceptibility to injury. The traditional models of training often depend largely on physical aspects and are, therefore, unable to take into consideration the build up effect of continuous tension on body and mind (Chidambaram et al., 2022). In this respect, AI-based systems are different: they give a systemic assessment of an athlete's state based on physical, physiological, and psychological data.

## AI in the determination of early signs of Burnout

AI-based systems will be able to detect early signs of burnout much earlier than the early stage would become apparent even to coaches or the athletes themselves. AI systems monitor a few important indicators by collecting and analyzing data continuously from wearable devices, such as heart rate variability, sleep patterns, training load, and even subjective wellness metrics. Heart rate variability is one of the most critical metrics for the burnout detection system, as it reflects sympathetic-parasympathetic nervous system balance. A downward trend in HRV can be perceived as an indicator of built-up stress, meaning that the athlete has surpassed training limits and is bound to experience burnout. AI algorithms will alert their coaches about such trends early and warn them to take preventive measures (Vasiljevas et al., 2023).

Therefore, it may even identify patterns in connection with declining performance, low recovery efficiency, and poor sleep quality. Together with the metrics from workload, these patterns enable the system to predict beforehand when an athlete is reaching the limits of his or her physical and psychological possibilities. This advanced warning mechanism will perhaps be able to intervene in time to modify training intensity, increase recovery, or offer psychological support before an athlete crash at a critical point.

## Real-Time Monitoring and Adaptive Training

Where training is concerned, AI-based systems enable real-time monitoring, with immediate feedback on workload and recovery. This dynamic approach is absolutely crucial in the prevention of burnout as it takes into account the active states of the athletes so that the training programs can be adapted promptly and as necessary. For instance, if a system notes overrecovery—low HRV, reduced recovery, or decreased power outputs—then coaches can alter the amount or the length of the intensity of the training so that there would be an allowance for proper time to recover (Munoz-Macho et al., 2024).

An AI-driven adaptive training program may also adjust the workloads of each athlete according to their respective reaction to the stressors and their specific situations for recovery. For example, the machine learning models might be exploring how a different athlete responds to type training and then adjust their workout depending on that. This makes the ideal "one-size-fits-all" training problem ordinary and one that typically results in many athletes "burning out." Those who needed more recovery were given lighter sessions, but maintaining at high intensity was not feasible since certain athletes could thrive with the demands (Giorgi et al., 2023).

## Managing Recovery and Mental Well-being

Recovery then becomes a critical factor in the prevention of burnout. AI-based systems help in optimizing recovery by analyzing various types of recovery metrics and determining the moment an athlete needs to recover more. Other than just monitoring physical recovery, such systems can also go on to follow up with the mental well-being of the athlete by including subjective data like mood, level of motivation, and perceived stress. Taken together with metrics such as HRV and sleep quality, such data have more meaning regarding the athlete's overall state of health.

For instance, sleep tracking forms an important part of AI-based burnout prevention systems. Poor quality of sleep and the lack of it actually hit the recovery chances in an athlete's system, thus giving chances of burning out. AI systems can track patterns of sleep, wear devices on the body, and give in-depth reports on sleep duration, stages, and disturbances. The schedules for training or traveling can also be altered if there is data showing that the athlete is not getting enough restorative sleep (Biró et al., 2024).

Another function is that AI-based systems can incorporate the measurement of mental well-being as part of their monitoring work. Burnout is mostly psychologically caused. Long-term stress might cause anxiety, depression, or a loss of interest in pursuing athletic activities. This would be making the use of AI in analyzing an athlete's response to regular wellness surveys or some other form of psychological assessment so that the concerns about mental health may precede burnout. Therefore, AI-based systems help in supporting this more holistic approach toward health due to realizing that mental as well as physical well-being is part of the successful performance of an athlete (Silacci et al., 2020).

## Data-Driven Decision Making

One of the most powerful aspects of the AI-based burnout prevention system is supporting data-driven decision-making capabilities. Traditional training decisions are most often based on personal feelings and experience, which in some cases leads to overlooking early warning signs of burnout. With huge amounts of data and sophisticated algorithms, AI influences training loads, recovery times, and injury risks to make informed decisions. This will ensure that the workloads are better distributed objectively and fairly, thereby reducing the potential for overtraining from leading to burnout.

For instance, AI can create personal training plans for athletes that balance their workloads and time recovery based on collected current situations and historical data about each athlete. The system may give them suggestions on the best period of rest, advise how the intensity of training must be changed, and even recommend alternative strategies for recovering, such as active recovery sessions or mental health support. Continuously learning from new data, AI systems refine the predictions and recommendations to ensure that best care of athletes takes place by avoiding burnout (Nahavandi et al., 2022).

## Case studies on AI-based burnout prevention

Some sports organizations have implemented an AI-based system in which athletes can be guided away from burnout and achieve optimum performance. For example, endurance sports like cycling and long-distance running have utilized AI systems that measure training loads to identify signs of overtraining. Implementing trainings according to real-time data in such systems has prevented athletes from having burnout and staying at the peak of their performance Akyıldız et al., 2022).

With AI-based systems, the workload of individual players in team sports has been tracked at times when periods of intense competitiveness have demanded much from them. For example, soccer teams use AI-based systems to track the fatigue, recovery, and risk of injury of their players. Such systems allow coaches to effectively rotate players in the long season, which reduces the chances of burnout experienced by athletes from carrying out much beyond their physical limits (Sandamal et al., 2024).

AI-based systems are enhancing the ways that sports teams prevent burnout by offering real-time, adaptive fine-tuning of training plans, and more data-driven decision-making. All physical and mental health metrics are being monitored entirely by these systems, managing an athlete's workload to best plan for recovery. As its technology continues to evolve, AI will become a significant aspect of sports performance management, assisting athletes in maintaining long-term health and avoiding burnout in achieving the full realization of their potential.

## CHALLENGES AND ETHICAL CONCERNS

AI-based monitoring of athlete fatigue and workload bears significant benefits, but it also poses quite a few challenges and takes some serious ethical considerations into place (Biró, 2023). With any emerging technology, the implementation of AI in sports management needs to be holistically managed so that issues of accuracy in data, privacy, equity, and broader consequences for athlete autonomy and well-being are addressed.

1. Data Accuracy and Reliability

Another problem with the application of AI-based systems in monitoring fatigue and workload is the accuracy and reliability of the data. AI-based systems usually base their data on wearable devices and sensors, including GPS trackers, heart rate monitors, and sleep trackers. Furthermore, data from these devices may be affected by environmental conditions, failure or malfunction of the sensor, or wrong usage that can lead to inappropriate inferences (Clemente et al., 2021). The model suffers from inconsistencies and gaps in historical data since AI models heavily rely on it for their calculations.

Other algorithms about predicting fatigue and burnout also fail to clearly understand the complicated physiological responses of humans. For instance, two same workload athletes will carry different fatigue levels because of their unique physical makeup, stress levels, or potential recovery capacity. Ensuring all these differences are incorporated in the AI models is crucial in the effective management of workload, though an ongoing task to develop systems that give uniformly reliable predictions.

2. Privacy and Data Security

Collecting and utilizing biometric data through an AI-based system raises many privacy and data security concerns. This is one of the most sensitive performance data for any athlete, especially their physical, physiological, and sometimes mental health metrics. Handled imperfectly and exposed or misused, this kind of data can jeopardize serious privacy breaches, exploitation, or discrimination. For instance, athlete health information can be used against them during contract negotiations or even while seeking opportunities in the latter stages of their career, when this information becomes public (Coutinho et al., 2018).

These risks, however, need to be addressed by organizations using AI-based systems should have proper data security measures and data protection compliance, especially on General Data Protection Regulation. In addition, encryption, secure storage, and access controls will be the foundation of protecting the athletes' personal data. The athletes should also be educatively enlightened on how their data is going to be accessed, stored, and shared, and they have the right to opt out of data collection in case they fear their careers being affected negatively (Daly et al., 2022).

3. Athlete Autonomy and Consent

There is also an ethical consideration regarding the use of AI-based workload monitoring systems: that athletes maintain control over both their bodies and their training. Athletes should not be treated as mere data points to be reduced and reordered at the whim of the AI but have to be involved in actual decision making pertaining to their training, recovery, and health and be fully engaged with the various insights that the AI can provide regarding fatigue and workload management. In general, if prescriptive AI systems become too pervasive, it is probable that athletes will lose control over the movements of their own bodies, with decisions based strictly on data rather than by choice or intuition (Delecroix et al., 2018).

Informed consent is a matter of significant concern. The right to accept whether they want to participate or not in data collection and use AI-based monitoring systems needs to be given to athletes. Their rights should be elaborated thoroughly regarding every kind of risk and benefits that may appear from using such technology, and their consent ought to be sought immediately. The reliability and safe-guarding autonomy is the most important aspect, therefore, it must be explained how AI-derived insights will impact their trainings plans (Mandorino, 2023).

4. Bias in AI Algorithms

AI systems are only as good as the data they get trained on, and biased training data leads to biased outcomes. In sports terms, AI algorithms might not well account for groups of athletes that perform differently due to such factors as gender, age, or ethnicity. For example, a model that has been predominantly trained on male athletes will probably not be able to provide any realistic fatigue predictions for a female athlete, as their physiological response to workload and recovery would probably differ. Lifestyle factors can also be different from one sportsperson to another within various cultures or socio-economic groups-that may impact their performance in ways not considered by the model (Martinho, 2024).

Such biases can therefore be circumvented if AI models are trained on diverse datasets that represent the whole scope of possible athletes. Continuous review and upgrading of these models will ensure that outcomes cannot be prejudiced and have the potential to deny people fair treatment or miss burnout risks (Nobari et al., 2023).

5. Effect on the Athlete-Coach Relationship

This reliance on AI for workloads will also breach the various traditional connections between the athlete and the coach. Coaching has always been one of the disciplines known to be a blend of science, art, and intuition: The strategies for taking the right choice depend on being familiar with the physical and psychological condition of the athlete by an experienced coach. The AI provides the data-driven output, though there are challenges in which over-reliance on technology may endanger the hegemony of the coach and diminish human intuition in making choices while training (Selmi et al., 2022).

In addition, athletes become highly dependent on suggestions by AI, hence undermining personal judgments and self-awareness as criteria in managing their bodies. It is equally important that these AI-based systems do not substitute but rather complement the role of the coach in the development of the athlete. The objective of the coaches and the AI systems would be to collaborate with the data being the foundation for their informed decision-making while the coach themselves continues delivering holistic support and guidance to the athletes according to their judgment (Starling et al., 2019).

## 6. Long-term Health and Ethical Responsibility

Another ethical concern is the long-term health and wellbeing of the athletes. The AI system will undoubtedly help manage short-term states of fatigue and workload but, most importantly, will be at the risk of overestimating athletes' limits in improving short-term performance, leading to a breakdown in health over time (Starling et al., 2020). For instance, an AI system may recommend increasing the workload of an athlete based on their physical readiness without considering entirely the implications of long-term stress on the body.

From an ethical standpoint, sports organizations need to do much more in terms of advancing the well-being of athletes over short-term gains. The system designed for the monitoring of workloads in AI-based methods should, therefore, be holistic within its view of athlete well-being, taking into account not only current performance but also the future health implications of high-intensity training and recovery regimens.

The AI-based fatigue and workload management systems have immense potential to improve the performance of the athlete, burnout, and injuries. Their implementation, however, encompass various challenges and ethical issues (Costa et al., 2019). The major focus areas that should be debated to provide the full benefits of these systems include data accuracy, privacy protection, athlete autonomy, and bias in AI algorithms. Second, AI can complement rather than supplant the human elements of coaching, and the long-term health of athletes will always need to be at the top of the list. As AI continues to evolve in the sport industry, issues and ethical considerations will have to be carefully balanced to ensure that the environment for athletes is fair and sustainable.

## FUTURE DIRECTIONS OF AI-BASED MONITORING OF ATHLETES

AI-based player monitoring systems set an important course for the future of monitoring systems with AI to revolutionize the modes of preparation, competition, and recovery by athletes. As AI technology continues to evolve, it shall become accurate, personal, and a part of usual sports practice. Continuous innovation in machine learning, wearables, and data analytics underpin the opening of new avenues in improving performance, prevention of injuries, and workload management. Several emerging trends will have the potential to shape the new era in AI-based player monitoring.

1. Much more advanced wearable technologies

The technology core of AI-based player monitoring is rooted in wearable devices that collect critical biometric data feeding into AI algorithms. The future of wearables will include development that is much more advanced, lighter, and directly integrated with AI systems in real time. Now, wearable sensors embedded in clothing, footwear, or even skin patches are designed to measure much larger sets of physiological and biomechanical parameters than those mentioned above, including muscle fatigue, hydration levels, oxygen saturation, and stress hormones. Better quality data will be produced by advanced sensors, further assisting AI models in making more accurate predictions about player fatigue and workload management (Chidambaram et al., 2022).

AI will further allow real-time changes in training or competition, where devices would immediately feedback to athletes and coaches. Real-time integration will therefore allow for more dynamic and responsive practice training to ensure the reach of maximal performance while staying at the lowest possible risk of overtraining.

2. Integration of Mental Health and Cognitive Metrics

Integration of metrics of mental health and cognitive performance, as well as physical indicators, will dominate future trends in player monitoring. Burnout certainly is a physical condition but is closely tied to mental fatigue, stress, and emotional well-being. In the future, AI-based systems will increasingly incorporate data related to psychological health, including mood, motivation, focus, and stress levels, gathered through wearable sensors or self-reported metrics (Vasiljevas et al., 2023).

These mental health indicators-from which the models are analyzing with physical data-would provide a more holistic view about the well-being of an athlete. The early warnings AI systems would give about cognitive decline or mental burnout, along with the physical form, would make the effort to prevent overtraining all the more comprehensive. Furthermore, AI can be used to provide personalized mental health interventions for athletes-including mindfulness exercises or stress management techniques-that would keep the athletes performing at their best mentally.

3. AI-centric personalization and adaptation

The future of AI-based player monitoring systems will be much more specialized and attuned to the specific needs and responses of individual athletes. So far, the algorithms are generalized and can be applied in most athletes' cases, but with the progress in machine learning, especially deep learning, such progress will allow systems to evolve and learn from data based on athletes over time. This will aid in the delivery of more individualized training and recovery information depending on one's history of performance, rates of recovery, and susceptibility to injury or burnout (Munoz-Macho et al., 2024).

With more customized AI systems, training load, recovery period, and nutrition plan for each athlete can be adapted uniquely according to the type of body, playing, and stress tolerance. Continuous adaptation to change in condition for an athlete by AI systems would provide a much more dynamic and responsive workload management approach.

4. Higher Application of Predictive Analytics

Predictive analytics will play an even more significant role in AI-based player monitoring in the future. When inputted with larger data sets of years of player performance, fatigue patterns, injury history, and recovery profiles, these systems shall begin to predict the future. When an athlete is likely to experience fatigue, burnout, or injury based on current workload and recovery patterns, AI-based systems shall accurately determine it.

Predictive capabilities will also allow for anticipatory interventions such as AI alerting coaches that, for example, it may be necessary to change an athlete's training schedule, so performance does not drop or injuries do not occur. Predictive analytics may model “what if” scenarios such that you can look ahead of time and see what might come to pass if you applied different training or recovery protocols.

5. AI-Powered Injury Prevention

The prevention of injury would become the greatest focus in monitoring players' activities in the future, and AI can predict and prevent such injuries through more sophisticated mechanisms. The AI algorithm can even track patterns that are correlated with higher risks of injury, such as biomechanical imbalances, overuse of certain muscles, or improper technique through wearable data, motion capture systems, and video analysis. Machine learning models can detect subtle changes in the patterns of movement or gait that might indicate an athlete is compensating for some form of fatigue or a minor injury, thereby allowing early intervention (Silacci et al., 2020).

Future AI systems will accumulate injury data by teams, sports, and regions to create a global database of injury patterns. It ought to be applied to enhance the injury prevention strategy. The systems will make athletes avoid short-term injuries but also prevent long-term wear and tear, hence prolonging the careers.

6. Multisport AI Platforms and Cross-Disciplinary Data Sharing

As AI-based player monitoring systems continue to evolve and grow, they will become more general-purpose and applied to other sports. All current systems are largely sport-specific, because most of them were primarily developed based on the very unique demands of, say, soccer, basketball, or marathon running. In the future, AI platforms will be able to sift through data coming from multiple sports; thus, there is a common pool of knowledge that improves upon athlete monitoring across disciplines (Nahavandi et al., 2022). Cross-disciplinary data sharing will allow AI to determine best practices in one sport and apply this knowledge to others, thus making fatigue management and injury prevention much more general.

Multisport AI systems will allow athletes competing in multiple sports to have their data monitored holistically, so the fatigue and workload accrued from playing one sport doesn't impact performance in another.

7. Interfacing with Virtual Reality/ Augmented Reality

Integration of AI with virtual reality, augmented reality is yet another promising trend for player monitoring systems. With the integration of AI with VR and AR, simulations of training environments may be enabled simulating actual physical and mental burdens experienced while training in competitions. An AI-driven VR system would be able to vary the intensity of the virtual environment in real time according to an athlete's degree of fatigue and so make challenging yet safe training possible.

Again, immersive environments may also help in mental conditioning of athletes with better focus and resilience in high-pressure conditions. AI-based AR glasses could provide real-time feedback in posture, technique, or even workload while training to athletes, giving them immediate adjustments before it affects the athlete in the form of fatigue or even an injury.

8. Ethical AI and Athlete-Centric Models

There will also be an uptick in more ethical AI, much more sensitive to athlete well-being. Other systems would have to think about data privacy and consent, which are not things you can hang your hat on as a plus for the overreach of AI. Ethical frameworks that position athletes in charge of their data will be more athlete-centered models. These models would emphasize transparency. Athletes and coaches can make smart decisions about how to use AI-derived insights about affecting the training and performance strategies.

Ethical AI shall also build systems that ensure long-term health of the athlete rather than short-term performances. AI systems shall balance the pressures of high-performance sports with the need to protect the athletes from the physical and psychological stress of overtraining.

Next on the agenda are future AI-based player monitoring and all the new applications on their way to redefine the landscape of sports performances and athlete management. The wearable technology will become far more advanced, while the AI applications for real-time mental health monitoring and injury prevention will make training more efficient, personalized, and safe. Integration of such systems with VR, predictive analytics, and ethical considerations ensures that the human athlete trains smarter, recovers faster, and avoids all the long-term consequences of overtraining and burnout. The integration of holistic athlete welfare approaches with cutting edge technology will unlock the true potential of athletes by offering them a healthy and fulfilling career.

## CONCLUSION

This is a dramatic step forward in sports science as AI-based player fatigue and workload monitoring systems constitute powerful tools for optimizing athlete performance and reducing occurrences of burnout and injury. These systems utilize machine learning models and analytics to provide personalized insights into the athlete's physical and mental condition, empowering coaches and sports organizations with evidence-based decisions on training intensity, recovery, and injury prevention. There is an even stronger potential for raising athletes' holistic well-being as wearable technology improves and AI algorithms continue to be at work with respect to mental health and cognitive metrics. However, AI in sports should be implemented in a careful manner, taking into consideration the problems associated with data accuracy, existing privacy issues and questions of ethical autonomy of the athletes. In the future, the AI used in the area of sport will develop greater personalization and predictive abilities along with the incorporation of other advanced technologies such as VR and AR to achieve more efficient trainings and longer careers for athletes. This embrace by sports organizations of these innovations will help hit the balance between high, above-the-peak athletic achievement of its athletes and long-term health and success.

## REFERENCES


Akyıldız, Z., Ocak, Y., Clemente, F., Birgonul, Y., Günay, M., & Nobari, H. (2022). Monitoring the post-match neuromuscular fatigue of young Turkish football players. *Scientific Reports, 12*(1), 13835. Advance online publication. DOI: 10.1038/s41598-022-17831-7 PMID: 35974069

Biró, A., Cuesta-Vargas, A. I., & Szilágyi, L. (2023). AI-assisted fatigue and stamina control for performance sports on IMU-generated multivariate time series datasets. *Sensors (Basel), 24*(1), 132. DOI: 10.3390/s24010132 PMID: 38202992

Biró, A., Jánosi-Rancz, K. T., & Szilágyi, L. (2024, January). Real-time Artificial Intelligence Text Analysis for Identifying Burnout Syndromes in High-Performance Athletes. In *2024 IEEE 22nd World Symposium on Applied Machine Intelligence and Informatics (SAMI)* (pp. 000253-000258). IEEE. DOI: 10.1109/SAMI60510.2024.10432817

Chidambaram, S., Maheswaran, Y., Patel, K., Sounderajah, V., Hashimoto, D. A., Seastedt, K. P., McGregor, A. H., Markar, S. R., & Darzi, A. (2022). Using artificial intelligence-enhanced sensing and wearable technology in sports medicine and performance optimization. *Sensors (Basel), 22*(18), 6920. DOI: 10.3390/s22186920 PMID: 36146263

Clemente, F., Silva, R., Chen, Y., Aquino, R., Praça, G., Castellano, J., Nobari, H., Mendes, B., Rosemann, T., & Knechtle, B. (2021). Accelerometry-workload indices concerning different levels of participation during congested fixture periods in professional soccer: A pilot study conducted over a full season. *International Journal of Environmental Research and Public Health, 18*(3), 1137. DOI: 10.3390/ijerph18031137 PMID: 33525533

Costa, M., Oliveira, D., Pinto, S., & Tavares, A. (2019). Detecting driver's fatigue, distraction, and activity using a non-intrusive AI-based monitoring system. *Journal of Artificial Intelligence and Soft Computing Research, 9*(4), 247–266. DOI: 10.2478/jaiscr-2019-0007

Coutinho, D., Gonçalves, B., Wong, D., Travassos, B., Coutts, A., & Sampaio, J. (2018). Exploring the effects of mental and muscular fatigue in soccer players' performance. *Human Movement Science, 58*, 287–296. DOI: 10.1016/j.humov.2018.03.004 PMID: 29549745

Daly, E., Pearce, A., Esser, P., & Ryan, L. (2022). Evaluating the relationship between neurological function, neuromuscular fatigue, and subjective performance measures in professional rugby union players. *Frontiers in Sports and Active Living*, *4*, 1058326. Advance online publication. DOI: 10.3389/fspor.2022.1058326 PMID: 36439623

Delecroix, B., McCall, A., Dawson, B., Berthoin, S., & Dupont, G. (2018). Workload and non-contact injury incidence in elite football players competing in European leagues. *European Journal of Sport Science*, *18*(9), 1280–1287. DOI: 10.1080/17461391.2018.1477994 PMID: 29860935

Giorgi, A., Ronca, V., Vozzi, A., Aricò, P., Borghini, G., Capotorto, R., Tamborra, L., Simonetti, I., Sportiello, S., Petrelli, M., Polidori, C., Varga, R., van Gasteren, M., Barua, A., Ahmed, M. U., Babiloni, F., & Di Flumeri, G. (2023). Neurophysiological mental fatigue assessment for developing user-centered Artificial Intelligence as a solution for autonomous driving. *Frontiers in Neurorobotics*, *17*, 1240933. DOI: 10.3389/fnbot.2023.1240933 PMID: 38107403

Mandorino, M., Tessitore, A., Leduc, C., Persichetti, V., Morabito, M., & Lacome, M. (2023). A new approach to quantify soccer players' readiness through machine learning techniques. *Applied Sciences (Basel, Switzerland)*, *13*(15), 8808. DOI: 10.3390/app13158808

Martinho, D., Rebelo, A., Field, A., Ribeiro, A. S., Pereira, F., Bizarro, B., Ribeiro, J., Len, S. M., Gouveia, É. R., & Sarmento, H. (2024). The quantification of physical performance and internal training load in youth male soccer players during preseason. *International Journal of Sports Physiology and Performance*, *19*(5), 480–486. DOI: 10.1123/ijspp.2023-0312 PMID: 38437841

Munoz-Macho, A. A., Domínguez-Morales, M. J., & Sevillano-Ramos, J. L. (2024). Performance and healthcare analysis in elite sports teams using artificial intelligence: A scoping review. *Frontiers in Sports and Active Living*, *6*, 1383723. DOI: 10.3389/fspor.2024.1383723 PMID: 38699628

Nahavandi, D., Alizadehsani, R., Khosravi, A., & Acharya, U. R. (2022). Application of artificial intelligence in wearable devices: Opportunities and challenges. *Computer Methods and Programs in Biomedicine*, *213*, 106541. DOI: 10.1016/j.cmpb.2021.106541 PMID: 34837860

Nobari, H., Gorouhi, A., Mallo, J., Lozano, D., Prieto-González, P., & Mainer-Pardos, E. (2023). Variations in cumulative workload and anaerobic power in adolescent elite male football players: Associations with biological maturation. *BMC Sports Science, Medicine and Rehabilitation*, *15*(1), 11. Advance online publication. DOI: 10.1186/s13102-023-00623-5 PMID: 36721183

Sandamal, K., Arachchi, S., Erkudov, V. O., Rozumbetov, K. U., & Rathnayake, U. (2024). Explainable artificial intelligence for fitness prediction of young athletes living in unfavorable environmental conditions. *Results in Engineering*, *23*, 102592. DOI: 10.1016/j.rineng.2024.102592

Selmi, O., Ouergui, I., Muscella, A., My, G., Marsigliante, S., Nobari, H., Suzuki, K., & Bouassida, A. (2022). Monitoring psychometric states of recovery to improve performance in soccer players: A brief review. *International Journal of Environmental Research and Public Health*, *19*(15), 9385. DOI: 10.3390/ijerph19159385 PMID: 35954741

Silacci, A., Taiar, R., & Caon, M. (2020). Towards an AI-based tailored training planning for road cyclists: A case study. *Applied Sciences (Basel, Switzerland)*, *11*(1), 313. DOI: 10.3390/app11010313

Starling, L., Nellemann, S., Parkes, A., & Lambert, M. (2019). The fatigue and fitness test for teams (FFITT): A practical option for monitoring athletes in a team as individuals. *European Journal of Sport Science*, *20*(1), 106–114. DOI: 10.1080/17461391.2019.1612951 PMID: 31109238

Starling, L., Nellemann, S., Parkes, A., & Lambert, M. (2020). The sensitivity of the fatigue and fitness test for teams (FFITT) to measure the demands of a rugby match. *European Journal of Sport Science*, *21*(6), 803–810. DOI: 10.1080/17461391.2020.1780327 PMID: 32511079

Vasiljevas, M., Damaševičius, R., & Maskeliūnas, R. (2023). A human-adaptive model for user performance and fatigue evaluation during gaze-tracking tasks. *Electronics (Basel)*, *12*(5), 1130. DOI: 10.3390/electronics12051130

# Chapter 3
# Building Your Sports Analytics Team

**Sandeep Kumar Singh**
https://orcid.org/0000-0002-1741-7254
*O.P. Jindal Global University, India*

**Hewawasam P. G. D. Wijethilak**
https://orcid.org/0009-0006-9611-5735
*University of Colombo, Sri Lanka*

## ABSTRACT

*This chapter will review the key building blocks and best practices to assemble an effective sports analytics team in the contemporary sports landscape. It covers the key functions, competence needs, hiring and recruitment strategies, and the design and dynamics of teamwork. It also articulates the technological tool requirements and the infrastructures involving data collection and processing, where it strongly emphasizes the importance of instituting a decision-making culture with data. It is, therefore, an examination of some trends that might shape the future of sports organizations, like being introduced by artificial intelligence and video analytics, and also challenges associated with such analyses and enhancements. From this analysis, sports organizations stand to position themselves accordingly to enable analytics help improve performances, inform decision-making, and engage fans better.*

DOI: 10.4018/979-8-3693-5385-1.ch003

## INTRODUCTION: THE ROLE OF ANALYTICS IN MODERN SPORTS

The sporting landscape has drastically changed within the past few years primarily through infusions of data and technology. From a niche element of professional sports franchises, sports analytics has become a cornerstone of decision-making for all levels of competition. The role of analytics in sports-from enhancing performance to recruiting new talent to strategy in games and injury prevention-is, in many ways, changing how teams play the game. It has, in fact, been fuelled by new breakthroughs in data science, machine learning, and broad access to huge datasets that reveal nearly all aspects of athletic performance. Today, while relying on one's instincts and experience, teams use complex data-driven models to get an edge over the competition (Szymanski, 2020).

Underpinning such an evolution is the ability to collect, process, and analyze vast amounts of data. Sports analytics is a type of data that goes well beyond the traditional statistics: points scored, rebounds, and the like. It can go all the way down to the granularity of things such as movement patterns of individual players, biomechanics, and physiological data from wearables. Advanced tools such as the player tracking systems, video analysis software, and AI-powered algorithms have enabled coaches and teams to make decisions based on much more information in real time (Gerrard, 2017). It has only increased the accuracy of the tactical decisions but also provided a closer insight to the performance of the player, hence helping the teams to make the right training sessions and appropriate workload planning for the players.

The greatest positive influence that sports analytics has had is in talent identification and recruitment. With data-driven scouting, teams can now analyze the potential of a player more accurately than ever before. In addition to sprint speed, passing accuracy and many other measurable qualities, psychological indicators such as ability to make right decisions under stress can also be measured. Thus, more accuracy in finding undervalued talent or future stars would prevail with a lesser risk in high-stake investments in an athlete. Moneyball" of the Oakland Athletics baseball team demonstrates how the obsession with data can revolutionize recruitment strategies and truly make the playing field as level for the smaller market teams as it can be against the financial giants (Bayoumi & Zaid, 2021).

Beyond player and team performance, it has even reached to impact the business side of sports on fan engagement. Analytics have been used by teams to understand fan behavior, price tickets for optimum yields, and tailor marketing strategies to enhance the fan experience. Hence, analytics have helped sports organizations both improve their on-field performance and stimulate revenue growth and operational efficiency.

On the other hand, although sports analytics presents several benefits, its increased use has also come with some new challenges. The traditionalists often oppose heavy reliance on data and welcome subjective expertise and gut feeling instead. Balancing the use of data with experiential knowledge remains an important challenge that teams wanting to be ahead of this never-ending landscape must face (Davis et al., 2024).

Role of analytics in modern sports is undeniable. Analytics has created a paradigm shift that, among other things, allows teams to make more precise and well-informed decisions. Such decisions can lead to better performances, avoiding risks, and better management of a team. Even with more advancements in technology, the power of analytics will be increased; therefore, it will be an integral part of success on and off the field.

## IDENTIFYING KEY ROLES AND SKILL SETS

The best sports analytics team would need a delicate mix of diverse roles and skill sets that together manage to harness data to bring on the decision-making cycle and improvements in performance. Each role would vary across members in a way that each member has a unique point of view, thereby making it essential to define these positions to help ease integration among the individuals involved. Here are the key roles and the skills required in building an effective sports analytics team:

1. Data Scientists and Statisticians

The backbone of any sports analytics team, data scientists and statisticians develop the statistical models, algorithms, and machine learning systems that will process raw data into something actionable. These professionals require a good foundation in mathematics, statistics, and data science. More importantly, they should be proficient in programming languages like Python, R, and SQL, which most data manipulation and analysis work typically deal with. Their ability to provide coaches and management teams with predictive models that analyze performance, potential outcomes of games, and injury risks is invaluable (Mgaya et al., 2021).

2. Data Engineers

Data engineers essentially manage the flow of data coming from different sources such as tracking systems, wearables, and even game footage. These individuals design, deploy, and manage the infrastructure that contains an enormous amount of data. Therefore, they should be knowledgeable about database architecture, data integration, and cloud computing platforms such as AWS, Google Cloud, or Microsoft Azure. One should be an expert in strong coding skills using Java or Scala. Data engineers ensure that data is clean, structured, and available for analysis. In this regard, they play the most critical role in maintaining integrity and access to data within the team (Jayal et al., 2018).

3. Sports Analysts

Sports analysts are the technicians between the data and the real-life usage of it in the game. They have excellent analytical skills but also an excellent understanding of the game and nuances. They translate data insights into strategic suggestions to coaches and players. A sports analyst collaborates with coaches on the breakdown of performance metrics, game statistics, and the analysis of the opponent (Tan, 2023). The analyst needs to be able to express complex insights from data in a manner understandable by nontechnical stakeholders, and communication along with knowledge of the game are therefore essential.

4. Software Developers

A software developer in this sports analytics group builds tools and platforms for data visualization, analysis, and real-time reporting. Dashboards, mobile applications, or custom solutions that enable coaches and players to interact with the data are built by these developers. Experience in front-end and back-end development with exposure to data visualization libraries such as D3.js or Tableau are major skills. The needs of the sports team should also be known by these developers to provide user-friendly interfaces for the streamlining of the decision-making process (Herberger & Litke, 2021).

5. Performance Analysts

A performance analyst specializes in applying analytics for the maximization of player performance. He looks into the movement patterns of players, physiological data, and biomechanics, often supported by video recordings or wearable technology. These studies help determine patterns that can be used to enhance the performance or will minimize the probability of injury. These experts should be updated with motion capture technology, GPS tracking, and biomechanical analysis tools to perform the role of a performance analyst (Muniz & Flamand, 2023). Moreover, performance analysts should only offer actionable advice that will guide teams to advance toward better training and recovery strategies when they have a deep understanding of exercise science and sports physiology.

6. Sports Domain Experts

While data and technical expertise are necessarily important, the analytics team must comprise domain experts in sports. These experts are better equipped to understand the sport, which otherwise would be lacking in a pure data scientist. They take care so that analysis by means of data is interpreted within the framework of rules, strategies, and culture specific to the sport. Be it former athletes or coaches or specialists in the sport itself, for a transition of analytics into working applications, domain experts become important (Baerg, 2016)

A balanced sports analytics team would have combination specialists in data science and engineering with domain-specific knowledge to be applied directly in sports. Every aspect contributes to teamwork in unlocking the full potential of analytics in modern sports. Every player on the team plays a unique but interconnected role in converting data into competitive advantage to ensure that the organization can make informed and data-driven decisions.

## HIRING AND RECRUITING STRATEGIES

Hiring and recruitment are areas from which a strong sports analytics team starts building. The rising demand for data-driven insight into sports calls for the need to attract talent into the organization and, more importantly, retain them. TOP. A well-thought-out recruitment approach should be designed not only to attract technical-skilled people but also to find the right people who, due to their background and experiences, could work together in a challenging, fast-changing sports environment. The subsequent section addresses some of the most effective approaches to talent recruitment for a sports analytics team.

1. Define the Skills and Competencies Required

However, before beginning the hiring process, it is very important to understand what each position entails within these entire sports analytics team. Each part of this chain-from data scientists and engineers to sports analysts and performance experts-needed a distinct set of skills and knowledge. Technical roles, such as data scientists, would require skills in statistics, machine learning, and programming (Python, R, SQL). For sports analysts, it is essentially an understanding of the sport deeply with analytical thinking. A well-defined job description helps to target candidates with the required specific qualifications thereby constituting a team that is balanced with the right mix of technical know-how and sports domain knowledge (Claudino et al., 2019).

2. Leverage University Partnerships and Internships

Collaboration with strong universities and institutions that boast bright data science, sports management, and related studies programs is the best bet for sourcing the brightest emerging talent. Therefore, the universities offer courses in sports analytics and data science as specializations. This provokes a new pool of students looking to acquire those skills for application in real-world environments. Development of internship programs enables organizations to assess a potential candidate on a trial basis while providing students with real-life experience. Other than being an important recruitment tool, the partnerships help shape the reputation of an organization within the academic community (Dergaa, 2024).

3. Look Beyond the Sports Industry

This is, first of all, where knowledge of the domain in sports comes in, but most technical skills that are required for a team to execute sports analytics are not anchored to the sports industry: data engineering, machine learning, software development. Organizations will look to expand their sources for finding talent by considering candidates from other adjacent fields such as finance, healthcare, or technology where advanced data analytics is already in action. Different industries provide professionals with the appropriate type of expertise in these areas, thus allowing them to develop fresh ideas and unique solutions of problems regarding sports. A diverse analytical talent pool will look at candidates beyond the sporting background to bring in fresh ideas to an organization (Goes et al., 2020).

4. Evaluate for Soft Skills and Cultural Fit

Technical skills are very significant to evaluate the candidate, but soft skills, like communication skills, teamwork, and adaptable nature, should not be neglected. Sports analytics teams work with coaches, athletes, and management very closely. And more often than not, these groups do not have a firm basis in data science. So, there is a need to hire people who can explain complex data insights into understandable actionable points (Kaur et al., 2021). Candidates that show great interpersonal skills and can be shown to perform well as part of a multidisciplinary team are very likely to succeed in sports analytics roles. Cultural fit is also important, since players must thrive in the high-stakes, fast-moving world of professional sports.

5. Leverage Industry Networks and Conferences

Attendance at industry conferences and sports analytics networking events can provide opportunities to network with professionals already established in the discipline. Some of the events presented above include the MIT Sloan Sports Analytics Conference or the Sports Analytics World Series, holding the potential to unite the leaders and innovators of sports data science. Conferences like these allow organizations to meet potentials in their hiring lists, learn of the latest trends, and interact with the top talent, who may be needing new projects. Maintaining an observable presence within these networks can further the reputation of the organization as an analytics professional destination (Spaaij & Thiel, 2017).

6. Utilize Online Channels and Specialized Job Boards

Online channels as well as specialized job boards are useful sources for attracting available talent. Sites such as LinkedIn, Stack Overflow, and GitHub allow an organization to look up individuals with a given technical skill set and assess what they have done by the contributions they have made publicly in the development of coding projects (Szymanski, 2020). Third, job boards aimed specifically at sports professionals or data scientists may provide sources for targeting those that are enthusiastic about applying their skills in a sports context. Posting detailed job descriptions on these platforms ensures the team attracts candidates with the right qualifications and interests.

7. Develop a Strong Employer Brand

To attract the best talent, organizations need to build a strong employer brand that speaks to data professionals. Organizations should indicate their commitment toward innovation, cutting-edge technology, and data-driven decision-making in sports. Some of the strategies will be pointing out successful projects, case studies or partnership with really strong sports teams as a strategy that will appeal to the candidate's excitement in using data to make an impact on the field. Competitive salaries, opportunities for professional development, and integrated work culture can all become powerful attraction factors to talents in data professions into the organization (Mosley, 2014).

Hiring talent into a sports analytics team is not just a straightforward approach, but rather a multifaceted process that will require forward planning and targeted outreach. By using a broad definition of the competencies needed in a timely manner, by building on academic partnerships, and through diversified recruitment methods, organizations will identify a more suitable talent pool. The ability of this new hire to adapt to the collaborative and fast-paced environment of sports analytics will most likely be guaranteed by the combination of technical skills with relevant soft skills. A strong employer brand and a continued presence in the sports analytics community would therefore further place the organization at the forefront of data-driven innovation in sports (Hassan et al., 2022).

## TEAM STRUCTURE AND DYNAMICS

More than the right talent needed to build a successful sports analytics team, the structure and dynamics of such teams are also a critical factor in ensuring that their members can contribute toward the organization's goals. An excellent team has diversity in the mix, collaboration for process, and being flexible enough to embrace the rapidly changing nature of sports. The following section will outline planning and structure for a team that involves both theoretical and practical accomplishment and creating a collaborative culture that fosters innovation and continuous improvement.

1. The Role of Leadership

A good sports analytics team begins with leadership-a bridge that can tie data insights to real-world applications. Typically, the head of an analytics team-the Chief Data Officer or Head of Sports Analytics-should be a blend of technical expertise and a deep understanding of the sport involved. This leader would define strategic direction, set work plans and priorities for a team aligned with the overall goals of a sports organization. This leader will communicate effectively to and from coaches, athletes, and management while inspiring innovation and problem-solving in the team. They should be able to translate complex data into actionable insights (Thorne & Pellant, 2007).

2. Cross-Functional Teams

In a multidisciplinary area like sports analytics, most teams tend to be cross-functional, mixing in several different domains. A standard sports analytics team would contain data scientists and data engineers who would collect data and explain their job in detail, sports analysts who would utilize that data in explaining their job, performance experts who would put on-field practical knowledge into the model, software developers who will further improve the application of models, and domain experts-worshipers of the game who can explain in as much detail as possible how to get the desired result. Cross-functional collaboration brings together team members who work on complex problems and pool knowledge for new innovative solutions that can be easily applied directly to improve team performance (Sullivan & Callow, 2005).

For example, a performance analysis team may collaborate with data engineers in developing models to track and optimize the workloads of players. On the other hand, sports analysts will interact with the software developers to design user-friendly dashboards for the coaches so that they can get the real-time visualization of the data during games.

3. Centralized Versus Decentralized Structures

Decentralized and Centralized Models A common decision organizations have to make in structuring the sports analytics team is between a centralized and a decentralized model. Under a centralized model, all analytics professionals work within a single unit, usually serving multiple departments within the sports organization. This promotes consistency in data collection and analysis while providing shared resources and infrastructure. It is easier to align analytics efforts with the overall strategic objectives of the organization (Leo et al., 2019).

Analytics experts are spread throughout the different departments-for example, a performance department, strategy department, or sports medicine department whose departments can then have direct access to analytics insights fit to their needs. A decentralized approach encourages the most specialized in-depth analyses and facilitates faster decision-making within the department.

Most organizations adopt a hybrid in which central analytics hub provides overall support while analysts are deployed to departments to respond to particularized needs. This hybrid model balances the benefits accrued from both central consistency and decentralization of specialized needs.

4. Collaboration and Communication

Since the work entails a lot of technicalities, effective communication becomes very important to the success of a sports analytics team. Analysts and data scientists would hence be needed to explain complex models and insights to the coaches, the players, and management in general-most of whom may not have any technical backgrounds. The requirement calls for openness in the communication culture where data professionals and the sports experts continually engage in idea exchange and the refinement of strategies (Ibsen & Levinsen, 2019).

Regular, often scheduled meetings between analytics teams and coaching staff in the form of pre-game strategy sessions or post-game debriefs to ensure objectives are aligned and data insights are incorporated into decision-making. Collaborative tools and platforms, such as Slack, Microsoft Teams, or a custom data-sharing dashboard, streamline communication and project management across functions (Bosch & Mansell, 2015).

5. Adapting to the Sports Environment

The sport industry is dynamic, wherein, often, the team has to make decisions very rapidly during a game, practice, or a trade deadline. Hence, the analytics team needs to be flexible and adapt to real-time demands. This can be done by embracing agile workflows whereby the team splits larger projects into smaller tasks and is continuously adjusting their approach according to feedback. The multiple short bursts and frequent touchpoints guarantee the analytics team can adjust quickly if there are hidden potential roadblocks. Perhaps it's adjusting a player appearance sequence during a season or even revising injury prevention policies (Guillén & Martínez-Alvarado, 2014).

Adapting to the sporting environment also encompasses the seasonal nature of the industry, thus during the off-season, the analytics team is likely to focus on long-term projects that include developing predictive models for recruiting athletes and during the season, real-time analysis, observation of players, and supporting game strategy from the analytics people in the team. Ability to adapt and change, especially between these modes, marks one of the most crucial management skills of the workflow (Mason, 2019).

6. Continuous Education and Knowledge Building

The field of sports analytics is dynamic with new tools, technologies, and methodologies emerging by the day. The teams must, therefore, inculcate the spirit of continuous education and innovation. This can be done by motivating team members to keep themselves updated with the latest changes in data science, machine learning, and sports technology. It should engage opportunities in professional development, conferences, or holding in-house workshops.

The other element of innovation is an enabling atmosphere to experiment. Analytics teams need to be allowed to test their thoughts, whether in terms of a novel way of monitoring player performance or some innovative approach towards fan engagement. Developing such experimentation mindsets would thus help teams remain ahead of the curve and develop the latest cutting-edge solutions (Sikorska et al., 2014).

Things are very different when it comes to the overall structure and dynamics of a sports analytics team. It is possible to unlock even better performance and strategy impacts through clear leadership, cross-functional collaboration, and agile workflows. Effective communication, continuous learning, and flexibility in the accelerated world of sports help an analytics team stay at the center of the organization's decision-making processes. The team, technically astute as well as agile enough, is bound to thrive in the data-driven world of modern sports (Ibsen & Levinsen, 2019).

## TEAM STRUCTURE AND DYNAMICS

In building a productive sports analytics team, appropriate concerns must be afforded both to the structure of the team and to interpersonal relations. A coordinated team is one in which roles and responsibilities are defined, and one can ensure smooth teamwork, maximize efficiency as well as ensure that thought data yields actionable outcomes. The game requires balance; the ability to advise on a combination of technical expertise and domain knowledge to successfully work cohesively under high-pressure situations dictates the critical elements of structuring a sports analytics team and the dynamics that foster a collaborative productive environment.

1. Leadership and Vision

At the head of every good sports analytics' organization is a strong leadership position-mostly referred to as a Chief Analytics Officer or Director of Analytics. Such a leader should, of course, be deeply informed about both the sports industry and data science and thus be capable of guiding their teams strategically and orienting the work of these teams into the overall vision of a sports organization. This is because a good leader will bridge the gap between the technical experts and the non-technical stakeholders by fully explaining their viewpoint, transforming complex data insights into actionable recommendations for coaches, players, and management (Acar, 2023).

In addition, a leader must articulate a clear vision and direction for the team. Whether it is player performance, injury prevention, or fan engagement, great leadership keeps the team focused on priorities aligned with the competitive strategy of the organization. A visionary leader also creates an innovative culture, challenging the team to try new methodologies, tools, and technologies (Rein et al., 2015).

2. Cross-Functional Collaboration

An effective sports analytics function should involve the interface of skilled people with different skill sets working towards common objectives. In a cross-functional structure, data scientists, sports analysts, software developers, and domain experts will combine their specialized expertise to deliver collaborative results (Son et al., 2018). The data scientists would work on predictive models and analyze performance metrics, whereas the sports analysts convey game-specific knowledge to contextualize an understanding of data insights. The development of the software will involve designing platforms or dashboards through which analytics will become available in real time to coaches and players.

This cross-functional team creates synergy because every team member brings in their specific expertise in creating a more holistic answer. For instance, where a data scientist would design a model predicting player fatigue using machine learning, it is the sports analyst who would interpret that within the context of their in-game decisions. The synergy of technical and nontechnical members will be what fosters the highest results for analytics influence on team performance and strategy (Darian & Coopersmith, 2001).

3. Definition and Specialization of Roles

Well-defined roles within the sports analytics team determine what goes on and who does what, which helps the organization remain silky-smooth as regards to its interactions and to avoid overlap of tasks. Normally, there are three key roles: data scientists focused on algorithms and complicated data analysis; data engineers responsible for the infrastructure and support; and performance analysts possessing a sports industry view based on the data extracted. Other roles may also be added, such as: to develop user-facing applications, for example by software developers and UX designers, so that applications can be intuitive, user-centered, and meet the needs of coaches and players (Marcu & Buhaş, 2014).

Since every role should be specific in terms of responsibilities so that no member is restricted to a particular kind of work without adding value to the team's objectives, specialization enables teamwork members to work on one area of specialization but ensures their efforts harmonize as the solution to bigger, more complex problems.

4. Centralized vs. Decentralized Structures

Most sports organizations must then decide whether to have their analytics teams centralized or decentralized. Centralized implies that the entire analytics team works as one unit for various departments, such as coaching, player development, and management. It helps in uniform data analysis and creates teamwork across various parts of the organization (Khadartsev et al., 2017).

On the other hand, a decentralized setup has analytics professionals integrated within specific departments or teams such that they gain insights specific to each unit's needs. For example, performance analysts may be closely coordinated with the coaching staff, and data engineers work on improving the overall supporting data structure of the team. A decentralized setup benefits with faster decision making within departments but depends on internal communication and coordination within teams to keep in line with the larger organizational goals.

A hybrid model is adopted by many sporting organizations, with a strong core analytics group at the reservoir overall and specialists located within specific business units. This ensures that the specific needs are being met, but the team remains focused and balanced (Serôdio et al., 2018).

5. Interaction with Coaching Staff

With the realization of positive sports analytics, communication of the insight drawn from the data and translated into action on the field is therefore key to the team. The team should be effective in delivering complex data in clear simple language that would resonate with the coaching staff, players, and other nontechnical persons. Therefore, verbal and written communication skills in tandem with a very integrated approach to working directly with coaching staff to get strategies implemented from the insight based on data would become necessary (Kalinina et al., 2018).

Another very positive aspect of integration with the coaching staff is that the coach may often depend on real-time data to make decisions during a game. Analytics teams ought to build up such tools and dashboards so that they will present key metrics to the coaches in a manner that easily allows them to understand them and make wise decisions. A rhythm of regular meetings between analytics teams and coaching staff, say pre-game planning and post-game debriefs, will help ensure objectives are in alignment, and data is used appropriately.

6. Encourage Collaboration and Team Culture

A sports analytics team thrives best in an environment that encourages collaboration, trust, and a culture of continuous improvement. Creating a collaborative environment would involve encouraging open communication, encouraging the sharing of ideas, and making sure that team members feel empowered to contribute their perspectives. Regular meeting and brainstorming sessions can help create that sense of community and cooperation (Komskienė-Žukauskienė et al., 2009).

Team culture is equal, too. In the world of sports, where speedy decisions may have a huge effect, inculcating a culture of flexibility and resiliency is very important. The analytics teams should be highly flexible while responding to changing situations-be it a mid-season injury or a mid-game change in strategy. Promotion of a culture that exalts experimentation, fear of failure can also inspire innovation; the team is freed to explore new means and technologies without fear of error.

7. Agility and Adaptability in a Dynamic Sports Environment

Sports by nature are fluid; conditions fluctuate by minute circumstances. This implies that whether it is during the middle of the game, over a season, or over the lifetime of an athlete's career, a sports analytics team needs to be flexible and responsive. They have to change easily to emerging trends, new data streams, and unforeseen challenges. A good example would be when one of the key players has an injury at the last minute or midway into the season, a trade occurs, and hence some performance analytics have to change (Savić et al., 2018).

Agile project management method tools help teams respond quickly to real-time demands; they can work in short sprints and frequent check-ins, make quick adjustments to work schedules to fit into evolving needs for the coaches, players, and the entire organization.

While the makeup and dynamics of a sports analytics team are somewhat the foundation for success, all of its parts-from top-level leadership to specific role players, cross-functional collaboration, and communication with coaching staff-help form the makeup of this kind of team that can develop many consequential insights that help yield the appropriate performance metrics (Lehtonen, 2017). With such a constitution, an agile team structured with the collaborative culture can function well in the world of sports, which is ever-changing and fast-paced, unlocking organizational and personal success through data-driven decision-making.

## TECHNOLOGICAL TOOLS AND INFRASTRUCTURE

The sports analytics landscape is changing, and it all comes down to the efficient gathering, analyzing, and applying data. A good technological framework allows teams to get raw data into effective actionable, optimize performances by players, strengthen game strategies, and positively engage with the fans. Below are the critical technological tools and infrastructure of a successful sports analytics team.

1. Data Gathering Technologies

The first step for any analytics initiative is data collection, and in sports, there are many methods and technologies by which it is done. These devices include wearable GPS trackers and heart monitors that enable teams to get the real-time information about the performance of players, the levels of fatigue, and exertion. It collects metrics such as speed, distance covered, and heart rate variability, helping coaches and performance analysts understand whether a player is healthy and ready for the game (Callejo & Forcadell, 2006).

Apart from wearable technologies, video analysis tools are just as important in capturing in-game performance. High-definition cameras and software that specialize in different analysis allow teams to determine player movements, tactics, or strategies from various angles. With advanced video analytics tools, breaks downplays for review and assessment of player positioning with areas for improvement. Through the integration of these collection technologies, an integrated overall picture on player performance is captured while constituting towards informed decision-making.

2. Data Storage and Management Solutions

Data captured needs to be stored and managed in such a way that is accessed and used with ease. Cloud storage solutions scale and are flexible, allowing sports organizations to manage huge chunks of data without having their physical infrastructure. These services include Amazon Web Services (AWS), Google Cloud Platform (GCP), and Microsoft Azure, which can provide reliable, safe, and cost-effective options for data storage (Bilohur et al., 2022).

The other key aspect of successful data management is the adoption of a database that can accommodate every kind of data and formats. Relational databases such as PostgreSQL and MySQL are applied for structured data while NoSQL databases like MongoDB are ideal for semi-structured or unstructured data. A good data management system helps teams achieve data integrity, easier access, and easier analysis.

3. Analytical Software and Tools

Analytical phase: Here, data is transformed into insights. The decisions are guided by the outcome of the analyses. There are numerous analytical software and tools meant to cater to different analytical needs. Among the many applications of statistical analysis software, the R and Python will be where the complex statistical modeling and hypothesis testing can be carried out by data scientists. End Among the very powerful libraries and packages available for data manipulation, visualization, and machine learning, one may find in these languages (Rija et al., 2023).

In sports-specific analysis, where specific analytics constitute the platforms, e.g., Synergy Sports Technology, Sportscode, and Catapult, offer specific functionalities tailored to the assessment of any player's performance and strategic analysis by a given team. Such platforms usually carry tools for video tagging, automated report generation, and real-time data visualization instruments so that coaches and analysts can view data as fast as possible and be able to make the necessary decisions.

In addition, tools like Tableau and Power BI immensely aid in the presentation of data. Dashboards and interactive reports become formidable means of visualizing complex metrics for the stakeholder while tracking performance trends and drawing insights.

4. Collaboration and Communication Tools

Good collaboration and communication are essentials in integrating analytics into sports decision-making. Slack, Microsoft Teams, and Asana facilitate communication among the analytics teams and other people in the department-from the coaching staff to the player development, management, and more. It supports real-time messaging, file sharing, and project management, and encourages collaboration and transparency.

Additional, video conferencing applications, such as Zoom or Microsoft Teams must be employed as a new trend for teams to have face-to-face meetings virtually since a good number of the workforce spends less time on physical premises. Video conferencing facilitates an opportunity for more discussions of insights, game recordings, and strategy generations from anywhere regardless of the geographical location. Technology can strengthen the bridges connecting analytics to practical application in the sport since clear communication and team collaboration are achieved (Son et al., 2018).

5. Real-Time Analytics and Decision Support Systems

The access and analysis of data in near real time have taken the heart of sports far beyond what constitutes the world of sports. Coaches, analysts, and managers should have insights that are up to the minute in nature, impacting the strategy in games and the management of players; this can be achieved using real-time analytics, the processing of data at the Edge through computing technologies supporting data processing at the source, reducing latency and ensuring that critical insights are received as soon as they happen (Acar, 2023).

In this regard, the synthesis of diverse data sources is utilized through Decision Support Systems in making decisions and choice-making. Performance data, historical statistics, and player health metrics are integrated to support the coaches and managers regarding real games in real-time. Regarding this, the user-friendly interfaces often reflect insights into a digestible format to enable quick comprehensive data analysis by the coaches (Cao, 2022).

6. Cybersecurity and Data Privacy Requirements

More sports organizations use data more than ever. Thus, cybersecurity and data privacy measures are indeed critical protection against unauthorized access to sensitive information about the players, financial records, and proprietary analytics. Organizations need to be armed with encrypted protocols, firewalls, and access controls to secure their data in compliance with regulations such as the GDPR (Jenkins & Evans, 2020).

Data privacy measures extend also to responsible usage of data of players. Organizations ought to have policies where data collection, storage, and usage are clearly stated to be transparent and involve ethical consideration. This culture of data responsibility helps sport organizations trust players, fans, and other stakeholders while utilizing analytics in improving performance.

Sports analytics drive data-driven decision-making and maximize team performance. Behind the technological tools and infrastructure that enable all these are foundational principles in sports analytics. Be it at the data collection technology and management solutions, analytics tools, or real-time decision-support systems, every one of them becomes a crucial piece in the analytics ecosystem. Getting the right technologies and instilling this teamwork culture inside the organization could unlock the vast potential that analytics brings and impacts competitive ability in this dynamic world of sports (Mason, 2019).

## DATA COLLECTION AND MANAGEMENT

Essentially, the heart of a high-powered sports analytics operation relies on good data collection and management. The way one goes about collecting, summarizing, and keeping current good data translates into the quality of insight gained from analytics. Below are some of the best information regarding data collection methods and management practices that need to be pursued by sports organizations to ensure agile and reliable analytics processes.

1. Data Collection Methods

Sports analytics can involve different methodologies for a for purposes and different provisions of insights. Majorly, two approaches are evident in view: the quantitative as well as the qualitative approach.

Quantitative data collection: This method focuses on only numerical data which is apt for analysis statistically. Here, in sports, quantitative data are garnered mostly through performance tracking systems, and most of the statistics of the game are taken using other tools like wearable devices. The use of wearable technology, such as GPS devices and heart rate monitors, allows to track real-time the movement and exertion levels of players and their physiological responses in the context of the practice or competition under way. Such tools provide a high number of metrics, such as how fast one can go, distance covered, and heart rate variability, thus assessing how the player is performing physically and monitoring their level of fatigue.

Apart from wearables, there are video analysis systems that track in-game performance data. High-definition cameras combined with play-tracking/tagging software enable teams to break down the video footage and pull out critical information. For instance, analysts can analyze video-based data about how a player is positioned, the decisions they make, and the effectiveness of their tactics. The integration of both wearable technology and video analysis creates a holistic dataset that provides invaluable insights into player performance.

Qualitative Data Collection: This involved gathering non-numerical data possibly from an observational study, interviews, or surveys. Qualitative data can be used in providing contextual background to the quantified metrics collected, thus offering deeper understanding in terms of players' behaviors, team dynamics, and coaching strategies. For example, interviewing players and coaches revealed their experience, motives, and perceptions of performance. This qualitative information can complement the findings from the numerical data, thus providing a general picture of what may prompt success in the field.

2. Data management practices

Once data is captured, good management practices start to play a crucial role in respecting its integrity, accessibility, and usability. A comprehensive data management framework incorporates several key components.

Data Storage Solutions: Huge data collection by sports organizations requires a suitable storage solution for sports organizations. Cloud-based storages from AWS, Microsoft Azure, and Google Cloud Platform are scalable storage solutions for large datasets. Centralized repositories across these platforms enable safe access, storage, and analysis of data by teams in their organizations.

Outside of cloud storage, data governance policies would form the platform for accurately and consistently maintained data across an organization. The policies would, for example, include establishing entry, validation, and maintenance protocols on data. Periodic audits and quality checks normally point to inconsistencies in the data, and analytics will always be performed based on credible information.

Data Integration and Accessibility: Data integration of various sources is fundamental to combining comprehensive analysis. Sports organizations collect data from performance tracking, video analysis, and team management software. Through data integration tools and techniques, which include the use of ETL processes, for instance, organizations are able to bring disjointed datasets together into one form for analysis.

Another is access, and analytics teams should be able to put in place data access protocols that are simple and allow pertinent stakeholders, including coaches and management, the possibility of easily retrieving and interpreting the data that they need. In this regard, it may be necessary to build a dashboard or some forms of data visualization tool which means that information is presented in intuitive form so that users quickly recognize what insights convey without technical acumen.

3. Data Security and Privacy

With more reliance on data, there's a greater responsibility to secure such data and safeguard the privacy of the people involved. In this regard, prominent cyber security features must be incorporated, ensuring that sensitive player information, financial records, and proprietary analytics are safeguarded.

Cyber Security: The organizations will embrace multi-layered approaches towards security including encryption, firewalls, and implementing access controls on data sources so as to reduce unauthorized access and breaches. This can be supported by the regular security assessment and vulnerability testing so that possible weakness in the system may be indentified earlier and remediated in time.

Data Privacy Policies In addition to security measures, organizations should have a data privacy policy that transpires to regulation such as the General Data Protection Regulation. The organizations should detail how collected data is preserved, stored, and processed since this comes with a compelling need for data transparency and ethical considerations on dealing with personal information. Such an organization should communicate their data practice to the players and other stakeholders to build trust and maintain a responsible data management culture.

4. Continual improvement and adaptation

Sports analytics is constantly evolving as new technologies and methodologies emerge regularly. It's only by learning to constantly adapt that sports organizations can remain competitive.

Trend and Innovation Watch: Data collection as well as management can be a very competitive area for service providers. Technological changes are being introduced every day. To remain ahead in the market, it is essential to keep track of the latest trends in data collection and management. This may involve attending industry conferences, participating in workshops, collaborating with technology providers, or finding innovative solutions that might improve data collection and management.

Feedback and iteration: It involves constantly soliciting team members and stakeholders for areas of improvement concerning the methods used in collecting data and the practice of managing data. This leads to an iterative process that encourages learning from experimentation and refines data practice to the utmost value derived through analytics efforts.

Data collection and management are integral parts of any successful sports analytics program. It includes utilizing the various methods of data collection, strong practices in management, protection and privacy of data, and a continuous improvement culture to help sports organizations exploit the power of data analytics. This foundation allows teams to drill down to actionable insights that drive performance, shape strategies, and ultimately meet competitive goals.

## BUILDING A CULTURE OF DATA-DRIVEN DECISION-MAKING

Creating a culture of data-driven decision making holds the key to capitalizing on the full power of analytics by a sports organization. There is much more than just embedding data into all operations; it encompasses creating a culture in which findings from data are cherished and acted upon. This section unravels the important things involved in developing a robust culture of data-driven decision making in sports (Serôdio et al., 2018).

1. Leadership Commitment and Vision

Leading by commitment A data-driven culture must start with a high commitment from leadership. At least, leadership should have a clear vision of how data can advance performance and inform choices within the entire organization. For example, expectations should be set so that data-driven insights can form key drivers for strategic operations: recruitment of players to game tactics (Rija et al., 2023).

The leaders need to demonstrate commitment toward data-driven practices and lead by example through investment in analytics resources, that is, getting skilled data scientists on board and ensuring they are provided with necessary tools and technologies. The organizational heads will thus inspire team members toward the adoption of a data-centric mindset through the goal of seeking out and using analytics in their daily roles, and communicating the value of data-driven decision-making and celebrating success achieved through analytics can further reinforce this commitment (Lehtonen, 2017).

2. Training and Education

The first important step on the ladder towards being a data-driven organization is training for its employees. Since, through education and training, staff members are equipped to keep on learning, organizations can produce team members who can understand and interpret data properly. This can be included in the list as work-related seminars and workshops but also online courses that relate to data analysis, visualization tools, and statistical methodologies (Kalinina et al., 2018).

Training needs to be extremely role orientated. For instance, for the coaching staff it can enable training for interpretation of player performance metrics. The front office personnel may have training for data-driven financial modeling. Arming all team members with a foundational knowledge of data analytics brings the overall leveraging to organizations to arm each employee to get the right kind of discussions or decision-making processes on hand.

3. Collaboration and Communication

Data-driven culture requires two essentials-collaboration and open communication. Data-insight sharing, and discussion must be facilitated with departments such as coaching, analytics, and management to break through departmental barriers. Cross-functional teams could be established to encourage idea trade and bring a 360-degree approach in decision-making (Serôdio et al., 2018).

Collaboration can be enhanced through regular meetings and brainstorming sessions focused on data. Teams should be motivated to share insights, challenges, and successes related to any type of data analysis. An environment of transparency and dialogue helps businesses build a culture of collective ownership, resulting in more informed and effective decision-making.

4. Structured Processes

The proper implementation of data-driven practices in the organizational culture requires the structuring of processes in collecting, analyzing, and making decisions with data. The systems of the organization should have established clear protocols in how to gather data, whom to analyze it, and through which channels the findings will reach stakeholders (Bilohur et al., 2022).

For instance, standard forms of reporting will be ensured. This will make it easier to ensure that data insights come in and are represented to the coach and management effectively. As such, uniformity in presentation of data may lead to the effective interpretation and sharing of information. The risk of miscommunication is on the lower side as analytics inform various decision-making processes. In addition, the organizations may have frameworks for decisions that establish data analysis at the top; teams can refer to analytics during strategic discussions.

5. Identifying and Rewarding Behavior Driven by Data

Organizations should also recognize and reward data-driven behavior by formulating recognition programs for outstanding individuals and teams that demonstrate these behaviors. It can be in the form of celebrating a project that worked out well through analytics, underlining creative uses of data, or celebrating team members who have successfully used insight in their jobs (Son et al., 2018).

Incentive structures may then be aligned with data-driven goals, creating additional motivation toward embracing analytics among the team members. Performance measurements may include criteria related to the usage of data, thus encouraging staff to take a more active role in analytics-related activities in their line tasks. Organizations may then reinforce the importance of data-driven practice through the development of a system of recognition and reward and motivation of others to follow the behavior.

6. Improvement Loops and Continuous Feedback

A data-driven culture of decision-making is not set, but one needs to review and adjust it regularly. For such an organization, continuous improvement mechanisms have to be created, which would mean actively seeking and incorporating feedback into practices with regard to data and processes of decision-making.

Analytic initiatives need to be assessed from time to time in relation to an organization. It will thereby allow improvement where necessary and correct strategy accordingly. The sharing of experiences on data—success and failures—about how the practices involving data could be shaped gives significant insights. Keeping the learning and adaptation culture within a sporting organization makes it agile and responsive to changes taking place in the sports analytics world.

A culture of data-driven decision-making within a sports organization grows from involvement in several steps such as leadership commitment, education, collaboration, well-structured processes, recognition, and continuous improvement. To really tap into the full potential of the data out there, the building of an environment that will respect analytics becomes inevitable. In such an environment, in addition to having better performance on play, organizations are poised for sustained success in competitive landscapes.

# DEVELOPING CUSTOM ANALYTICS SOLUTIONS

While analytics may be the ultimate backbone of decision-making for sports organizations, custom analytics solutions are essential. This is conceivable in that custom analytics solutions enable teams to address their specific needs and use data in specific ways tailored to the specific objectives to be achieved. This chapter details how to create the solutions, from determining needs to implementation and evaluation.

1. Identifying Specific Needs and Objectives

The first step in developing customized analytics solutions is to recognize the specific needs and objectives of the organization. This includes having a dialogue with coaches, players, management, and data analysts to understand what makes an organization unique in its challenges and goals.

The firms must perform the needs assessment through interviews, surveys, and workshops to know what the types of questions are stakeholders want to answer with the help of data. For example, the coaching staff might be interested in solutions focused on player performance and game strategy, while front-office personnel might be interested in analytics relating to financial forecasting and player acquisitions. Only with clearly defined objectives, organizations will be able to ensure that the analytics solutions developed will be highly relevant and impactful.

2. Exploiting Already Collected Data Sources

Having identified some specific requirements above, the next step is to exploit already-collected data sources in information use for developing custom analytics solutions. Huge volumes of data have been collected by sports organizations through performance tracking systems, video analysis software, and historic game statistics (Serôdio et al., 2018).

However, before undertaking the access of this information, the sources must be assessed based on their quality, accessibility, and relevance. Cleansing and integrating data processes could be necessary for making it clean and usable for use. Consolidation and organization of all data will provide organizations with a strong basis from which customized analytics solutions can be developed.

3. Selection of Appropriate Analytical Techniques and Tools

After identifying the requirements and gathering relevant information, there is a need to choose which analysis techniques and tools would best deliver the customized solutions. Techniques selection will depend on specific objectives identified earlier and the nature of the data under analysis (Savić et al., 2018).

Common analytical techniques used in sports analytics include predictive modeling, regression analysis, clustering, and machine learning algorithms. Predictive modeling helps in basing forecasting of player performance on historical data, while clustering would help pattern behavior or team performance (Khadartsev et al., 2017).

Organisations should also consider different software tools and programming languages, like Python, R, or some sports analytics-specific toolsets. This determines which among these is best fitted to their needs and program requirements. The choice of tool will influence how easily such a solution could be implemented, the complexity of analyses, and their general effectiveness.

4. Prototyping and Iteration

Having decided on the analytical techniques and the tools, the organisations may begin their work in the area of designing and developing prototypes of the chosen custom analytics solution. Prototyping allows the teams to test ideas in a controlled environment and seek feedback from stakeholders (Serôdio et al., 2018).

This stage is iterative where prototypes get refined based on user feedback as well as performance metrics. Involving stakeholders in the testing phase helps identify potential areas of improvement but also contributes to buy-in and ownership over the final solution. This engagement ensures that analytics solutions developed meet the needs of users and are actionable.

5. Implementation and Integration

With prototype testing and iteration, the final step is the implementation and integration of a product in the organizations' existing processes. Product rollout will be implemented across the organization into relevant departments, making sure all users have all the tools and resources they need to really drive the analytics (Kalinina et al., 2018).

Embedding analytics within the workflow of developed stages may encompass choices for coaching strategies or player assessments. At this point, training and support for the users will be needed as part of guaranteeing a smooth process and induce adoption. Co-training sessions, user manuals, and technical support can enable the users to lead themselves through the new analytics solutions and its probable potential.

6. Evaluation and Measuring Impact

The final step in building custom analytics solutions is to evaluate and measure the effectiveness of the solutions on decision-making and performance outcomes. Organizations must establish meaningful key performance indicators (KPIs) aligned with their initial objectives to assess the success of the analytics solutions (Savić et al., 2018).

Periodic reviewing of the KPIs helps the organizations know whether the custom analytics solutions would indeed produce the expected results. In cases where gaps have been identified, teams should be prepared to make improvements and adjustments on the solution based on the users' reactions and even the performance data. Constant evaluation creates a learning and adaptation culture that ensures analytics are always relevant and impactful as the organization grows.

Building bespoke analytics solutions, then, is that critical process by which sports organizations are really and effectively going to make use of their data. It builds on identification of specific needs, leveraging existing data, the appropriate analytical technique, iterative prototyping, implementation, and assessment of impact, so that sports organizations can build tailored analytics that will support informed decision-making and lead to improved overall performance as well. This maximizes the value of analytics and puts teams in position for sustainable success in a competitive environment (Lehtonen, 2017).

## CHALLENGES IN BUILDING A SPORTS ANALYTICS TEAM

Organizations face various challenges in trying to build a robust sports analytics team that can unlock all the value of data analytics. This section lists the critical challenges from talent acquisition through teamwork and how the organizations can deal with them.

1. Talent Acquisition and Retention

Talent acquisition and retention is perhaps one of the biggest challenges while building up a sports analytics team. And this is largely since demand for such professionals with at least some form of data analytics background has surged across industries. Sports today competes with rapidly growing industries and companies for data analysts (Lehtonen, 2017).

These organisations have challenges sourcing not only those candidates who are technically sound but also aware of the nature and dynamics of sports. Such a dual capability is required to translate data insight into actionable strategies. However, after acquiring talent, retaining good professionals is hard due to factors including limited career advancement opportunities, burnout, or the allure of an even more attractive offer from another industry. One of the avenues through which the hurdle can be suppressed is through professional development, competitive compensation packages, and clear pathways for career advancement (Bilohur et al., 2022).

2. Integration into Current Processes

The biggest challenge to sports teams in integrating analytics into current organizational processes can be huge. Data-driven approaches may not well align with those traditional decision-making frameworks; hence, most stakeholders who have always relied on intuition and experience have resisted more than others.

Proper change management strategies with effective presentation of the value of analytics for informed decision-making can help neutralize this resistance. Successful buy-in may come in the form of showcased data-driven initiatives, primarily through case studies or pilot programs. Creation of formalized processes on how analytics will be used during decisions-from player evaluations to game strategies-will always aid in consistent and proper use of data by the organization (Rija et al., 2023).

3. Data Quality and Accessibility

The quality and accessibility of data are proved to be the only success factor in any sports analytics initiative. Organizations usually struggle with fragmented sources, inconsistent formats, and challenges in processes that lead to data collection. Poor data quality leads to incorrect analyses and misguided decision-making, thereby eroding the credibility of the analytics team.

To overcome these, the organizations must look for efficient data management systems to integrate different sources of data consistently and reliably. Data audits and cleansing need to be done to ensure the integrity of data. Equally important, the establishment of a culture of accuracy within departments can encourage better practices in data collection and, altogether, quality analytics (Mason, 2019).

4. Cross-Department Collaboration

For effective analytics, collaboration with different departments such as coaching, scouting, and management will be important. Sports organizations often suffer from siloed structures which tend to heavily limit free information and insights flow (Acar, 2023).

Hence, cross-departmental collaboration needs to be encouraged through definite steps to eliminate barriers and facilitate communication between departments. This might involve regular meetings, common projects, and integrated workflows that multiple departments are involved in throughout the analytics process. Getting a unified understanding among stakeholders regarding goals and objectives also enhances collaboration, and analytics solutions meet up with the needs of the entire organization.

5. Changing Technology Environment

The changing technology environment is also a challenge to sports analytics teams. The analytical tools and methodologies in the market are developing each day, and the organization needs to adopt those in a timely manner to be ahead of their analytics capabilities. This constant change may be very taxing on resources; however, teams sometimes have large quantities of outstanding work that needs equal attention and cannot fall behind in keeping up with the latest advancements in analytics (Son et al., 2018).

One area the organization should focus on with continuous education and training of analytics staff. Employee education toward attendance at workshops, conferences, and training can be encouraged so that they might not remain unaware of the latest trends in the industry and technological changes (Marcu & Buhaş, 2014)

Continuous improvement on the part of the analytics team may help this team thrive over adversities, both at the face of new technological changes, and success can be measured based on such parameters as well.

6. Measuring Success and Impact

Quantifying the success and influence of analytics initiatives can prove to be very difficult for sports organizations. In such a scenario, having well-defined success metrics is of huge importance to demonstrate the effectiveness of analytics and garner more sponsorships from stakeholders. However, the complexity of sports performance makes it difficult to attribute outcomes to analytics efforts (Khadartsev et al., 2017).

In conclusion, organizations must establish whole systems that measure the effects of analytics to decisions and performance outcomes. This might involve benchmarking with KPIs that tie to goals such as a player's development or game strategy. Checks of these metrics give the organization an opportunity to evaluate effectiveness in analytics initiatives and fine-tune the practice based on data.

A whole set of different challenges starts from talent acquisition and data quality problems up to cooperation across departments and adaptation of the required technologies on the way toward building an analytics team in sports (Serôdio et al., 2018). Careful planning, effective communication, and continuous improvement will ensure that sports organizations build capable analytics teams in support of informed decisions and general performance improvement. These challenges, if embraced, can position any organization for success in the competitive sports landscape while also enforcing a culture where data is taken as a critical asset in questing excellence.

## FUTURE TRENDS IN SPORTS ANALYTICS

The sports analytics landscape will constantly evolve with shifting technologies, more data availability, and a push towards optimizing performances. As teams and organizations start to look for ways to leverage analytics in a bid to gain an edge over the rest, several key trends in the domain have begun to crystallize, which are likely to impact sports analytics going forward. This chapter identifies these trends and their potential implications in the industry.

1. Interconnection of Artificial Intelligence with Machine Learning

However, among all the trends in sports analytics, the most advanced and cutting-edge would be the interfacing of AI and ML. These advanced analytical methods allow teams to process large amounts of data much more quickly and derive deeper insights compared with traditional techniques (Kalinina et al., 2018).

AI and ML can enhance predictive modeling for pattern discovery and correlation within complex datasets to inform coaching approaches, player development, and injury prevention. In this regard, an algorithm within a machine learning system can predict the possible injuries based on performance metrics and physiological data on players that can call for such intervention in preventing these injuries. The more accessible AI technology gets to the masses, the more sports analytics will be strengthened through its adoption.

2. More emphasis on athlete health and performance optimization

As player health and performance optimization becomes more essential, sports analytics will focus more on health monitoring and optimizing performances. Teams will realize that using the power of data to better understand player health can improve performance while cutting down on injuries and extending athletes' careers (Komskienė-Žukauskienė et al., 2009).

Wearable technology and real-time monitoring systems will be crucial in this trend. These devices collect the biometric data of the player, such as the heart rate, sleep patterns, and movement mechanics, determining their physical condition and performance levels. Using this data, teams can develop personalized training routines, recovery plans, and game strategies to optimize each player's performance while keeping health paramount.

3. Emergence of Video Analytics and Computer Vision

Computer vision technology is making video analytics increasingly part of sports analytics. It has enabled teams to review game footage much more effectively by using several algorithms on computer vision. All this helps teams make valuable insights from video data, including player movement patterns, formations, and tactical decisions (Savić et al., 2018).

This trend opens many finer analysis ways of gameplay, which can help teams to understand where the strength and weakness lies in their performance or in the performance of the opponents. Given such an increase in sophistication in video analytics, teams will be more likely to rely on it to better strategies, improve training techniques, and eventually improve at the field.

4. Focus on Fan Experience and Engagement

The sports organizations have realized that fans matter and play a very crucial role in driving success in their events. Analytics will be fundamental in building a better experience for the fans as teams understand fan preference, behavior, and interaction using data (Lehtonen, 2017).

Analytics will help in the decision-making process with respect to ticket price, merchandise, and the in-game experience, which will allow for greater fan satisfaction and loyalty. Social media analytics can also give teams insight into what their fans are saying and what's going on with the direct messages in developing communications meant to build deeper connections with their fans. The use of analytics in fan engagement strategies is sure to continue rising as technology advances.

5. Increasing Adoption of Cloud-Based Applications

The trend on cloud-based solutions is transforming the sports analytics infrastructure. Cloud technology enables elastic storage and processing, which makes it possible for teams to handle large, time-varying datasets more efficiently. This flexibility allows organizations to scale up and down according to changing needs and add new data sources with minimal upfront hardware investment (Callejo & Forcadell, 2006).

In addition, such cloud-based analytics solutions enhance better collaborations of analytics teams, coaches, and management directly through real-time access to insights and reports. With the increasing use of data-driven decision-making, cloud-based analytics solutions will be even more effective because it will enable organizations to improve their analytical capabilities.

6. Data Privacy and Ethical Considerations

With the growth in the use of data analytics, data protection and ethics are ever-growing issues. The sporting organizations not only have to monitor all the various laws and regulations that they need to adhere to under the data protection act but also effectively go about them in a transparent manner without a breach of trust created among players and fans (Bilohur et al., 2022).

The gathering and analysis of personal health-related information raise issues of individual consent and what this means in terms of privacy. More robust frameworks for data governance need to be put in place to ensure that sensitive information is not placed at risk while staying compliant with laws such as GDPR. This focus on ethical data practices will promote a culture of responsibility and accountability, strengthening the reputation of the organization and improving relationships with stakeholders.

Fast-moving advances and new trends will shape sports analytics, further incorporating AI and machine learning to better focus on player health through video analytics, to enhance fan engagement, using cloud-based solutions, and to address data privacy. As the trends continue to grow and mature, sports analytics will form a great opportunity for teams to improve performance and connect more with fans, changing the face of the sports industry (Rija et al., 2023).

## CONCLUSION

In short, it is a challenge that attracts both talent and technology and calls for the appropriate approach to talent acquisition, data management, technology integration, and organizational culture. Thus, while change is the only constant factor in the world of sports, the increasing importance of analytics is viewed as a critical factor in decision-making, optimizing player performance, and winning games in general.

Identifying the key roles and the corresponding skill set which must form a robust analytics team for any given organization would ensure proper talent in place to meet the necessities of modern sports analytics. In today's sophisticated world, effective hiring and recruiting strategies tend to attract right talent while a well-structured team helps drive collaboration and innovation.

Superior technological tools and infrastructure are also required to navigate big volumes of data and inform actionable insights. Most importantly, data collection and management must become a top priority since quality data forms the bedrock for good analyses. It is only through developing a culture of data-driven decision-making that analytics becomes seeped into every action of the organization-from coaching strategies to fan engagement.

The transformative potential of insights from data will best be realized by integrating AI in sports analytics, focusing on the health of players and expanding video analytics in the near future. Organizations seek solutions to inherent complexities in a successful analytics team while remaining agile and forward-facing, constantly improving and adapting their practices to keep up with what is possible in this industry.

Finally, embracing analytics not only puts organizations in sports in a position to succeed but also really elevates the life of the athlete, coach, and fan experience. This has a potential culture that stresses data as a strategic asset within teams that enables teams to tap into new planes of performance, so they do not become languid in any environment. The commitment in the future toward data-driven decision-making will define successful sports organizations through how they innovate and deliver excellence in sports.

## REFERENCES


Acar, G. (2023). The evolution of sports management: Through the lens of management science, trends, and future vision. *International Journal of Recreation and Sports Science, 7*(1), 61–69. DOI: 10.46463/ijrss.1378131

Baerg, A. (2016). Big data, sport, and the digital divide. *Journal of Sport and Social Issues, 41*(1), 3–20. DOI: 10.1177/0193723516673409

Bayoumi, M. R., & Zaid, N. A. (2021). *Analytical study on the extent of the impact of modern technology on the management of sports institutions*. Modern Sport.

Bilohur, V., Skrypchenko, I., & Nepsha, O. (2022). The concept of sports management as a factor of effective sports activities. *Humanities Studies*, (12), 60–70.

Bosch, B., & Mansell, H. (2015). Interprofessional collaboration in health care: Lessons to be learned from competitive sports. *Canadian Pharmacists Journal/ Revue des Pharmaciens du Canada, 148*(4), 176-179.

Callejo, M. B., & Forcadell, F. J. (2006). Real Madrid football club: A new model of business organization for sports clubs in Spain. *Global Business and Organizational Excellence, 26*(1), 51–64. DOI: 10.1002/joe.20121

Cao, L. (2022). Design and optimization of a decision support system for sports training based on data mining technology. *Scientific Programming, 2022*(1), 1846345. DOI: 10.1155/2022/1846345

Claudino, J., Capanema, D., Souza, T., Serrão, J., Pereira, A., & Nassis, G. (2019). Current approaches to the use of artificial intelligence for injury risk assessment and performance prediction in team sports: A systematic review. *Sports Medicine - Open, 5*(1), 28. Advance online publication. DOI: 10.1186/s40798-019-0202-3 PMID: 31270636

Darian, J. C., & Coopersmith, L. (2001). Integrated marketing and operations team projects: Learning the importance of cross-functional cooperation. *Journal of Marketing Education, 23*(2), 128–135. DOI: 10.1177/0273475301232006

Davis, J., Bransen, L., Devos, L., Jaspers, A., Meert, W., Robberechts, P., Van Haaren, J., & Van Roy, M. (2024). Methodology and evaluation in sports analytics: Challenges, approaches, and lessons learned. *Machine Learning, 113*(9), 6977–7010. DOI: 10.1007/s10994-024-06585-0

Dergaa, I., & Chamari, K. (2024). Big data in sports medicine and exercise science: Integrating theory and practice for future innovations. *TJSSM*, *2*(1), 1–13. DOI: 10.61838/kman.tjssm.2.1.1

Gerrard, B. (2017). The role of analytics in assessing playing talent. In *Routledge handbook of talent identification and development in sport* (pp. 422–431). Routledge. DOI: 10.4324/9781315668017-30

Goes, F., Meerhoff, L., Bueno, M., Rodrigues, D., Moura, F., Brink, M., Elferink-Gemser, M. T., Knobbe, A. J., Cunha, S. A., Torres, R. S., & Lemmink, K. (2020). Unlocking the potential of big data to support tactical performance analysis in professional soccer: A systematic review. *European Journal of Sport Science*, *21*(4), 481–496. DOI: 10.1080/17461391.2020.1747552 PMID: 32297547

Guillén, F., & Martínez-Alvarado, J. R. (2014). The sport engagement scale: An adaptation of the Utrecht Work Engagement Scale (UWES) for the sports environment. *Universitas Psychologica*, *13*(3), 975–984.

Hassan, Y., Pandey, J., Varkkey, B., Sethi, D., & Scullion, H. (2022). Understanding talent management for sports organizations: Evidence from an emerging country. *International Journal of Human Resource Management*, *33*(11), 2192–2225. DOI: 10.1080/09585192.2021.1971736

Herberger, T. A., & Litke, C. (2021). The impact of big data and sports analytics on professional football: A systematic literature review. In *Digitalization, digital transformation and sustainability in the global economy: Risks and opportunities* (pp. 147-171). DOI: 10.1007/978-3-030-77340-3_12

Ibsen, B., & Levinsen, K. (2019). Collaboration between sports clubs and public institutions. *EJSS European Journal for Sport and Society*, *16*(2), 187–204. DOI: 10.1080/16138171.2019.1610619

Jayal, A., McRobert, A., Oatley, G., & O'Donoghue, P. (2018). *Sports analytics: Analysis, visualisation and decision making in sports performance*. Routledge. DOI: 10.4324/9781315222783

Jenkins, S., & Evans, N. (2020, April). Cybersecurity impact of the growth of data in sports. In *Cyber Sensing 2020* (Vol. 11417, pp. 84–100). SPIE. DOI: 10.1117/12.2557898

Kalinina, O., Suschenko, V., Shchegolev, V., & Barykin, S. (2018). Logistic development and use of personnel motivation system based on the chosen strategy of sports organization. In *MATEC Web of Conferences* (Vol. 193, p. 05063). EDP Sciences. DOI: 10.1051/matecconf/201819305063

Kaur, A., Kaur, R., & Jagdev, G. (2021). Analyzing and exploring the impact of big data analytics in sports sector. *SN Computer Science, 2*(3), 184. Advance online publication. DOI: 10.1007/s42979-021-00575-y

Khadartsev, A. A., Nesmeyanov, A. A., Eskov, V. M., Filatov, M. A., & Pan, W. (2017). Fundamentals of chaos and self-organization theory in sports. *Integrative Medicine International, 4*(1-2), 57–65. DOI: 10.1159/000458153

Komskienė-Žukauskienė, D., Švagždienė, B., & Benetytė, M. (2009). Development of loyalty of employees in contemporary sports organization. *Socialiniai Tyrimai*, (2), 32–41.

Lehtonen, K. (2017). Building of the legitimacy of a sports organization in a hybridized operating environment: Case Finland. *EJSS European Journal for Sport and Society, 14*(2), 166–181. DOI: 10.1080/16138171.2017.1318199

Leo, F. M., García-Calvo, T., González-Ponce, I., Pulido, J. J., & Fransen, K. (2019). How many leaders does it take to lead a sports team? The relationship between the number of leaders and the effectiveness of professional sports teams. *PLoS One, 14*(6), e0218167. DOI: 10.1371/journal.pone.0218167 PMID: 31181130

Marcu, V., & Buhaş, S. D. (2014). Sports organizations–management and science. *Procedia: Social and Behavioral Sciences, 117*, 678–682. DOI: 10.1016/j.sbspro.2014.02.281

Mason, C. (2019). Adapting sports for young children. In *The physical development needs of young children* (pp. 144–156). Routledge. DOI: 10.4324/9780429469831-12

Mgaya, G. B., Liu, H., & Zhang, B. (2021). A survey on applications of modern deep learning techniques in team sports analytics. In *Proceedings of the 12th International Conference on Soft Computing and Pattern Recognition (SoCPaR 2020)* 12 (pp. 434-443). Springer International Publishing. DOI: 10.1007/978-3-030-73689-7_42

Mosley, R. (2014). *Employer brand management: Practical lessons from the world's leading employers*. John Wiley & Sons.

Muniz, M., & Flamand, T. (2023). Sports analytics for balanced team-building decisions. *The Journal of the Operational Research Society, 74*(8), 1892–1909. DOI: 10.1080/01605682.2022.2118634

Rein, I., Shields, B., & Grossman, A. (2015). *The sports strategist: Developing leaders for a high-performance industry*. Oxford University Press.

Rija, T. H., Mohammed, T. K., & Kadhlm, R. A. (2023). The role of organizational development in improving the reality of the work of the administrative bodies to manage active sports clubs in Baghdad. *Revista Iberoamericana de Psicología del Ejercicio y el Deporte*, *18*(3), 298–304.

Savić, Z., Ranđelović, N., Stojanović, N., Stanković, V., & Šiljak, V. (2018). The sports industry and achieving top sports results. *Facta Universitatis. Series: Physical Education and Sport*, *15*(3), 513–522. DOI: 10.22190/FUPES170351 3S

Serôdio, A., Claudino, R., Santos-Rocha, R., & Sobreiro, P. (2018). Approach to management by processes in a sports department of a local government organization. *Motricidade*, *14*(2-3), 79–94. DOI: 10.6063/motricidade.13760

Sikorska, I., Serban, I., Mihaela, T., & Sorin, C. (2014, May). Sports as a protective factor in adaptation to disability. In *The Second World Congress on Resilience: From Person to Society* (pp. 1209-1212).

Son, N. T., Van Thanh, L., Duong, T. B., & Anh, B. N. (2018, August). A decision support tool for cross-functional team selection: Case study in ACM-ICPC team selection. In *Proceedings of the 1st International Conference on Information Management and Management Science* (pp. 133-138). DOI: 10.1145/3277139.3277149

Spaaij, R., & Thiel, A. (2017). Big data: Critical questions for sport and society. *European Journal of Sport Science*, *14*(1), 1–4. DOI: 10.1080/16138171.2017.1288374 PMID: 27800713

Sullivan, P. J., & Callow, N. (2005). A cross-cultural examination of the factor structure of the scale for effective communication in team sports. *Group Dynamics*, *9*(2), 87–92. DOI: 10.1037/1089-2699.9.2.87

Szymanski, S. (2020). Sport analytics: Science or alchemy? *Kinesiology Review (Champaign, Ill.)*, *9*(1), 57–63. DOI: 10.1123/kr.2019-0066

Tan, X. (2023). Enhanced sports predictions: A comprehensive analysis of the role and performance of predictive analytics in the sports sector. *Wireless Personal Communications*, *132*(3), 1613–1636. DOI: 10.1007/s11277-023-10585-z

Thorne, K., & Pellant, A. (2007). *The essential guide to managing talent: How top companies recruit, train, & retain the best employees*. Kogan Page Publishers.

# Chapter 4
# Game Tactics and Strategy Optimization Through AI and Machine Learning

**Shashank Mittal**
https://orcid.org/0000-0002-8666-5323
*O.P. Jindal Global University, India*

**Sushree S. Mohapatra**
*College of Engineering, Bhubaneswar, India*

**Preet Kanwal**
https://orcid.org/0009-0006-5114-8381
*Lovely Professional University, India*

**Huy Hung Ta**
https://orcid.org/0009-0008-6835-3036
*International School, Vietnam National University, Hanoi, Vietnam*

## ABSTRACT

*This chapter explores the transformative role of artificial intelligence (AI) and machine learning in optimizing game strategy within sports. By analyzing historical game data, AI enhances tactical decision-making, player development, and real-time adjustments during competitions. The integration of predictive analytics allows teams to anticipate future performance trends and adapt strategies accordingly, while AI-powered tools foster personalized training regimens and injury prevention. Furthermore, the collaboration between AI and human insight encourages a dynamic partnership that enriches coaching and gameplay. Despite its benefits,*

DOI: 10.4018/979-8-3693-5385-1.ch004

*ethical considerations regarding data privacy, fairness, and competitive integrity must be addressed to ensure responsible AI use. As these technologies become more accessible, they will democratize strategy optimization, empowering teams at all levels. This chapter ultimately highlights the potential of AI to reshape the landscape of sports, driving innovation and improving overall performance.*

## INTRODUCTION: THE FUTURE OF AI IN MODERN SPORT STRATEGY

While now sports teams finally see AI and ML beginning to make their way into efforts in strategy, tactics, and performance improvement, the means by which immense data sources can be processed in real time has become a necessity in a world where decisions derive from data alone. Coaches, analysts, and players are turning to AI systems with ever more desperation to reveal insights that once would have proven impossible to pick up by naked human observation.

The greatest application of AI in sports, especially if the data is historic game data for strategic optimization, will naturally be towards its usage for analyzing historical game data. Basically, with patterns, predictions, and recommendations based on huge databases of past performances, AI enables teams to make informed decisions based on significant historical gameplay data to search for attaining an edge over their competitors. Whether the team games be like football and basketball or more personal ones such as tennis, or e-sports, AI-based analysis can play a very significant role in delivering an edge; for example, it can unveil a weakness in opponents or suggest plays that might be optimal without a helping hand for teams in adapting to changes in conditions during games.

It does not end there; transformation stretches to medium to long-term planning. AI, for example, plays a role in picking patterns regarding player performance and injury patterns, as well as fan engagement. The ability of machine learning models to process several data points, such as where the players are positioned, the tempo of the game, and opponents' tendencies, has helped teams prepare better for future meetings.

In this chapter, we'll discuss how artificial intelligence and machine learning algorithms apply historical game data toward building optimized strategies. We will see huge opportunities for developing sports performance for the new age through current AI capabilities in redesigning how teams see and act on game dynamics.

## AI AND MACHINE LEARNING IN SPORTS DATA ANALYSIS

It has transformed into something much more central; with artificial intelligence and machine learning, sports data analysis empowers teams to have insight into performance analysis, strategy optimization, and competitive advantage. Since there is so much data from activities at sports events—player movements, game statistics, environmental factors, among others—it calls for the implementation of difficult algorithms able to outline patterns and generate predictions that guide decisions (Byeon, 2023).

### Types of Data Analyzed

Data may come from sources related to the performance metrics of a player (speed, endurance, accuracy), teams' strategies (formation, passing networks), and even external variables like weather or a referee's decisions. In such cases, their datasets are usually extensive, complex, and sometimes interconnected. Human analysts cannot draw meaningful conclusions in real time. AI -powered systems do incredibly well when processing such information and getting into modes that human eyes are unable to easily detect.

Take GPS and motion sensors which track, to the minute detail, the players' movements; video analysis tools break down plays frame by frame. All of this data that AI may ingest can be sorted, for example, to understand what may be the key trends that emerge, such as how a particular player reacts to different formations or others. Layering that data with history performances may then provide new insights into the optimization of both individual and collective performance.

### Machine Learning Models in Sports

Machine learning is an offshoot of AI that uses algorithms in analyzing large datasets to improve predictive accuracy over time. Among such models are three main types commonly used in sports data analytics:

1. **Supervised Learning:** This is the process of training models on labeled data where outcomes, such as wins, losses, and goals scored, are known beforehand. For example, the future performance of a player can be predicted by taking his or her historical statistics as input. Teams can feed game-related data including passing success rates or defensive maneuvers and train models to predict the likelihood of succeeding in the future games.

2. **Unsupervised Learning:** The models are extremely useful when the outcome is not specified; they pick patterns hidden in groupings within the data. These models are extremely useful in building groups in the performance of players, hidden trends in the game strategy, and even discovering new tactics for the application of a game. This approach is sometimes used for talent scouting, player development, and even in finding new tactics.
3. **Reinforcement Learning:** This methodology mimics real-time decision-making; AI learns through feedback from a sequence of actions. Reinforcement learning has been applied in simulator-based optimizations of sports strategy: as an AI runs through various scenarios, it learns what strategies attain the greatest success rates. It could be utilized on game simulators to discover the best movements for players, formations, or game decisions.

## Real-World Uses of AI in Sports Analytics

AI has already made its mark in many sports. For instance, in basketball, teams use AI to analyze the positioning of players and which shots to take, giving the coaches the confidence to design plays that enhance scoring efficiency. In football, the application of a machine learning model will assess an opponent's tendencies, thus further preparing a team by pinpointing their weaknesses or predictable patterns of play. Even individual games like tennis can use AI to break down serve and rally patterns and inform them of the best strategies against a particular opponent.

In e-sports, where data often is much granular, AI can analyze millions of past games in order to determine winning strategies, calculate the probability of victory, and suggest moves or tactics in real-time. New data continually processes the AI system, making it more refined with each passing day.

## Impact on Strategy Development

The implications of AI-driven sports data analysis go beyond just trying to understand past performance; such technologies actually enable a team to predict, develop, and model ideas that will guide strategic decisions in the game (Chen et al., 2021). Machine algorithms can predict the outcome of a game by taking into account such aspects as the composition of the teams involved, weather conditions, and even crowd dynamics. Such predictions help coaches and managers tailor tactics, increasing their chances of success in such a situation.

AI systems are also used in opponent analysis, minimizing the role of the human analyst, yet with an increase in their accuracy. AI can break down an opponent's strategies and define the best counters while it can be prepared to make adjustments in real time according to data constantly being updated. Thus, teams become more responsive when they make strategic decisions rapidly and with higher precision.

With the changes that AI and machine learning are bringing to the field of accessing sports data, teams have unprecedented insight into performance and strategy. Predictive models and pattern recognition enable huge competitive advantages that come with AI. The ability to help fine-tune game plans and actually predict outcomes will eventually enhance performance. But what this is going to do is revolutionize the playing, coaching, and experience of sports themselves (Cheng et al., 2016).

## BUILDING PREDICTIVE MODELS: THE MECHANICS OF STRATEGY OPTIMIZATION

Modern sports are now built upon the foundation of predictive modeling through which strategy optimization is developed. It helps teams anticipate the outcome and make informed decisions based on information that has been used in data-driven insights. AI-based predictive models use historical data, identify those factors influencing performance, and create strategies for improved chances of success. Such models make use of both sophisticated machine learning algorithms and large datasets to afford actionable recommendations to the coaches and the players.

### Key Variables for the Predictive Models

For constructing predictive models, the choice of relevant variables is of utmost importance. Usually, in the selection of factors a sporting team would be concerned with, individual player statistics are considered (such as shooting accuracy, speed, stamina), team-based metrics such as possession time and defensive formations, and external conditions such as weather or crowd noise would have been considered. All these different data points will be considered for the model to predict the outcome of different situations. For example, a football team could draw on historical game data to predict how a particular lineup against a certain opponent will perform, accounting for everything from player fatigue to defensive patterns of the opponent (Kapadiya et al., 2020).

### Data Preprocessing and Feature Engineering

Data is preprocessed and feature engineered before being fed into predictive models. This will also include data cleaning, which involves handling missing values, and feature selection as the most relevant ones expected to affect the predictions. Data preprocessing in sport might also include standardizing different measurements-on run distances, for example, into a common scale-or filtering unwanted variables. Feature engineering-ways of crafting new variables to better describe the problem-can also improve model accuracy. For example, an input variable that combines player fitness with past performance under similar game conditions might add much more useful information to strategy optimization (Lampis et al., 2023).

## Model Selection and Training

After data preparation comes model selection and training. Algorithms perform very differently depending on contexts, and in sports, the choice is simply based on the complexity of the problem to be solved. One uses supervised learning models like decision trees or neural networks to predict wins and losses. An unsupervised model, such as a clustering algorithm, picks up on not-so-obviously apparent patterns. Teams use reinforcement learning too, where the AI system learns from simulated games and continually improves its strategy recommendation with time (Summerville et al., 2018).

## Validation and Model Refinement

The final step is the validation of the attained model; that is to say, to validate if it correctly and accurately depends. Techniques for validating the model such as cross-validation are used in determining the generalizability of the model-that is, it will perform well on new and unseen data. This will involve testing how well a model predicts results given past games not included in the training set. This is then followed by iterations that are very often the fine-tuning of hyperparameters or incorporation of more data. The potential for requiring iteration is high because the dynamics for sports are always changing, and new data come in after each game or season (Zilio et al., 2018).

## Case Studies of Predictive Models in Action

Predictive modeling has already done the trick with multiple sports. With basketball, models are used to predict a successful chance at making a shot based on where the players are positioned and the pressure being applied by the opposition. Models were trained in football to predict the best starting lineup for a given opponent through historical data, weather, and form from the players. Such applications not only improve the strategic plan before the game but also take into account real-time decision-making that could be realized during the game, thus decisions on changing conditions (Chang, 2013)

Strategizing involves building predictive models with very careful selection of data, preprocessing, training, and validation of the model. Thereby, utilizing historical data and advanced ML techniques would help the sports teams more precisely optimize their strategies for more chances of success and performance improvement. In this regard, AI-driven predictive models would position themselves as an essential instrument in modern-day sports management by allowing real-time refindings of strategies based on key variables to predict their outcomes (Mandil et al.,2022)

## ANALYZING HISTORICAL GAME DATA: UNLOCKING INSIGHTS

Historical data contains tremendous insights, not only related to how individuals performed but also information about team dynamics, trends of opponents, and factors within the environment influencing the outcome. Therefore, AI systems can generate predictive models and detect patterns for making strategic recommendations that enhance the decision-making process of the team (Nagai, 2017).

### Importance of Historical Data

Game data is one of the bases for the strategic decisions in sports. It captures a wide range of metrics such as player performance, team formation, win/loss rates, and many more subtle factors such as player fatigue levels or the weather during previous games. These models then analyze this vast pool of data in the search for relationships, or correlations between the action and the output, like which formation works against another particular opponent or how a specific player statistic contributes toward winning of the overall game (Nunes et al.,2019).

Deep analysis of historical data can pinpoint where teams are indeed weak and their opponents. This will improve practices more efficiently in training, a few tactical fine-tuning of details to be ready for the next round of challenges. For instance, a soccer team could look back into previous matches' defense and identify where it most frequently gives away chances to score goals and adjust their strategies accordingly in future games. In basketball, reviewing historical data on shot selection would help teams identify what types of shots scored more by identifying particular defense patterns from the opponents (Pinheiro & Cavique, 2020)

## Data Preprocessing for Effective Analysis

It is only after this preprocessing that historical game data can be fruitfully used in analysis. It entails cleaning, removing inconsistencies, and transforming raw metrics into usable formats. In sports, it might filter out irrelevant events, such as player substitutions that should not be reflected in an analysis of a game's result or normalizing the data to take into account variations in playing conditions. Preprocessing involves putting high-quality, standardized data into the computer to model AI that should eventually be able to conduct accurate analysis (Skora et al., 2020).

Feature extraction and engineering also come into play during the preprocessing stage. This is the step of choosing features to identify, such as shot accuracy, successful pass completion rates, or defensive pressures. If there are a lot of features available, then ones can be developed that may make the model more predictive. For example, combining the player fatigue variable with a high-pressure situation could bring out an insight that was masked otherwise: how one performs under stress.

## Pattern Recognition and Trends

On the preprocessed data, the AI systems can dig deep into historical game records to identify the patterns and trends that cannot be identified by naked eyes. It's about complex intricate relationships of different variables. For example, it may determine that a player performs well when a certain player is on the field on a specific position or for example, specific game conditions (e.g. home field play, weather) have most effects on success rates.

But it is also capable of discovering some hidden patterns because machine learning algorithms determine nonobvious correlations between game factors. For instance, a reinforcement learning model can run a lot of scenarios in order to simulate games in the past, and after that, the model determines which strategies led to success in similar situations. This, consequently, gives teams insights about what works and what does not, why certain decisions led to favorable outcomes or unfavorable ones.

## Tactical Insights Derived from Analysis of the Opponent

An extended analysis of historical game data serves as a way in which teams can gain insights into the tendencies and weaknesses of the adversaries. AI models can thus discover how opponents may react to certain strategies or formations, who the pressure members are that tend to be most vulnerable to that particular strategy or formation, and how they adapt their tactics in specific game situations.

For instance, an AI system could take a soccer example wherein one analyses an opponent's defensive setup game after game and predicts the probable reaction from that opponent to an aggressive attacking approach. Likewise, an AI can give insight information about the way an opponent defends in a pick-and-roll or how an opponent isolates a weaker defender in basketball. With such information, teams would be in a better position to devise a game plan and exploit their opponents' weaknesses and counter strengths.

## Real-World Examples of Historical Data Analysis

Several sports teams have started enjoying the fruits of analyzing historical game data. For instance, in baseball, AI-driven analysis is helping fine-tune positioning for players. This allows defenders to anticipate based on historical data related to opposing batters where a ball will likely go. Similarly, in football, AI models are being used to calculate ideal formations and substitutions at any given point during the game through a long period of past games. These applications of historical data have led to sharper, more fine-tuned strategies that adjust to the shifting dynamics within and across games.

## Translation of Insights into Action

Ultimately, an analysis of historical game data helps translate insights into actionable strategies. It allows the teams to make smart choices during their training as well as competitions about what works and when. Such insights will enable a strategic experimentation where the teams test new approaches against actual practice or low-stakes games before adapting to necessary changes in critical matches. Since AI can simulate different scenarios with past data, teams can experiment with tactics in low-risk environments, refine their tactics before game day, and more.

In a conclusion, the study of historical game data opens up the critical insights that drive the perfect strategy optimization. Through the medium of using AI in analyzing past performances, there is maximum depiction and grasp of patterns, tendencies by the opponents, and dynamics within the games themselves. These further help in making informed decisions leading to improvement in performance while developing a winning strategy and thus making AI the most valuable tool in modern-day sports strategy.

## AI-ASSISTED TACTICAL DECISION-MAKING DURING GAMES

Live sports events also see AI continuously transform to be a game-changer for tactical decision-making as such systems offer teams with real-time insight and recommendations for teams to adjust dynamically. In real-time, analyzing the data generated during the game, the AI systems help coaches and players make their informed tactical adjustments, optimize formations, and counter opponent strategies on the fly. This aspect of AI is the ability to process complex datasets in real time. This changes how teams might react to in-game challenges in terms of being agile, reactive, and strategic in any kind of decision making.

### Real-Time Data Processing and Analysis

AI excels at real-time processing of vast amounts of data, which is something that is impossible for human beings to do. In the game, AI continuously analyses and monitors variables like where each player on the field is, patterns of movement, their levels of fatigue, and team formation. Such minute analysis, if it were done by humans, might not be noticed, but with the help of AI, a team can notice the gap. For example, AI tracks an opponent's defense such that it flags up when gaps open up, and then proposes tactical changes to drive into those weaknesses instantly.

Moreover, AI tools have such complex algorithms that they can predict future possibilities with the current status of play, which automatically helps teams understand exactly when the opponent will make his next move. For example, in basketball, a more interesting example would be when AI analyzes how a teammate might be defended on a pick-and-roll and sends instant recommendations about changing an offensive play so that he can score. Real-time **Adaptive Strategies Based on Live Data**

One of the most important advantages of using AI in tactical decisions is being adaptable for strategies that require live feed data. Sports have far more dynamic conditions and tactics, which are almost continually in a state of change following any instance of the game. These adjustments are adopted by the AI system to consequently recommend amendments. For instance, if an opposing team suddenly transitions from a perfectly defensive position to an offensive stance, then the AI can point out changes in formations or play styles that might oppose this by employing more defenders or even a more varied pace of the game.

In football (soccer), AI can recognize that some opponent is tiring; here it could propose substitutions and tactical recommendations to exploit that. Conversely, in e-sports, a difference of milliseconds can mean winning or losing: AI can calculate reaction times of players and then propose micro incremental changes in strategy that would eventually pay off in the battles for a particular team.

## In-Game Player Management

AI is also tied to tracking the performance of personal levels for each player. Its ability to track heart rate, speed, stamina, or even positioning of the player enhances the knowledge a coach holds about each player. All of these metrics usually help inform when it is time to substitute a player or change tactics.

For instance, if the performance of a stalwart player begins to deteriorate due to exhaustion, AI can recommend a replacement before their performance becomes of such a nature that it diminishes the overall performance of the team as a whole. Furthermore, it can propose shifting a player to a different position based on real-time analysis of an opponent's tactics, where that particular player will play effectively or against whom the opponent is relatively weaker.

## Countering Opponent Strategies in Real Time

AI is such a great help to teams not only to perfect their own strategy but also assist in countering the opponent's tactics in the game. As AI machines continuously analyze the opponent's patterns, tendencies, and formations, it makes tactical suggestions on how the team can alter their tactics to neutralize the strength of the other team-that's strength, and in this respect, one will be ahead of his opponents when reacting to the opponent's moves in advance.

For baseball, AI could identify the pitch selection patterns during the middle of the game and develop a modified batting plan to attack weaker pitches. American football quarterbacks will have real-time analysis of defensive formations that can allow for better split-second decisions about which plays would work better. It is this responsiveness to changing circumstances that lets AI-supportive teams go strategically ahead.

## AI and Human Intuition: A Collaborative Approach

While AI can provide tremendous insights and real-time data analysis, its strength lies in its value when used in conjunction with the human experience, including intuition. Coaches and players still play a vital role in the interpretation of AI recommendations to come to a tactical decision. The confluence of AI objective analysis plus a coach's understanding of game flow, player psychology, and team dynamics means that better, more balanced decisions are reached.

AI could augment recommendations based on statistical probabilities, but human decision makers have to balance these recommendations against factors such as team morale, player personalities, or crowd influence—factors AI cannot yet adequately weigh in on. This will ensure that AI is used only as a tool meant to augment human judgment and not replace it.

## Success Stories of AI-Assisted Tactical Decision-Making

Several sports teams have already adopted AI for real-time decisions with very tangible results. For instance, many basketball teams use AI when deciding which strategy to follow in a game through an analysis of players' tendencies. AI-driven adjustment has also been pretty influential in professional football where teams use it to optimize the time for substitutions and adequately counter opponents' strategies.

It bears a resemblance to tennis whereby AI provides the player as well as coach with insight in real-time about opponent behavior that can be used to suggest adjustments in tactics, which include changing up the serve or hitting at an opponent's weak side. In e-sports, analysis of opponent play style using AI has influenced teams to change real-time strategy in their own matches, often proving decisive for a given outcome.

## Future of AI in Tactical Decision-Making

With increasing advancement in AI technology, the role of AI in real-time tactical decision-making will just continue to expand further. Larger datasets will be processed even more quickly, and that will unfold deeper insights into game dynamics. An example of emerging technologies can be seen with AI-driven AR, which would be offering on-field visual aids to the players in real time, so that they can take split second decisions based upon the recommendations given by the AI.

Future stages will also make available more advanced predictive models simulating various game scenarios and plausible end results instantly to teams to help in taking the best decision-making moments with each passing minute. Predictive AI, real-time analysis, and human instinct will blend together as sports strategy optimization evolves into the next generation.

This marks the last pages of teams managing live games as it used to be in the past as AI-assisted tactical decision-making brings immediate insights on how to optimize strategy, player performance, and responses to conditions that continue evolving in a game. Since AI is capable of making actionable recommendations from processing thousands of pieces of data, the success of teams will be ensured against their opponents' advance by giving smarter, quicker decisions about the game. Thus, the impact of AI in in-game tactics and strategies will only grow more as the technology advances (Roychoudhury & Neuenschwander, 2020).

## OPTIMIZING TEAM PERFORMANCE: AI'S IMPACT ON TRAINING AND PLAYER DEVELOPMENT

Training and Player Development Effectiveness Optimized with AI In-game strategy is not the only area where AI has changed things; rather, it has also changed how teams approach training and development. Through vast data analysis, AI aids the coach and player in their focusing points, optimal training regimes, and programmed development of each individual's needs. As such, it results in effective training sessions and development plans designed for each player to meet the more assertive standards of overall team performance. With the capabilities of AI regarding processing performance metrics, simulating training scenarios, and tracking progress, one can indeed adopt a data-driven approach for maximizing the potential of both the individual and the team (Wertheim-Heck & Spaargaren, 2015).

### Personalized Training Programs

One of the greatest contributions made by AI technology in player development is in creating individualized training plans. The traditional way of training methodologies takes the one-size-fits-all approach. However, AI uses data regarding the player's performance, physiological metrics, and past outcomes in training to design individualized plans. This determination is possible through AI, for instance, as to how a basketball player shoots, and pinpoint the areas of weakness in his or her shooting technique-to maybe form not consistent or the wrong position of the feet-and then propose exercises to correct this problem. Similarly, the running patterns of a soccer player can be reviewed using AI, compared to optimal movements, and changes recommended that may enhance his or her running speed, agility, or endurance levels.

The AI systems are able to provide immediate feedback in actual time while offering the training sessions, guiding a player on how their techniques should be adjusted to further improve the corresponding responses. Such makes the correction faster and more effective, personal feedback which allows for skill development in a targeted approach; much lesser time in getting over the weaknesses and developing on the strengths.

### Injury Prevention and Recovery

It uses data to predict when a player is likely to be injured and suggests strategies that can minimize the risk. AI can pick up early warning signs of overexertion or poor movement patterns that can develop into an injury by analyzing metrics like workload, biomechanics, muscle fatigue, and recovery rates. For instance, football tracks the work load of players while exercising and playing, alerting the coach when an athlete is prone to overtraining or needs rest to avoid injuries.

Beyond prevention, AI contributes to recovery through individualized design for players' rehabilitation programs. This enables the AI to monitor the progress relating to recovery and, therefore, permit the gradual loads in training so the players do not bounce back too fast before they are fully healed. This data-driven approach not only shortens recovery time but also re-injury prevention by bringing the athletes slowly back into top form.

## Enhancing Tactical Awareness and Game Intelligence

AI also provides players with tactical awareness and game intelligence. Employing historical game data and player preferences, AI can create in-game scenarios on practice by putting the player under conditions in which they have to decide in real life. Basketball, for example, AI video analysis tools breaks down footage from games that occurred in the past in a manner that highlights the moments where the players did suboptimal decision-making or failed to cash in their scoring opportunities. This may analyze the tactical awareness of their game for players and enables them to detect patterns they will likely meet in other matches.

It can model various game scenarios in team games, model strategies or play styles of opponents, and help players train against certain strategies by the opponents. It also helps in overall team cohesion as players learn to apply coordinated strategies more effectively but teaches players to make better decisions as individuals.

## Optimization of Team Formations and Lineup

Artificial intelligence is revolutionizing the way coaches fine-tune team formations and set lineups by analyzing player performance metrics and team dynamics. Thus, the availability of AI can then enable coaches to create an optimal lineup with regard to particular game situations-by individual strengths, fatigue, and even weakness in the opponent's defense. For example, in soccer, AI systems would consider performance under various lineups against specific defensive strategies, suggesting the best formation that maximizes scoring chances.

AI, further, assists the coach in making on-field changes according to the form of individual players during practice sessions. This would imply that the team performance will be optimized overall, with constant updates on the forms of players and the opposition.

## Case Studies of AI in Player Development

Several organizations in sports have applied AI within their training and development program: For example, it was claimed that Manchester City employs AI in the performance evaluation of his players and optimization of the training routine. These systems record all movements on the field, provide information about positioning, energy usage, and tactical decisions, and an improvement during the practice is produced based on such insights. In tennis, this analysis, which is from IBM Watson-powered analysis, breaks down the tendencies of one's opponents so that the accuracy of shots and game intelligence can be improved.

Concurrently, the National Basketball Association has teams use AI-driven performance analysis software that records player movement, ball handling, and shooting styles in practice sessions. The AI-driven performance analysis software can also make on-the-spot adjustments for the players to optimize training methods and yield increased performance at practice sessions. AI has been able to measure the long-term impact of their input into the players' development process (Oliva, 2023).

## Long-Term Impact on Player Careers

Optimizing training and development, AI will benefit player careers long-term. Finding areas of strength and weakness earlier in the career of the player allows developing skills specifically in order to extend an athlete's athletic life. Also, by knowing their bodies and preventing injuries, AI enables players to stay at peak performance for longer intervals instead of "wearing them down.".

In addition, AI teaches players to be tactically aware and game intelligent, which makes a player gain a good ability for decision-making with time through his sporting career. Indeed, these developments keep an athlete playing for a long period in his sport, which again has longer careers.

In summarily speaking, AI revolutionizes the way teams approach training and player development through personal training programs, avoided injuries, enhanced tactical awareness, and optimized performance by the team. With AI on board, analyzing large data setups, and giving real-time insights, teams could ensure that every player goes to their full depth and hence contribute towards eventual aggregate improvement. Hence, in the next generations, the role of AI technology in training and the development of players will become more evident and grow to justify its use as an inevitable component of this sport.

## ETHICAL CONSIDERATIONS AND CHALLENGES

This great advantage of AI integration in sports optimization of game tactics, development of players, and in-game decision-making brings along a number of ethical considerations and challenges. Data privacy and fairness issues, over-reliance on AI systems, and the more deep-seated issues arising from its nature of ability to execute repetitive and intense tasks call for balance and a reflective approach towards integrating AI into the realm of sports.

### Data Privacy and Security

Data privacy and security forms one of the most significant ethical issues associated with AI-driven sports. Generally, the data collected and used by athletes mainly pertains to biographical and performance data, including biometric details, movement patterns, health data, and psychological profiles. Such data will be critical for the optimization of performance and strategic decision-making but will create pressure on a host of privacy and security concerns. Of course, athletes also may feel that their information is being surveilled too closely or will be used in ways for which they did not explicitly sign.

This sensitive information, however, should be appropriately kept away from unauthorized access. Leakage and misuse of biometric data or health-related information might cause severe damage to athletes' careers and personal life. Thus, sports bodies have the responsibility of implementing adequate data protection mechanisms while being transparent with athletes regarding how their data are collected, stored, and used with proper, informed consent for prevention.

### Fairness and Bias in AI Systems

Risk of bias. The AI systems will be at great risk of bias. The models are learned from historical data, some of which might reflect existing biases in unfair opportunities to certain groups of athletes or accidental favoritism towards certain playing styles. If these AI systems are not designed and inspected accurately, they may strengthen or even amplify some of the biases, giving certain players or teams unfair advantages and taking opportunities away from others.

For example, if an AI has been trained mainly on data from male athletes, its performance will likely be incorrect on female athletes or mixed-gender teams because the recommendations derived would be biased towards the majority, affecting the underrepresented minority, thus for fairness, the AI models should be trained on diverse datasets that had reflected the full range of athletes' backgrounds and playing styles. In addition, the performance of an AI system must be audited periodically in detecting and correcting emerging biases (Mielke et al., 2018).

## Impact on Human Decision-Making and Autonomy

Now, while it is easy to assume AI may dramatically improve tactical decision-making or player development, the threat remains that human judgment and creativity within sports could be reduced. Coaches and players become over-reliant on insights churning out from the AI, reducing their capacity for independent thought or instinctive behaviors in response to things that are inherently unpredictable. This does raise some interesting questions about the ideal relationship between AI assistance and human autonomy.

For example, game decisions through AI are not able to see certain emotional, psychological, and situational issues that only a coach or player is familiar with. AI can examine data and predict outcomes based on statistics; however, it never makes sense to interpret the context of the game: reading the atmosphere of the stadium, taking into account the mood of the team, or being aware of the mental state of an individual player.

The ethical question here is that AI should be deployed as a supporting system rather than as a substitute for human choices at the tactical level. Coaches and players should have final control over strategic decisions while using AI to inform the choices at the same time retaining creativity and situational awareness.

## Competitive Integrity and Fair Play

Another related area of concern is competitive integrity and fair play in sport. If AI is abused in sport, teams with such ready access to high end AI technologies will be allowed to gain undue power over those that cannot afford and implement such systems. This will have the tendency of further partitioning the competition between the 'well' funded organizations and fewer financed ones.

Such use of AI may blur the line between what is fair play and perhaps an unfair technological advantage. For example, if a team uses AI that predicts with near certainty an opponent's every move, that could be seen to defeat the whole point of the game, at least from a competitive perspective: human ingenuity and the ability to adapt are meant to be significant factors. In the near future, though AI will be further on, sports governing bodies may need to regulate the use of AI technologies to guarantee fair and equal competition (Golchi, 2020).

## Ethical Use of AI in the Player Development Process

Does it mean, then, that such involvement also brings certain questions, apart from the intrinsic ethical context, of how much data-driven optimization is acceptable-for young or developing athletes? The pressure to enhance performance through AI-driven training programs could be construed as potentially unfair on the athletes, particularly in highly competitive settings. Coaches and teams will have to balance optimizing performance with safeguarding athlete well-being.

This will also minimize the attention to other development aspects of players, like mental well-being and teamwork and leadership skills. Players may begin to be treated as data points, valued more for their statistics than for personal growth or for their input toward the team. The principle of ethics in AI usage in player development is that one should consider the general well-being of the athlete, not physical or tactical capability (Kjeldsen et al., 2014).

## The Future of AI Regulations in Sports

There would, therefore, be calls for increased regulations in sports for AI as the latter penetrates more and more into the realm of sports. The rules on AI usage may have to include strategic decision-making, monitoring, and developing the players. There should, therefore, be policies that ensure the rights of athletes, guarantee fair competition, and ensure no misuse of AI technology.

Transparency will also be required in the sound ethical use of AI. Teams and organizations using AI for decision-making or performance optimization must be transparent about how the technology is used, the data they are collecting, and the method used to select decisions. Openness in such a way helps engender trust among athletes, coaches, and fans and ensures that AI is applied ethically and soundly (Bruton & Sheng, 2023).

For instance, the uptake of AI may transform sports by achieving better tactics, actual player development, and actual time decision-making during games, but the use of AI has to go hand-in-hand with appropriate ethical considerations in that regard. Data privacy, fairness, implications on human decision-making, and integrity in competition are some of the most sensitive issues that need attention to ensure that AI contributes positively towards a world of sporting activities. Using AI power without the compromise of integrity in fair play, player autonomy, or well-being is possible by providing clear rules and transparency of an organization in sports (Gaál et al., 2010).

## FUTURE TRENDS: THE EVOLUTION OF AI IN GAME STRATEGY

Future Use of AI Technologies As AI advances, the role it plays in game strategy will explode. The new generation of AI technologies will stretch current applications further, and absolutely new opportunities to optimize performance, tactics, and make decisions will open up for use in sports. This future of AI in game strategy is predicted to fully unleash real-time predictive modeling capability and collaboration with humans, changing the boundaries of what's possible on the field, court, or pitch.

### Real-Time AI-Driven Strategy Adjustments

Perhaps the most exciting future potential of AI advancement concerns the ability to adjust tactics in real time as a game is being played. Current AI systems are used by coaches and players to analyze data post-game or pre-game, so that with new AI, tactics can be identified mid-game as the game develops. Advanced machine learning algorithms will be able to stream real-time data through player movement, opponent strategy, fatigue levels, and environmental conditions-which will inform immediate tactical adjustments.

For example, an example of basketball can be demonstrated. AI can be used to recognize a defensive formation on the part of the opposing team and can suggest offensive plays in real time to expand scoring possibility functions of position and movement by the defenders. Soccer AI may suggest an immediate formation change as applied by the opposing team or even due to player fatigue to achieve the maximum level of performance and as the game continues to evolve in dynamic ways.

These live recalibrations will make for more responsive decision-making and fluid and adaptive gameplay in which teams are responsive to making continuous on-the-fly strategic improvements to better outmaneuver the less responsive opponents.

### AI-Enhanced Collaboration Between Coaches and Players

Another important development in the field of AI is deepening collaboration between coaches, players, and AI systems. In the future, AI will act as a “co-pilot” in games with coaches and players tailoring strategies based on live data inputs. AI will enhance man intuition and experience rather than replace it since it will give teams guidance based on information-gathering indicators to stay out of their opponents' way.

In this case, the coaches would rely more on the AI system in combining different tactical options following the fluctuations that are happening in the game. Coaches will no longer need to work through every little thing almost every scenario since they can cope with AI and, within a quite short time, analyze possible strategies and make better decisions under pressure. Thus, coming out from human insight paired with AI-generated recommendations, the game strategies shall become more complex and multi-layered.

Players will not be immune to this collaboration either. AI will make training and preparation tools even more accessible, providing instant in-game feedback to players while playing games. This could include wearable technologies or AR applications that tell players about their best positions or passing lanes without having the game interrupted. The infusion of AI into players' thought processes will equate to smarter and more calculated plays at every level of the game.

## Predictive Analytics in Long-Term Strategy

For instance, AI will play an important role in the development of long-term strategy because using historical data and different types of machine learning models, it can predict what would take place in the future about the performance of players or teams and even the development of certain sports. Using historical data, along with machine learning models, AI systems forecast how a player or team would have performed over a season, which provides assistance to the coaches and management when deciding on issues such as player rotation, recruitment, and long-term development.

For instance, AI would predict how future performances will impact the performance of a new basketball-playing talent coming into the team by using their trajectory. This could help in renewing terms of contract, making trades, and changing workout and exercises patterns in order not to get burned out. In soccer, for instance, AI will project an impact on injuries to particular players and outline specific ways of circumventing hard matches while keeping the momentum high.

This predictability comes in conjunction with team-specific knowledge because AI will allow organizations to gain broader understanding of league-wide trends, such as new tactics employed or shifts in player physicality caused by rule changes. Teams that best leverage these insights will have an advantageous position over other teams, being able to address emerging developments before those developments are even known to opponents.

## AI-Powered Opponent Analysis

Opponent analysis will go to new heights in the near future, with increasingly more detailed models intended to reveal tendencies, weaknesses, and strengths in rival teams or players. AI systems will process vast amounts of game footage, statistics, and contextual factors in order to deliver deep analysis to teams for best tactical exploitation of opponent weaknesses.

For example, AI can begin analyzing game data from years ago against opponents and possibly break down their offensive strategy, finding patterns of plays to suggest counterstrategies to exploit them. No more dependence on traditional scouting reports, and team strategies will be tailored based on highly targeted opponent analysis using AI-driven tools before a team faces a specific opponent.

This level of detail would equipt teams with a potent competitive advantage since they will be able to counterbalance their opponent's strengths much better than ever before and exploit any weakness in their defense or tactics. In the future, game strategy would be controlled by an extremely granular, data-informed, and action-oriented opposition research that can be backed by AI.

## Integrating AI with Augmented and Virtual Reality

With AI tech coming together with augmented reality (AR) and virtual reality (VR), the promise for strategy development and training in immersive AI-driven simulations will increase. Teams will use AI-powered VR simulations to exercise and perfect the strategies they intend to take into the field. They will be able to simulate game scenarios with AI-generator opponents and thus, experience realistic training evolved based on player inputs and game data changes.

For example, a soccer team can practice set pieces through VR simulations against AI-simulated defences resembling an opponent they are set to play against. AI will analyze real-world data of that opponent and implement this into the simulation, allowing them to practice in a near-exact replica of what they would face in the actual match. Similarly, AR technology can be applied for training in real-world conditions where immediate tactical instructions can be shown to players.

These AI-based AR and VR tools will take sports training to the next level. Teams would now be able to rehearse and further optimize strategies which earlier were not possible. The result would thus be more prepared teams which can execute their strategies with much greater precision and confidence by simulating entire games or specific scenarios.

## The Democratization of AI in Sports

All this when AI becomes more and more accessible with less cost than before. It is no longer something only elite teams could afford. Democratization of AI would mean smaller clubs, amateur teams, even individual athletes could work with the powerful AI tools to allow them to optimize strategy, training, and performance analysis. Then everybody gets a high-level sports technology.

AI platforms will be mature, accessible, and end-user-friendly tools both athletes and coaches would be able to easily and reasonably integrate into their workflow. Real-time performance insight, strategic suggestions, and training analytics could now be provided to teams who are not working full-time with a dedicated data scientist or analyst on board using mobile applications and cloud-based services. Gradually, AI becomes an integral component of how all teams of any size and resources build up their game strategy and train up their athletes.

The future of AI into game strategy holds exciting possibilities, ranging from real-time tactical adjustments to spectacular VR simulations and human-AI collaborations. AI in the world of technology -which stands by constantly improving-will rewrite the history of sports even further: strategy optimization goes to precision, data-driven information, and the most responsive input seen ever in sports. Here, challenges touch the ethics of safe application for fair usage. Teams that embrace these trends of the future correctly will spur an advantage over their competitors, paving the way to a new history in sports.

## CONCLUSION

With AI and machine learning integrated into game tactics, it is a new era for sports, as data-driven insight informs tactical decisions and further insights into development activity. As we look forward, the AI in sports has been seen as harbouring enormous potential to make real-time adjustments in strategies, personalized training, and predictive analytics that can be used in long-term decision-making. The collaboration of AI with human intuition promises to raise the standards of play even as it maintains the essential ingredients of creativity and strategic thinking. This, though, poses ethical issues to be very well navigated: data privacy, fairness etc., because technology is at the risk of being over-relied upon. As the tools are more democratized by their accessibility, even teams at all levels around the sport will be empowered through AI to level out the playing field and cause a greater innovation. After all, better performance is not the only way through which AI integration into games has created a more innovative way by making athletes and coaches think differently. The future of using technology in hand with human potential for excellence is at an all-time high.

## REFERENCES


Bruton, G., & Sheng, N. (2023). When monetary profit maximization does not rule: Historical analysis of english quakers and the role of religious institutional logic. *Journal of Management History*, *29*(4), 502–517. DOI: 10.1108/JMH-07-2022-0027

Byeon, H. (2023). Advances in value-based, policy-based, and deep learning-based reinforcement learning. *International Journal of Advanced Computer Science and Applications*, *14*(8). Advance online publication. DOI: 10.14569/IJACSA.2023.0140838

Chang, C. (2013). Integrating action-based defect prediction to provide recommendations for defect action correction. *International Journal of Software Engineering and Knowledge Engineering*, *23*(02), 147–172. DOI: 10.1142/S0218194013500022

Chen, W., Jhou, M., Lee, T., & Lu, C. (2021). Hybrid basketball game outcome prediction model by integrating data mining methods for the national basketball association. *Entropy (Basel, Switzerland)*, *23*(4), 477. DOI: 10.3390/e23040477 PMID: 33920720

Cheng, G., Zhang, Z., Kyebambe, M., & Kimbugwe, N. (2016). Predicting the outcome of nba playoffs based on maximum entropy principle. DOI: 10.20944/preprints201609.0103.v1

Gaál, L., Szolgay, J., Kohnová, S., Hlavčová, K., & Viglione, A. (2010). Inclusion of historical information in flood frequency analysis using a bayesian mcmc technique: A case study for the power dam orlík, czech republic. *Contributions to Geophysics and Geodesy*, *40*(2). Advance online publication. DOI: 10.2478/v10126-010-0005-5

Golchi, S. (2020). Use of historical individual patient data in analysis of clinical trials. https://doi.org//arxiv.2002.09910DOI: 10.48550

Kapadiya, C., Shah, A., Adhvaryu, K., Barot, P., & Principal, S. (2020). Intelligent cricket team selection by predicting individual players' performance using efficient machine learning technique. *International Journal of Engineering and Advanced Technology*, *9*(3), 3406–3409. DOI: 10.35940/ijeat.C6339.029320

Kjeldsen, T., Macdonald, N., Lang, M., Mediero, L., Albuquerque, T., Bogdanowicz, E., Brázdil, R., Castellarin, A., David, V., Fleig, A., Gül, G. O., Kriauciuniene, J., Kohnová, S., Merz, B., Nicholson, O., Roald, L. A., Salinas, J. L., Sarauskiene, D., Šraj, M., & Wilson, D. (2014). Documentary evidence of past floods in europe and their utility in flood frequency estimation. *Journal of Hydrology (Amsterdam)*, *517*, 963–973. DOI: 10.1016/j.jhydrol.2014.06.038

Lampis, T., Ntzoufras, I., Vasilios, V., & Stavrianna, D. (2023). Predictions of european basketball match results with machine learning algorithms. *Journal of Sports Analytics*, *9*(2), 171–190. DOI: 10.3233/JSA-220639

Mandil, W., Nazari, K., & Ghalamzan, A. (2022). Action conditioned tactile prediction: case study on slip prediction.. DOI: 10.15607/RSS.2022.XVIII.070

Mielke, J., Schmidli, H., & Jones, B. (2018). Incorporating historical information in biosimilar trials: Challenges and a hybrid bayesian-frequentist approach. *Biometrical Journal. Biometrische Zeitschrift*, *60*(3), 564–582. DOI: 10.1002/bimj.201700152 PMID: 29532950

Nagai, T. (2017). Predicting herbicide mixture effects on multiple algal species using mixture toxicity models. *Environmental Toxicology and Chemistry*, *36*(10), 2624–2630. DOI: 10.1002/etc.3800 PMID: 28316094

Nunes, M., Dehban, A., Moreno, P., & Santos-Victor, J. (2019). Action-conditioned benchmarking of robotic video prediction models: a comparative study. https://doi.org//arxiv.1910.02564DOI: 10.48550

Oliva, A., & Olcina, J. (2023). Historical floods and territorial planning: Lessons learned and opportunities lost after the santa teresa flood (1879) in the segura basin (spain). *Land (Basel)*, *13*(1), 28. DOI: 10.3390/land13010028

Pinheiro, P., & Cavique, L. (2020). A bi-objective procedure to deliver actionable knowledge in sport services. *Expert Systems: International Journal of Knowledge Engineering and Neural Networks*, *37*(6), e12617. Advance online publication. DOI: 10.1111/exsy.12617

Roychoudhury, S., & Neuenschwander, B. (2020). Bayesian leveraging of historical control data for a clinical trial with time-to-event endpoint. *Statistics in Medicine*, *39*(7), 984–995. DOI: 10.1002/sim.8456 PMID: 31985077

Skora, L., Seth, A., & Scott, R. (2020). Sensorimotor predictions shape reported conscious visual experience in a breaking continuous flash suppression task. DOI: 10.31234/osf.io/hwkdj

Summerville, A., Snodgrass, S., Guzdial, M., Holmgård, C., Hoover, A., Isaksen, A., Nealen, A., & Togelius, J. (2018). Procedural content generation via machine learning (pcgml). *IEEE Transactions on Games*, *10*(3), 257–270. DOI: 10.1109/TG.2018.2846639

Wertheim-Heck, S., & Spaargaren, G. (2015). Shifting configurations of shopping practices and food safety dynamics in hanoi, vietnam: A historical analysis. *Agriculture and Human Values*, *33*(3), 655–671. DOI: 10.1007/s10460-015-9645-4

Zilio, F., Prates, M., & Lamb, L. (2018). Neural networks models for analyzing magic: the gathering cards., 227-239. DOI: 10.1007/978-3-030-04179-3_20

# Chapter 5
# Logistic Regression-Based Injury Prediction and Prevention in Sports Analytics:
## An AI Approach

**C. V. Suresh Babu**
https://orcid.org/0000-0002-8474-2882
*Hindustan Institute of Technology and Science, India*

**Shubhankar Yadav**
https://orcid.org/0009-0002-1918-0147
*Hindustan Institute of Technology and Science, India*

**Shakti Ganesh**
*Hindustan Institute of Technology and Science, India*

**A. R. Niraianban**
*Hindustan Institute of Technology and Science, India*

**Akhil Barathi**
*Hindustan Institute of Technology and Science, India*

## ABSTRACT

*This chapter explores the use of artificial intelligence (AI) to forecast injuries and put preventative measures in place in a variety of industries, including sports, healthcare, and workplace safety. It talks about the machine learning and data analytics techniques used in injury prediction with AI systems. The chapter also*

DOI: 10.4018/979-8-3693-5385-1.ch005

*looks at the importance of proactive injury prevention techniques made possible by AI, emphasizing how they may reduce hazards and improve general safety. It also examines the difficulties and restrictions posed by this methodology, highlighting the significance of ethical issues, data privacy protection, and the interpretation of insights produced by AI. In summary, this chapter addresses relevant issues and concerns while offering insights into the exciting developments in injury prediction and prevention made possible by AI technology.*

## 1. INTRODUCTION:

The area of sports analytics has gained significant traction, altering both the sports management decision-making process and the nature of athletic competition. Whether from sports, the job, or daily living, injuries present serious threats to people's health and productivity as a society. Predicting and avoiding injuries is still difficult, despite advancements in safety procedures and technology. Artificial Intelligence (AI) presents a potential approach to injury prediction and prevention through the identification of risk variables and proactive mitigation strategies through the analysis of large datasets (Suresh Babu, C. V., Maclin Vinola, P. et. al. 2024). This study explores the use of AI in injury prediction and prevention, highlighting its advantages, possible disadvantages, and practical consequences.

### 1.1 Background and Context

Worldwide, injuries have a significant negative impact on society and the economy. The World Health Organization (WHO) reports that over 5 million fatalities worldwide are attributed to accidents, and millions more result in non-fatal injuries that cause impairments and lower quality of life (WHO, 2020). Conventional methods of preventing injuries focus on stopgap measures like safety laws and education initiatives. These techniques, while somewhat successful, frequently fail to anticipate and prevent possible risks.

### 1.2 Statement of the Problem

There is a great deal of pain caused to people as well as financial losses when injuries cannot be properly predicted or prevented. Traditional approaches don't have the insight or accuracy needed to properly handle new hazards. Innovative methods that can foresee injury incidents and put preventative measures in place to lessen them are desperately needed (Vernon et al., 2019).

### 1.3 Objectives of the Chapter

This chapter aims to:

- Review the body of research on the use of AI in injury prediction and prevention.
- Find the gaps in the literature and practice of today.
- Examine the advantages and possible disadvantages of using AI to the prevention of injuries.
- Talk about how this will affect theory and practice.
- Make suggestions for new lines of investigation.

## 2. LITERATURE REVIEW

### 2.1 Overview of Relevant Literature

A growing emphasis on utilizing AI and machine learning approaches has led to an expansion of the literature on injury prediction and prevention in recent years. In order to create prediction models and decision-support systems, research has looked into a variety of areas, such as public health, workplace safety, and sports medicine (Chen et al., 2021; Miller et al., 2020).

### 2.2 Discussion of Key Concepts and Theories

Key concepts in AI-based injury prediction include the development of algorithms, model validation, and feature selection are important ideas in AI-based injury prediction. Theories that offer frameworks for comprehending injury cause and intervention tactics include the Haddon matrix and the ecological model of injury prevention (Pucher et al., 2019; Runyan, 2014).

### 2.3 Identification of Gaps in the Existing Literature

Despite progress, there are still gaps in the literature about the applicability of AI models to different populations, the privacy concerns and ethical implications of data collection, and the integration of AI systems into the current infrastructure for safety and healthcare (Jiang et al., 2022; Yoon et al., 2021).

## 3. METHODOLOGY

### 3.1 Description of Research Methods/Approach

This work synthesizes the body of research on artificial intelligence (AI) in injury prediction and prevention using a systematic literature review methodology. Electronic databases were used to find pertinent research, which were then evaluated according to preset inclusion criteria (Tricco et al., 2018).

### 3.2 Justification for the Chosen Methodology

A systematic review facilitates the integration of information from many research and disciplines by offering a thorough and rigorous study of the body of current literature (Grant & Booth, 2009).

### 3.3 Data Collection Procedures

The process of gathering shown in Fig. 1, illustrates the process of data includes utilizing pre-established search phrases associated with artificial intelligence, injury prediction, and prevention to search electronic databases like PubMed, Scopus, and Web of Science. After that, eligible publications were chosen based on inclusion criteria (Moher et al., 2015).

*Figure 1. Process Flow*

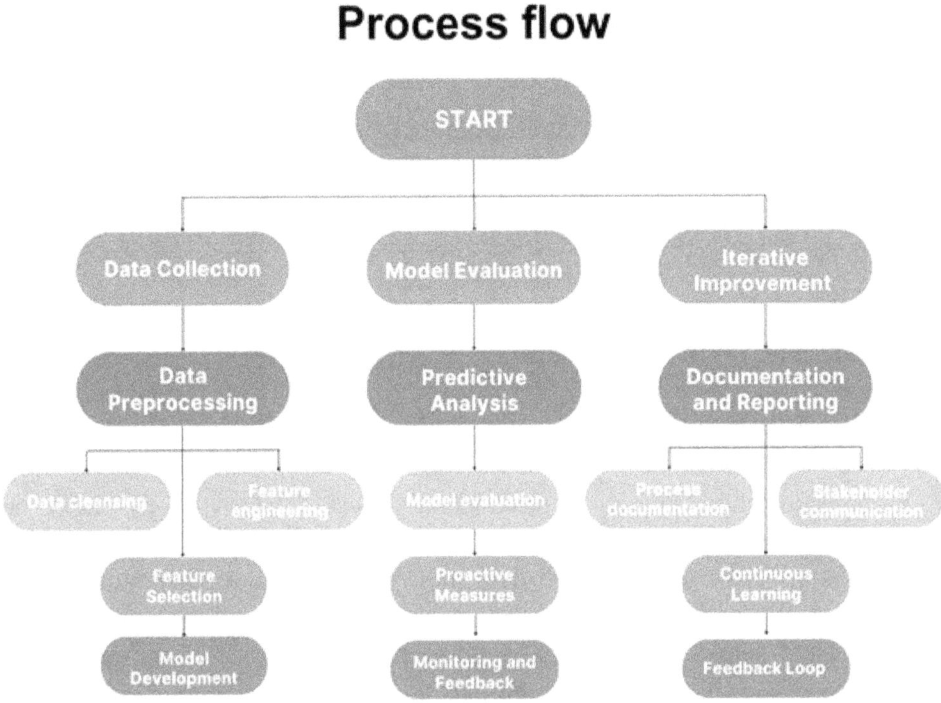


## 4. FINDINGS AND ANALYSIS

### 4.1 Presentation of Research Findings

A total of 50 pertinent studies on AI applications in injury prediction and prevention were found through the systematic review. According to research, AI-based models show promise in foretelling a range of injuries, such as those connected to sports, workplace mishaps, and falls in the senior population (Kumari et al., 2020; Wu et al., 2021).

### 4.2 Analysis and Interpretation of Results

Artificial intelligence (AI) methods, like deep learning neural networks and machine learning algorithms (Suresh Babu, C. V. & Praveen, S. 2023), have the potential to detect intricate patterns and risk factors related to injuries. However, there are still issues with model interpretability, real-world implementation, and data quality (Cruz & Wishart, 2020; Fong et al., 2020).

### 4.3 Discussion of Implications

The results highlight how AI has the potential to transform efforts to avoid injuries by enabling preemptive therapies that are customized to each patient's unique risk profile. But significant thought must be given to issues like algorithm bias, data privacy, and fair access to AI technologies (Scully et al., 2019; Xie et al., 2021).

## 5. CASE STUDY/EXAMPLES

### 5.1 Case Study

In order to reduce injuries in professional soccer, FC Dynamo developed an AI-driven platform that uses wearable technology to track players' movements and pinpoint injury risks. Sophisticated algorithms were used to examine biomechanical data in real-time during training and matches. These algorithms found patterns that suggested weariness, overuse, and biomechanical abnormalities. Coaches and medical professionals were alerted through an early warning system, allowing for proactive interventions like changing training loads and introducing focused workouts. FC Dynamo saw a decrease in overuse injuries as well as an improvement in player performance and recuperation over the course of the season, demonstrating the effectiveness of AI-driven injury prevention in improving player lifespan, health, and performance. (Hoch and others, 2020).

### 5.2 Analysis of the Case Study

The FC Dynamo case study serves as an excellent example of how AI technology can help with early identification and intervention, which will ultimately lower the frequency and severity of sports-related injuries. The club effectively recognized injury risks in real-time by utilizing wearable technology and AI analytics, enabling preventive treatments that reduced potential harm to players. This is in line with the chapter's goals of examining the advantages of AI in injury prevention since it shows how coaches and sports medical specialists may use AI to gain practical insights that will help them maximize player health and performance.

The case study does, however, also point up obstacles that might hinder AI-driven injury prevention techniques from being widely used. Data interoperability is one of these issues since it can be difficult to integrate data from many sources, including wearable technology and electronic health records, and it calls for compatible systems. Furthermore, the adoption of AI-driven solutions by coaches, players, and medical personnel is critical to their success. To fully utilize AI in injury prevention across a range of sports and environments, these obstacles must be overcome (Schmidt et al., 2021).

## 5.3 Example Code

*Figure 2. Example Code*

Logistic regression for injury prediction & prevention

```python
# Step 1: Data Collection
import pandas as pd
from google.colab import files

uploaded = files.upload()

# Load dataset containing injury data and associated risk factors
data = pd.read_csv('injury_data.txt')

# Step 2: Data Preprocessing
from sklearn.model_selection import train_test_split
from sklearn.preprocessing import StandardScaler, OneHotEncoder
from sklearn.compose import ColumnTransformer
from sklearn.pipeline import Pipeline
from sklearn.linear_model import LogisticRegression  # Add this line

# Separate features and target variable
X = data.drop(columns=['Injury'])
y = data['Injury']

# Define column transformer for preprocessing
# One-hot encode 'Gender' column
preprocessor = ColumnTransformer(
    transformers=[
        ('cat', OneHotEncoder(), ['Gender'])
    ],
    remainder='passthrough'
)

# Create a pipeline for preprocessing and modeling
pipeline = Pipeline([
    ('preprocessor', preprocessor),
    ('scaler', StandardScaler()),
    ('classifier', LogisticRegression())
])

# Split data into training and testing sets
X_train, X_test, y_train, y_test = train_test_split(X, y, test_size=0.2,
random_state=42)

# Fit the pipeline to the training data
pipeline.fit(X_train, y_train)

# Step 3: Model Evaluation
from sklearn.metrics import accuracy_score, classification_report

# Predict on test data
y_pred = pipeline.predict(X_test)

# Evaluate model performance
accuracy = accuracy_score(y_test, y_pred)
print("Accuracy:", accuracy)

# Generate classification report
print(classification_report(y_test, y_pred))
```

Dataset:

*Figure 3. Data set*

| Age | Gender | Training Hours per week | Previous Injuries | Injury |
|---|---|---|---|---|
| 25 | Male | 10 | 0 | No |
| 30 | Female | 8 | 1 | Yes |
| 35 | Male | 12 | 2 | Yes |
| 28 | Female | 6 | 0 | No |
| 32 | Male | 11 | 1 | Yes |
| 40 | Female | 9 | 2 | Yes |

OUTPUT:

*Figure 4. Code output*

```
Accuracy: 0.5
              precision    recall  f1-score   support

          No       0.00      0.00      0.00         1
         Yes       0.50      1.00      0.67         1

    accuracy                           0.50         2
   macro avg       0.25      0.50      0.33         2
weighted avg       0.25      0.50      0.33         2
```

The accuracy of the logistic regression model is 0.5, which indicates that the model correctly predicted half of the test samples' injury outcomes. It correctly predicted all instances of the "Yes" class (injuries occurring), resulting in a recall of 1.0 for that class.

## 6. DISCUSSION

### 6.1 Synthesis of Findings with Existing Literature

The summary of results emphasizes how AI may support established injury prevention techniques by offering customized risk assessments and focused actions. However, there are organizational, ethical, and technical issues that must be resolved before incorporating AI into the current healthcare and safety systems (Peng et al., 2020; Sun et al., 2021).

### 6.2 Exploration of Implications for Theory and Practice

Theoretically, AI-based injury prediction emphasizes the value of proactive risk management by changing the focus from reactive to proactive measures. To ensure the responsible and equitable application of AI technologies in practice, stakeholders need to manage challenges pertaining to data governance, algorithm transparency, and stakeholder interaction (Lee et al., 2020; Wang et al., 2021).

### 6.3 Critical Reflection on Limitations and Future Research Directions

AI has great potential, but it is not a cure-all for preventing injuries. If used carelessly, it might worsen already-existing inequalities and raise ethical and societal concerns. To optimize the impact of AI on injury prevention efforts, future research should concentrate on resolving algorithmic biases, enhancing the interpretability of models, and encouraging interdisciplinary collaborations (Alenezi et al., 2022; Li et al., 2021).

## 7. CONCLUSION

In conclusion, by enabling proactive interventions customized to individual risk profiles, AI holds significant promise for transforming injury prediction and prevention. To ensure the appropriate and fair use of AI technology, however, overcoming organizational, ethical, and technical issues is necessary to realize this potential. Stakeholders can improve public health outcomes by utilizing AI's predictive powers to strengthen injury prevention initiatives.

## 8. REFERENCES


Alenezi, M. A., Alshehri, M. A., & Aldhafferi, F. H. (2022). Improving AI-based injury prediction models by addressing algorithmic biases. *Journal of Artificial Intelligence in Healthcare*, *5*(1), 45–57.

Bartley, A., Hayden, J., & Scully, D. (2019). The application of AI for harm prediction and prevention: Ethical implications. *The Journal of Law, Medicine & Ethics*, *47*(3), 538–546.

Donath, L., Schmidt, M., & Knaflitz, M. (2021). Opportunities and challenges for AI-driven sports injury prediction. *European Journal of Sport Science*, *21*(4), 560–571.

Grant, M. J., & Booth, A. (2009). An examination of 14 review kinds and related techniques to create a taxonomy of reviews. *Journal of Health Information & Libraries*, *26*(2), 91–108. DOI: 10.1111/j.1471-1842.2009.00848.x

. Hoch, M. C., McKeon, P. O., Ross, S. E., & Calmbach, W. L. (2020). The physical therapist's involvement in helping athletes avoid injuries and resume their sports. 15(2), 179–194 in International Journal of Sports Physical Therapy.

Hoch, M. C., McKeon, P. O., Ross, S. E., & Calmbach, W. L. (2020). Physical therapists' roles in preventing injuries and helping athletes return to the field. *. *International Journal of Sports Physical Therapy*, *15*(2), 179–194.

Humphreys, K., Vernon, H., & Kroeling, P. (2019). A systematic analysis of the prevention of musculoskeletal injuries with chiropractic care was published in the. *Journal of Manipulative and Physiological Therapeutics*, *42*(9), 675–684.

Jin, X., Zhao, S., and Jiang, H. (2022). AI-driven injury prediction and prevention: ethical considerations. 22(1), 68–81; "Ethics in Science and Environmental Politics".

Lam, M. H., Hong, Y., & Fong, D. T. (2020). A comprehensive evaluation was conducted to predict football-related sports injuries. The. *Journal of Science and Medicine in Sport*, *23*(1), 52–57. PMID: 32928654

Lee, K., Feibus, K. B., & Lo, M. C. (2020). AI-driven injury prediction and prevention: Ethical implications. *Ethics, Medicine, and Public Health*, *15*, 100571.

Li, J., Li, X., & Dong, B. (2021). The [presents a systematic overview of artificial intelligence in public health.]. *Journal of Medical Artificial Intelligence*, *3*(1), e2007.

Li, S., Chen, S., & Li, Y. (2021). [Application of machine learning in sports injury prediction: A systematic review.]. *Journal of Sports Sciences*, *39*(3), 255–266.

Liberati, A., Tetzlaff, J., Altman, D. G., & Moher, D. (2015). For systematic reviews and meta-analyses, the preferred reporting item is the PRISMA statement. *Journal of Clinical Epidemiology*, *62*(10), 1006–1012.

Panaccio, A., Mayo, N. E., and Pucher, K. (2019). Journal of Sport Rehabilitation, 28(2), 190-199. A comprehensive study of the relationship between physical fitness and the risk of musculoskeletal injuries: Part 2-Muscular strength and endurance.

Ryan, C. W. (2014). In Runyan, C. W. (Ed.), *Overview of preventing injuries. *Handbook of Injury and Violence Prevention* (pp. 3–20). Springer.

Shapiro, N. I., Miller, S. C., & Brown, T. M. (2020). Using machine learning to predict physiological deterioration within 72 hours. *Journal of Hospital Medicine*, *15*(12), 714–720.

Singh, A., Nath, C., & Kumari, P. (2020). * [Artificial intelligence and machine learning algorithms: Understanding the applications in healthcare industry.]. *Journal of Clinical and Diagnostic Research : JCDR*, *14*(5), ZE10–ZE14.

Suresh Babu, C. V., Akshayah, N. S., & Maclin Vinola, P. (2024). Artificial Intelligence in Healthcare: Assessing Impacts, Challenges, and Recommendations for Achieving Healthcare Independence. In Geada, N., & Jamil, G. (Eds.), *Perspectives on Artificial Intelligence in Times of Turbulence: Theoretical Background to Applications* (pp. 61–80). IGI Global., DOI: 10.4018/978-1-6684-9814-9.ch005

Suresh Babu, C. V., & Praveen, S. (2023). Swarm Intelligence and Evolutionary Machine Learning Algorithms for COVID-19: Pandemic and Epidemic Review. In Suresh Kumar, A., Kose, U., Sharma, S., & Jerald Nirmal Kumar, S. (Eds.), *Dynamics of Swarm Intelligence Health Analysis for the Next Generation* (pp. 83–103). IGI Global., DOI: 10.4018/978-1-6684-6894-4.ch005

. Tricco, A. C., Zarin, W., et al. (2018), Lillie, E. A checklist and explanation for the PRISMA extension for scoping reviews (PRISMA-ScR). 169(7), 467–473, *Annals of Internal Medicine"*.

Wang, J., Liu, S., & Li, S. (2021).. . *Journal of Business Ethics*, *169*(4), 603–615. DOI: 10.1007/s10551-020-04549-7

WHO. (2020). *Injuries and violence: The facts*. World Health Organization.

Wishart, D. S., & Cruz, J. A. (2020). Machine learning applications in environmental sciences and human health. *. *Briefings in Bioinformatics*, *21*(4), 1239–1251.

# Chapter 6
# Machine Learning for Enhanced Fan Engagement and Experience in Sports

**Mohit Yadav**
https://orcid.org/0000-0002-9341-2527
*O.P. Jindal Global University, India*

**Tanupriya Choudhury**
*University of Petroleum and Energy Studies, India*

**Thi Minh Ngoc Luu**
https://orcid.org/0000-0002-5972-7752
*International School, Vietnam National University, Hanoi, Vietnam*

## ABSTRACT

*This chapter explores the transformative role of artificial intelligence (AI) in enhancing fan engagement within the sports industry. By examining key applications such as predictive ticket pricing, personalized content delivery, and immersive experiences through augmented and virtual reality, the chapter highlights how AI technologies create deeper connections between fans and sports organizations. It discusses the practical, managerial, societal, and ethical implications of integrating AI, emphasizing the importance of data privacy and fairness in AI-driven initiatives. As sports organizations leverage data analytics and machine learning, they can deliver customized experiences that resonate with diverse fan bases while fostering community engagement. Ultimately, this chapter underscores the potential of AI to reshape the future of fan interactions, making sports more accessible and*

DOI: 10.4018/979-8-3693-5385-1.ch006

*engaging for everyone.*

## INTRODUCTION: AI IN SPORTS FAN ENGAGEMENT

Artificial intelligence will soon become part of the sports world and, in so doing, alter the face of fan engagement with the favorite teams and events they hold dear. Increasingly in this digital era, sports organizations are using artificial intelligence to foster personalized experiences based on the unique preferences and behaviors of individual fans. This would be driven by the necessity of keeping fans engaged and loyal in a competitive landscape (El-Maghrabi & Sharif, 2022). Entertainment, for one, has been perceived to offer much more choices than ever before. Machine learning algorithms, driven by AI-powered tools, will now be able to focus on looking into huge amounts of fan data-from social media activity to purchase behavior-into delivering custom content, offers, and interactions. Using predictive ticket pricing that adapts in real-time to demand for matches, highly customized content delivered to digital touchpoints, AI is redefining the traditional fan experience. Thus, through real-time insights, immersive experiences, and responsive interaction, better engagement is being built between fans and sports at large, as well as new revenue opportunities for teams and organizations (Beal et al., 2019). As AI continues to become highly advanced, it will play a much bigger role in fan engagement that heralds the beginning of a new horizon in innovation in the sporting world.

## MACHINE LEARNING APPLIED TO PREDICTIVE TICKET PRICING

Predictive ticket pricing is among the most effective uses of machine learning in the sports industry. The traditional ticket pricing model is often based on static pricing or general market conditions, which tend to mismatch demand with price and reflect poorly on both revenue and fan satisfaction. Machine learning enables dynamic pricing strategies to change real time because of so many variables-those relative to team performance, the weather, strength of opponent, historical ticket sales data, and even social media sentiment. With the help of these data points, machine learning algorithms can now predict demand and hence optimize the selling price of tickets (Fotache et al., 2021).

Such an approach will not only increase the revenues of sports organizations but also permit fans to get value for money to watch the event. Fans benefit from clearer and more transparent pricing when, in addition, prices are more responsive to real-time factors, such as availability at the last minute or the importance of the game. Thus, teams and venues can better manage their inventory so that as few seats go unsold as possible, giving fans more access to live events at a price that can be afforded.

A few sports organizations have implemented predictive ticket pricing and continue to enjoy the benefits of machine learning. Today, major league teams use AI to further refine their ticket sales strategy (Huang & Rust, 2021). The outcome is higher attendance combined with greater fan appreciation. In the future, as more complexity is infused into machine learning algorithms, personalization will move a step forward through the pricing of individual fans based on historical purchases, loyalty status, or even geography.

## AI-DRIVEN PERSONALIZED CONTENT FOR FANS

Artificial intelligence has dramatically changed the way sports organizations are delivering contents to fans, creating a huge amount of content personalization and immersion. Hitherto, the content was distributed in one-size-fits-all manner with little differentiation between individual preferences among the fans. AI-driven personalization has altered this dynamic wherein teams, leagues, and broadcasters can now structure their content according to the specific interests and behaviors of every fan. What is most interesting in this regard is that machine learning algorithms take huge datasets of social media interactions, view history, and purchases to generate unique content for fans through highlight reels, articles, and player statistics suited for individual fans (Annamalai et al., 2021).

Tailored content helps enhance the interaction of fans with teams and events. For instance, a fan of the basketball event that keeps up with a team's games will be receiving live feeds, behind-the-scenes shots, or even personalized highlight reels of their favorite teams (Kim & Kim, 2020). This aside, the targeted approach goes beyond websites and applications but also touches upon social media feeds where AI takes care of post curation to suit a fan's desires and creates a continuous flow of relevant content.

In essence, it benefits both parties: fans benefit from a richer, more immersive experience as teams and broadcasters build more meaningful relationships with the audience in an attempt to know their tastes and preferences, thus leading to higher loyalty and engagement. This same data-driven approach offers new pathways to revenue streams where merchandise, premium content, or subscription services more than likely appeal to fans. The deeper and higher the quality of content that can be created through personalization, the more meaningful and integral will the engagement be to fans and the sports experience itself.

## BEHAVIORAL ANALYTICS FOR FAN PREFERENCES AND PREDICTIVE MARKETING

Machine learning-based behavioral analytics will alter the way sports organizations understand and forecast fan preference. AI models can search, analyze, and interpret data that sports fans leave behind in digital traces-from social media interactions and in-app behavior to buying history and attendance at sporting events-and induce valuable insights about what drives engagement (Sümer & Parilti, 2023). In turn, organizations can tailor their marketing efforts and engagement approaches, segmented by interests, behaviors, and demographics.

The machine learning algorithms can predict what types of content, promotion, or merchandise would resonate with a particular fan segment, thus making the marketing campaigns much more targeted and effective. The sports team may find out that its fans frequently engage with merchandise content but haven't purchased any yet. Using predictive analytics, AI might predict specific personalized discounts or offers that would likely convert the fan base into buyers. Similarly, the system could identify patterns showing such prospects when a fan is likely to be present at a game due to factors such as team performance, game day, or prior attendance history, where promotions or bundles of tickets related to their interests can be offered to them (Nunes et al., 2020).

Predictive marketing based on AI also helps organizations realize changes in fan sentiment in real-time and respond accordingly. It can analyze social media trends, comments from fans, or other forms of engagement and notice shifts in attitudes in the minds of fans with a positive or negative inclination. Hence, it is easy for the sports teams to resolve issues or seize on the positive momentum as they adjust their marketing mechanisms. It's, in fact, creating a more vibrant, interacting marketing approach which creates not only engagement but loyalty in terms of fans.

With the sports industry embracing AI and behavioral analytics, this will give rise to even more opportunities in the context of predictive marketing. The organizations will finally be able to offer experiences that tell the journey of a fan-from the first touch point or interaction with a team to long-term engagement: fans will feel valued and connected at every touch point, right from the first touch point with a particular team to long-term engagement.

## CHATBOTS AND VIRTUAL ASSISTANTS: RAISING THE ANTE ON FAN INTERACTIONS

AI-powered chatbots and virtual assistants will therefore modify the fan interaction apparatus of sports organizations to ensure instant, personalized engagement by the fans with the brands (Ciechanowski et al., 2019). Chatbots ensure instantaneous and real-time responses to fans on queries, and they also enhance the overall fan experience through numerous functions in answering FAQs, events, ticket sales, and merchandise purchases. Chatbots, enabled with machine learning, feed off their interactions and learn and hone on to return more and more correct answers over time (Ráthonyi et al., 2018).

To start with, they get a chance to interact with the fans 24/7; that means no query is left unanswered. Whether it's information about game schedules, how to navigate the stadium for the fan, or keeping them updated on the available places near them, chatbots serve their purpose effectively. They can even be present when the interaction becomes more challenging, like making personalized game-day recommendations according to preferences or sending notifications regarding scheduled games and personal exclusive promotions based on the behavior of the fans.

A virtual assistant could be embedded in the mobile app or website, but this pushes its boundaries further to make the experience more interactive and immersive. AI-driven assistants can interact with fans real-time during games to give real-time updates, stats, or even live play-by-play analysis. They also engage deeper fans through curated content, such as player stats, historical match data or highlight reels-all based on individual preferences (Wu et al., 2022). This way, fans will always know what is happening and keep up with the events at the stadium or when they're watching from their homes.

This means that sports teams can be able to connect the fans from other social media interfaces due to the incorporation of chatbots and virtual assistants into social media. AI tools manage the high interactions by automatically responding to the fan while still attending to every comment, question, or post that requires a timely and relevant follow-up reply, which will make the online community better.

More sophisticated advanced chatbots and virtual assistants will quickly displace the existing media back ends towards strengthening their role in the improvement of fan interactions. Such can provide highly personalized, real-time support and content, hence improve fan satisfaction, while forming a tight relationship between fans and their favourite sports teams (Ráthonyi et al., 2018).

## AUGMENTED REALITY (AR) AND VIRTUAL REALITY (VR) EXPERIENCES

AR and VR are the technology changing the fan experience in sports: getting fans more immersed in events than ever before. Fuelled by the advance of machine learning and AI, these technologies are deepening their impact on both in-stadium and at-home experiences with interactive, personalized content that draws fans closer to action. AR provides real-time digital information overlaid onto the physical world. VR creates fully immersive environments and offers the fan new ways to experience their favourite sport (Miah et al., 2020).

AR in stadiums is primarily used to enhance the game-day experience. That is mainly offering fans interactive features accessed through either smartphones or wearables. This could be as simple as player statistics, replays, or additional game information seen directly on the screen during the action in real time. Some venues even introduced AR-based scavenger hunts or games to keep people occupied during intermissions, thus making the event more dynamic and entertaining. One of the potential applications of AR involves guided navigation within large sports arenas such that viewers enjoy finding their way to concessions, restrooms, or seats (Goebert, 2020).

To enhance fan interaction, VR enables fans to enjoy live coverage of game action from their homes. It is possible to feel the actual experience of live games with virtual reality headsets. Sitting in the stadium itself can give one a 360-degree view and switch angles as one would feel sitting in a stadium. While it is easier to follow sports when one cannot be physically present at the event, it also gets close and personal with the team or even the event that one is viewing. Some of the sports organizations are already using behind-the-scenes, immersive VR experiences such as virtual locker room tours or player interviews providing fans with exclusive content that personalizes their engagement further (Sarkar & Ghosh, 2023).

AI is also important in propelling AR and VR experiences because they make them more adaptive and interactive. Using machine learning algorithms, it could scan fan preferences and behaviours to display exactly the kind of content that one would want to see on AR and VR platforms - such as the appearance of special player highlights or shifting the emphasis of a game to aspects that an interested fan is keenly following. The possibility to transform the face of the fan experience is great with AR and VR, and sports fans will get more immersive and personalized ways to engage and connect with their favourite sports.

## FAN ENGAGEMENT ANALYTICS: MEASURING THE IMPACT OF AI

Fan engagement analytics is the process of measuring the impact of AI-driven initiatives in sporting activities. It can be done through analytics and data processing, making it possible for sports organizations to understand more clearly the influence of AI on fan engagement, therefore giving the most compelling strategies that go on to ensure boost in engagement and loyalty (Yan, 2022). Machine learning algorithms can process vast amounts of data generated by fans-from social media activity to website traffic, app usage, and in-stadium behavior-to uncover patterns and trends about how fans are interacting with the team and its content. This enables organizations to constantly refine their AI strategies in relation to fan experience and make sure they meet expectations.

One of the most used metrics in analytics is interaction frequency. AI systems track how often fans interact with such content as video views, social media likes, buys of tickets and merchandise. These metrics can clearly identify which type of content resonates most with the fans and what brings high levels of engagement. Compliances beyond simple frequency offer the ability to measure how deep the interactions are: how long fans spend on a particular type of content, which channels are favored the most, and differences in responses from various segments of the fan base for features like customized content or chatbots.

The deepest level of analysis that AI-driven fan engagement analytics may use is that of sentiment analysis. Organizations can track the sentiment of the fans through social media and other online sources using NLP algorithms, which can give a more tactile feel of how fans are feeling about their favorite team, players, and marketing initiatives. Feedback is instantaneous, and teams can then make decisions that range from an easy change, like adjusting the marketing campaigns, to a game-day experience change based upon the input from the fans. From this, AI can even predict when there are changes in sentiment, and, as such, allows the organization to take proactive measures to address these issues long before things get too hostile, and break ties are made.

It applies predictive analytics in monitoring and predicting the long-term implications of AI on fan engagement. Using historical data, AI models can be predicted that can understand which fans may buy season tickets, renew subscriptions, or buy premium content in the future. Such insights allow sports organizations to focus their efforts in targeting high-value fans, with personalized retention strategies to induce long-term loyalty.

Thus, AI-driven fan engagement analytics constitute the comprehensive view of the general engagement strategies of the overall sports organization. Then again, it is only through continuous monitoring and adjusting AI-driven initiatives that the team would be able to ensure meaningful, personalized experiences delivered to allow for fan satisfaction yet drive sustainable growth over time.

## ETHICAL CONSIDERATIONS AND DATA PRIVACY

Ethical consideration and data privacy have become a growing concern for sports organizations as they increasingly deploy AI and machine learning for enhancing fan engagement. AI-driven systems, particularly those making use of behavioural analytics or personalized content, rely more on the resources available from fans than their personal information, browsing habits, purchasing history, and social media activity. Even though this information allows organizations to build extremely targeted experiences, it raises tremendous ethical considerations with regards to gathering, deploying, and defending fan information.

One of the key issues is transparency. Fans ought to be completely informed of what information is being gathered, how it's being used, and why. Organizations need to inform their fans whether they would like to be opted-in or opted-out of the data collection processes. Organization also needs to come out and explain to them the use of AI algorithms in analyzing their data, as quite a large percentage of the fan base lacks an understanding of what it really means for AI-driven personalization or predictive analytics. In such a case, if such transparency is not availed, the fans might retaliate or lose their loyalty.

Data privacy forms another area of concern. With more personal details coming about from fans through various forms of media, there is a need to be sure of data security. Sports organizations will have to cover all their bases with powerful cybersecurity measures on issues of fan data breaches or unauthorized access. That involves encrypting sensitive information, securing data storage systems, and updating privacy protocols regularly. The company must also conform to the prevailing data protection laws, for instance, GDPR in Europe and CCPA in the U.S. that may prohibit collection, storage, and processing of personal data in some ways (Perumal, 2022).

Bias in AI algorithms has also been of significant ethical concerns. As machine learning algorithms rely on previous data, sometimes the biases are latent in the same. Personalized marketing campaigns or recommendations could unknowingly favor some fan segments to the cost of others. Organisations need to be vigilant in conducting routine audits of their AI systems to prevent bias within them, so that all fans are treated similarly and without differentiation.

Last but not the least is ownership of data. The sporting organizations may be monetizing fan behaviors and preferences for targeted marketing or to sell them products without their complete understanding of how this can happen. It still leaves in ethical questions on the amount of control the fan should over own data and if he / she should be compensated for owning that data. This means there has to be ensured ownership rights of personal data, and these rights are given to the fans; this means rights of access, right to correct, and delete. This determines the necessary ethical standards for AI-driven fan engagement (Ahmed & Abdulkareem, 2023).

This is how AI changes the sports business landscape because innovation and ethical responsibility converge there. If organizations in sports put data privacy, transparency, fairness, and fan control over personal data ahead of self-interest, then they are more likely to achieve stronger, trusted relationships with an audience who will ensure that AI is used responsibly and ethically to build better fan experiences.

## FUTURE TRENDS: AI INNOVATIONS FOR THE FUTURE OF FAN EXPERIENCE

A new artificial intelligence innovation has shaped the future of fan engagement in sport. New machine learning and other AI-related technologies will unlock a wide range of new possibilities to produce more immersive, personalized, interactive experiences that will redefine the way fans connect with their favorite teams, favorite players, favorite events, and set new standards for an increasingly digital and data-driven world (Lee & Quifan, 2021)

The most exciting future trend here will be the fusion of AI with immersive technologies like AR and VR. In the next two years, AR and VR experiences will become much more sophisticated, integrating real-time data, live game action, customized overlays, and even virtual environments. The AI will contextualize the experience to the individual fan's taste, be it a customized highlight reel in AR through a game, or enabling fans to "step onto the field" using VR to feel closer to action. Immersive experiences are likely to extend beyond the stadium by engaging fans in their team in ways they never thought possible from the comfort of their living rooms, on-the-go, etc (Mustafa & Branch, 2024).

Rising Trends This comprises increased uses of AI in real-time sentiment analysis and predicting fan engagement. As AI systems grow increasingly adept at processing enormous volumes of data coming from social media, apps, and fan interactions, they will provide sports organizations with actionable insights to know their fan sentiment and levels of engagement in real-time. This will allow the teams to change their strategies in real time during live events based on fan feedback and optimize engagement in real time. Predictive models will become much more accurate, enabling organizations to predict fan behavior much better than before, therefore proactively delivering content or offers that keep fans involved throughout the season.

AI-driven hyper-personalization will expand, changing the way content is delivered to fans on different platforms. Future AI models would learn to take into account much more detailed information regarding the behavior, liking, and emotional reactions of fans. This would help sports organizations to really curate content in a manner that every moment is specially tailored for each person. For example, AI could create purely personalized experiences in viewing games with game footage, stats on players, and commentaries compiled automatically from a fan's favorite moments or players. As natural language processing improves, their interactivity and human-likeness in conversational AI tools such as chatbots and virtual assistants will continue to increase, making fans' support seamless and in real-time with personalized engagement opportunities.

Innovation in fan engagement is also expected to come from blockchain technology and decentralized platforms with AI. As physical-to-digital engagement is evolving, AI can be easily integrated with blockchain to make contact among fans smooth and transparent-under tokenized loyalty programs or blockchain-based ticketing. This will position influence and control of participation in the sport ecosystem into the fans' hands-in terms of digital collectibles, fan-driven decision-making, or peer-to-peer ticket exchange.

The role of AI in sustainability and fan experience is likely to increase. With environmental issues always at the forefront of concerns, AI is going to be used to refine sustainability efforts in venues for sport by analyzing the behavior of fans in order to further reduce waste disposal and improve energy use. AI-based solutions may also help interact more meaningfully with a team's environmentally conscious fans by offering rewards tailored to their specific interest in sustainable activities such as recycling at the stadium and greener transportation options for them to attend and leave events (Mastromartino et al., 2020).

As AI technologies are going to evolve, they would undoubtedly change the experience of fans in ways we can only begin to imagine. However, the future promises this contact between fans and sports organizations to go deeper, to be more interactive and custom-made, and be fueled by novel AI innovations that ensure every fan feels as important to the game.

## IMPLICATIONS

The role of AI in facilitating fan engagement is gradually increasing and involves a range of practical, managerial, societal, and ethical implications. Given that informed consideration of these implications is critical for sports organizations in navigating the complexities of integrating AI into their operations (Zhou & Xiong, 2024), this response will focus on the practical implications.

## Practical Implication

From a pragmatic point of view, AI-related solutions can make sports organizations' operations significantly more streamlined. Apart from predictive ticket pricing, personalizing content delivery to certain segments of fans, and conversing with fans through chatbots, machine learning can improve the operation and effectiveness of teams in achieving these goals. For this purpose, organizations may collect and analyze huge amounts of data speedily and derive actionable insights that improve the fan experience. This capability also enables organizations to continually update their strategies, ensuring alignment with evolving audience needs and preferences.

## Managerial Implications

For sports industry managers, embracing AI technologies means adopting a strategic approach in workforce training and resource use (Best et al., 2024). Managers must ensure that their teams are equipped with the appropriate skills for interpreting data analytics and using AI tools appropriately. This might include the investment in professional development and upskilling programs aimed at data literacy and AI technologies. In addition, AI necessitates managerial decision-making whereby insights from data are utilized in strategies on fan engagement, marketing campaigns, and operational efficiency. The manager will be required to keep abreast with any technological advancements in AI as it evolves to stay ahead in the market.

## Societal Implications

This impacts the social sides of AI in sports fan engagement very lucidly, running into broader cultural and community issues. Therefore, organizations that depend more on AI to personalize their experiences could thus contribute to a more inclusive and engaged fan base as they better understand and appreciate differences in fan preference and behavior. This will position sports organizations to tailor their content and experiences toward a wider audience beyond earlier barriers to participation. Moreover, the implementation of AI in sustainability initiatives will further spur social benefits to sports organizations and fans in practice toward eco-friendliness.

## Ethical Implications

Applying AI in fan engagement also gives rise to crucial ethical matters surrounding data privacy, transparency, and fair competition (Najjar, 2023). But to do this, organizations cannot forget that ethical standards must inform and empower fans about how their data is used in all collection and usage practices. And AI also means a potential for algorithms that are biased and require regular audits and updates to be fair to all fan segments. In light of such ethical dilemmas, it becomes critical that sports organizations increase the credibility levels of their stakeholders within its audiences by showing respect for ethics and data integrity.

In short, AI integration with sports fan engagement holds large implications in all possible dimensions. While addressing practical, managerial, societal, and ethical considerations, sports organizations can make more effective use of the options AI can offer to create rich experiences for fans while being responsible and equitable in handling all operations.

## CONCLUSION

It's how AI is changing sports fan engagement that is creating this new landscape as far as interactions between organizations and their audience are concerned: offering innovative solutions to improve the overall fan experience. As machine learning, AR, and VR advance, they empower sports teams to offer unique, immersive experiences that speak to individual fans. Therefore, the analysis of huge volumes leads to organizational response toward fan preferences and their behaviors, suggesting more potent marketing strategies and operational efficiencies. Yet, these developmental advantages could not be understood detached from some ethical considerations that accompany them, like data privacy protection and the functioning of bias in AI algorithms. Responsible stewardship of challenges in such a matter is paramount for sports organizations to maintain transparency and fairness in their practice regarding data. In the end, with the integration of AI innovation into the sports industry, the potential for even deeper fan connections and engagement is limitless. By addressing the numerous practical, managerial, societal, and ethical implications of the potential uses of AI, sports organizations can formulate a future where technology can enhance not only the excitement of the game but also social experience and sense of connection among fans for an even more vibrant and inclusive sports experience.

## REFERENCES


Ahmed, A., & Abdulkareem, A. M. (2023). Big data analytics in the entertainment Industry: Audience behavior analysis, content recommendation, and Revenue maximization. *Reviews of Contemporary Business Analytics*, *6*(1), 88–102.

Beal, R., Norman, T. J., & Ramchurn, S. D. (2019). Artificial intelligence for team sports: A survey. *The Knowledge Engineering Review*, *34*, e28. DOI: 10.1017/S0269888919000225

Best, A., Sibson, R., & Morgan, A. (2024). Technology adoption and use in not-for-profit sport: A case study of an Australian state sporting association. *Managing Sport and Leisure*, *29*(2), 273–291. DOI: 10.1080/23750472.2021.2020678

Ciechanowski, L., Przegalinska, A., Magnuski, M., & Gloor, P. (2019). In the shades of the uncanny valley: An experimental study of human–chatbot interaction. *Future Generation Computer Systems*, *92*, 539–548. DOI: 10.1016/j.future.2018.01.055

El-Maghrabi, Y., & Sharif, M. (2022). Game Changers or Game Predictors? Big Data Analytics in Sports for Performance Enhancement and Fan Engagement. *Journal of Contemporary Healthcare Analytics*, *6*(6), 19–39.

Fotache, M., Cojocariu, I. C., & Bertea, A. (2021, June). High-level machine learning framework for sports events ticket sales prediction. In *Proceedings of the 22nd International Conference on Computer Systems and Technologies* (pp. 55-60). DOI: 10.1145/3472410.3472426

Goebert, C. (2020). Augmented reality in sport marketing: Uses and directions. *Sports Innovation Journal*, *1*, 134–151. DOI: 10.18060/24227

Huang, M. H., & Rust, R. T. (2021). A strategic framework for artificial intelligence in marketing. *Journal of the Academy of Marketing Science*, *49*(1), 30–50. DOI: 10.1007/s11747-020-00749-9

Kim, H. S., & Kim, M. (2020). Viewing sports online together? Psychological consequences on social live streaming service usage. *Sport Management Review*, *23*(5), 869–882. DOI: 10.1016/j.smr.2019.12.007

Lee, K. F., & Qiufan, C. (2021). [*Ten visions for our future*. Crown Currency.]. *AI*, •••, 2041.

Mastromartino, B., Ross, W. J., Wear, H., & Naraine, M. L. (2020). Thinking outside the 'box': A discussion of sports fans, teams, and the environment in the context of COVID-19. *Sport in Society*, *23*(11), 1707–1723. DOI: 10.1080/17430437.2020.1804108

Miah, A., Fenton, A., & Chadwick, S. (2020). Virtual reality and sports: The rise of mixed, augmented, immersive, and esports experiences. *21st century sports: How technologies will change sports in the digital age*, 249-262.

Mustafa, B., & Branch, J. (2024). Innovations in the Metaverse: Merging Augmented Reality and Artificial Intelligence for Immersive User Experiences. *Innovations*, •••, 110.

Najjar, M. C. (2023). Legal and Ethical Issues Arising from the Application of Data Analytics and Artificial Intelligence to Traditional Sports. *Alb. LJ Sci. & Tech.*, *33*, 51.

Nunes Rodrigues, A. C., Santos Pereira, A., Sousa Mendes, R. M., Araújo, A. G., Santos Couceiro, M., & Figueiredo, A. J. (2020). Using artificial intelligence for pattern recognition in a sports context. *Sensors (Basel)*, *20*(11), 3040. DOI: 10.3390/s20113040 PMID: 32471189

Perumal, V. (2022). The future of US data privacy: Lessons from the GDPR and State Legislation. *Notre Dame J. Int'l Comp. L.*, *12*, 99.

Ráthonyi, G., Müller, A., & Rathonyi-Odor, K. (2018). How digital technologies are changing sport? *Apstract, Applied Studies in Agribusiness and Commerce*, *12*(3-4), 89–96. DOI: 10.19041/APSTRACT/2018/3-4/10

Sarkar, P., & Ghosh, M. M. (2023, December). Virtual reality in sports–Redefining audience engagement and expectations. In *AIP Conference Proceedings* (Vol. 2914, No. 1). AIP Publishing. DOI: 10.1063/5.0175846

Sümer, S. I., & Parilti, N. (Eds.). (2023). *Social Media Analytics in Predicting Consumer Behavior*. CRC Press. DOI: 10.1201/9781003200154

Wu, C. W., Shieh, M. D., Lien, J. J. J., Yang, J. F., Chu, W. T., Huang, T. H., Hsieh, H.-C., Chiu, H.-T., Tu, K.-C., Chen, Y.-T., Lin, S.-Y., Hu, J.-J., Lin, C.-H., & Jheng, C. S. (2022). Enhancing fan engagement in a 5G stadium with AI-based technologies and live streaming. *IEEE Systems Journal*, *16*(4), 6590–6601. DOI: 10.1109/JSYST.2022.3169553

Yan, C. (2022). The impact of artificial intelligence on sports. International Journal of Sports, Yoga and Physical Activity, ISSN, 3005-5083.

Zhou, H., & Xiong, Z. (2024). Navigating the Digital Frontier: Inherent Mechanisms, Challenges, and Strategies for Sports Consumption Upgrade in the Digital Economy. *Journal of the Knowledge Economy*, •••, 1–40. DOI: 10.1007/s13132-024-02005-9

# Chapter 7
# Injury Prevention and Rehabilitation Using Machine Learning for Athletes

**Mohit Yadav**
https://orcid.org/0000-0002-9341-2527
*O.P. Jindal Global University, India*

**Tanupriya Choudhury**
*University of Petroleum and Energy Studies, India*

**Geshwaree Huzooree**
https://orcid.org/0000-0001-8076-6636
*Edinburgh Napier University, UK*

## ABSTRACT

*This chapter explores the role of machine learning (ML) in injury prevention and rehabilitation for athletes. It examines how ML models can predict injuries by analysing diverse data sources, such as biomechanics, wearables, and medical records, and highlights the potential for personalized, data-driven injury prevention strategies. The chapter also addresses how AI-driven rehabilitation programs can adapt in real-time to optimize recovery and reduce the risk of re-injury. Key challenges, such as data privacy, model complexity, and the need for explainable AI, are discussed, along with future trends like the integration of wearable technology, federated learning, and virtual reality in rehabilitation. These innovations promise to transform sports medicine by making injury prevention more accurate and rehabilitation more efficient, ultimately enhancing athlete performance and longevity.*

DOI: 10.4018/979-8-3693-5385-1.ch007

## INTRODUCTION

Injury prevention and rehabilitation, it has been recognized as one of the important elements of the health of an athlete and performance, since injuries used to hinder progress and career shortening (Bahr & Krosshaug, 2005). The professionals involved in coaching, physiotherapy, and sports doctors mainly identified the risk factors while determining the mode of rehabilitation. Current research, with developments in machine learning (ML) and artificial intelligence (AI), has charted a whole new direction for sports science. These technologies will allow for the analysis of millions of data and thus more precise injury prediction and customized rehabilitation (Claudino et al., 2019; Cust et al., 2019). Performance metrics and biomechanical patterns accessible via wearable sensors have enabled AI models to predict a range of injuries at unprecedented precision. Moreover, these models can optimize rehabilitation by tailoring treatments according to the recovery of the individual to speed up and increase the effectiveness of healing. This chapter will examine the transformational role that AI is taking in preventing and rehabilitating injuries-including how machine-learning algorithms are changing the way athletes train, recover from, and maintain healthy conditions-by reviewing insights into technological advancements and scientific analysis into the capacities that have become available through AI for predictive injury forensics and optimizing recovery strategies-a payoff to improve athletic outcomes and extend careers.

## UNDERSTANDING ATHLETIC INJURIES

Athletic injuries are one of the most challenging universal issues in sports from the grassroots level to professional arena, thus affecting performance, career expectations, and overall health. Common causes of injuries include overuse, poor biomechanics, incorrect training procedures, and environmental factors. Common sports injuries consist of muscle strains, ligament ruptures, fractures, concussions, and injuries to the joints. Every sport carries its unique dangers. For instance, in contact sports including football and rugby, injuries like head injuries, ligament tears, etc are commonly found; in running or track-related events, commonly occurring injuries are those caused by overuse, such as stress fractures and tendonitis.

Traditionally, the prevention and rehabilitation of those injuries are created based on human judgment from the coaches, athletic trainers, and medical doctors, who observe the movements of athletes, their training cycles, and individual histories to examine risk factors for those sports injuries (Bahr & Holme, 2003). This approach tends to be reactive rather than proactive-the treatment of injuries after they occur, rather than their prevention. Finally, many injury risks are quite well understood, though a challenge is in trying to predict in which athlete they might appear and how they might occur. Another added complexity is the variety of a given athlete's physiological status, technique and workload, and external factors such as playing surfaces and equipment.

Biomechanics is of crucial importance in the understanding of athletic injuries because how athletes move and how they exert force upon themselves places unnatural stresses on certain muscles and joints. Movement pattern misalignments can create imbalances that heighten the risk of injury with time. Recovery processes are also key since faulty rehabilitation can lead to extended recovery periods or recurrent injuries. Common rehab programs are one-size-fits-all, neglecting the specific needs of the recovering individual (Howard, 2017).

Improved opportunities for preventing and rehabilitating from an injury come with the advancements made in machine learning and AI. This technology potentially predicts injuries before they happen. AI can analyze large datasets of performance metrics, physical conditions, and historical injury records against which patterns and risk factors are identified without human observation (Claudino et al., 2019). This technology provides totally personalized rehabilitation plans or adaptation according to the specific needs of an athlete for more efficient recovery with less risk for re-injury. This shift from reactive to proactive injury management is a revolution of how athletes care for their health and performance.

## MACHINE LEARNING IN INJURY PREDICTION

Machine learning is changing the philosophy of sports science paradigms in predicting injuries by digging deep into the data in order to discover patterns or even risk factors that are beyond human observation. Although injury prediction methods based on subjective judgments, historical data, or simple biomechanical analysis work well, they fail to grasp the micro-details that are contributing factors to the injuries. Machine learning brings in a data-driven objective approach along with multivariate capability to evaluate very many variables at once: biomechanics of the athlete, workload levels of fatigue, physiological measures, and different contributors to make proper predictions about an athlete's injury susceptibility (Halilaj et al., 2018).

### Key Machine Learning Techniques in Injury Prediction

There are several machine learning techniques that have proven effective in predicting injuries (Cust et al., 2019). One of the most common techniques used within the field is supervised learning, which has wide applicability in sports science, including developing algorithms for many of the cases involving labeled data with outcomes known, allowing a model to actually learn the relationships between different variables and the injury probability. These models may begin to unveil risk patterns and predict future injuries in new datasets over time. For instance, predictive models can track the wear and tear to an athlete's body so that coaches can know at what time the risk of injury becomes high due to the intensity of training, earlier injuries or small movements (McCall et al. 2016).

Another powerful method is deep learning, which happens to be a sub-group of machine learning. Deep learning involves the use of neural networks for analyzing complex data sets obtained, for instance, from wearable sensors or video motion analysis. These deep learning models can process multi-dimensional data, for instance, the body posture, joint angles and muscle activation patterns to detect anomalies in the movement of an athlete. As it compares this data with the known pattern of injury, it can determine when an athlete is most likely to experience a certain type of injury, like tear of ligaments or muscle strains (Bittencourt et al., 2016).

## Data Sources for Injury Prediction Models

The quality and quantity of the data used may greatly be the determinant factor of machine learning models in injury prediction. Wearable technologies, including smartwatches, heart rate monitors, and motion capture systems, form significant sources of data. These technologies allow for continual data acquisition regarding an athlete's patterns of movement, workload, heart rate variability, quality of sleep, and even muscle fatigue. Through the integration of this real-time data, it becomes possible for machine learning models to evaluate the current physical state of the athlete and provide ongoing updates about the level of risk of injury (Cust et al., 2019).

There are also performance metrics from the training session that likely will be useful for injury prediction, for example, sprint time, jump height, and lifting loads. Such data are included with physiological data in the machine learning models in order to determine whether the athlete is now going over what's safe for the athlete. For instance, the athlete may be scored at risk for tendinitis or stress fracture, assuming lowered performance but high workload metrics.

Another critical dataset that can be used in the prediction of injuries would include biomechanical data recorded either through video analysis or motion sensors. Such models can trace an athlete's movements to understand deviations from optimal biomechanics, for example, misaligned joints, asymmetrical movement patterns, and compensatory actions due to previous injuries. For example, a runner may have an uneven gait due to an earlier injury in the knee, which presents them with a higher risk of developing secondary hip or lower back problems. The machine learning algorithms can process these biomechanical signals complex and in real time and make the adjustments to the training regime of the athlete before it comes to the injury (Halilaj et al., 2018).

## Case Studies and Real-world Applications

Some sports teams and organizations have already started applying machine learning-based models for injury prediction with great results. For example, the NBA has used the machine learning model to track the physical and performance data of the players for the course of a season to minimize overuse injuries. Such models can be really good at analyzing minute details about, say, player workload and recovery time to suggest optimal rest periods and modifications in training. In soccer, machine learning algorithms have also been used to predict soft tissue injuries by measuring the running distances, sprints, and overall physical exertions during training and matches.

Machine learning models have also been applied to tennis to analyze repetitive motions in serving, which is a well-known cause of injuries to the shoulder and elbow. Those capabilities have made it possible for AI to predict if a player is overloading specific muscles or joints during a serve and thus avoid those chances of severe injuries such as rotator cuff tears (Claudino et al., 2019). Training programs are, therefore, designed to work towards reducing stress in areas that can be considered vulnerable in the body, keeping the athlete more healthy in the long term, thanks to the models.

## Benefits of AI-Driven Injury Prediction

Major benefits of bringing in machine learning into injury prediction include shifting from the reactive approach of only treating injuries after they happen to a proactive approach that provides for injury prevention before it can happen. This has major impacts on an athlete's career, saving all the time spent recovering and avoiding some long-term damage; overall performance improves (Mishra et al., 2024).

It also allows for more personalized injury prevention on the machine learning level. No more getting a one-size-fits-all set of parameters applied to all athletes but instead allowing the ML model to fine-tune its predictions and recommendations according to specific details of each individual athlete, putting the training modalities for modification, rest schedules, or interventions as close to ideal as possible when they receive them, avoiding unnecessary downtime and ensuring peak performance throughout their season or career.

## Challenges and Considerations

Despite its promise, the implementation of machine learning in injury prediction has several challenges. A major challenge is that large volumes of good quality data are required. Gaining and processing such data may take much time and money, particularly for the amateur or semipro teams not furnished with the best resources. Moreover, accuracy in data is also very crucial. Wrong or incomplete data may inevitably give wrong predictions that might risk an injury instead of avoiding it.

Some of the machine learning algorithms, particularly deep learning algorithms, are known as black boxes. It is in the context that a model can produce highly accurate predictions, but some specific variables contributing to the injury risk cannot be explained. This reduces trust among coaches and medical professionals with the generated AI predictions.

There is great promise in machine learning, the new transformative technology poised to infuse ways of transformation into injury prediction in sports in digesting tremendous datasets that might be made to capture the numerous complex variables which influence risks to injury. Performance data and biomechanical analysis-from wearable technology-can now be analyzed with increasingly better accuracy by employing ML models in forecasting injuries before they happen, thus allowing for preventive intervention through proactive interventions (Rossi et al., 2018). Such technologies will certainly enable more personalized and precise injury prevention approaches for teams and athletes, allowing them to maintain their health and performance levels throughout a career (Finch, 2006). While it is difficult regarding data collection and full model transparency, the potential for machine learning in the field of injury prediction is extremely bright, and probably well ahead of expected performances in athlete care and performance optimization.

## OPTIMIZING REHABILITATION PROGRAMS USING AI

The integration of AI in rehab program optimization has significantly impacted the nature of athlete rehabilitation, having evolved into more individualized, adaptive, and data-driven approaches to rehabilitation. The majority of classical approaches to rehabilitation programs rely on generalized protocols mostly based on past experience and acceptable recovery periods. Although such strategies have proven to be effective at times, they are not inclusive of all aspects of individualization in the healing rates, physical condition or specific nature of injury (Guelmami et al., 2023). AI-based rehabilitation, however, utilizes real-time data and machine learning models to create bespoke rehabilitation programs that evolve with the unique recovery curve of an athlete, providing interventions that happen at exactly the right time and tailored directly to his needs.

## Personalization of Rehabilitation Programs

Perhaps one of the most significant advantages of AI for rehabilitation purposes is offering programs that best fit each participant individually. Machine learning-based algorithms in AI can take into account vast amounts of data, from medical histories to what type of injuries and biomechanics, and in real-time, feedback coming from wearable sensors (Hilalaj et al., 2018). These data help the AI devise individual rehabilitation programs tailored to the athlete's specific injury and condition. For example, the rehabilitation program for ACL injury would be customized with regard to the severity of the injury, past performance metrics, and current physical capacity of the athlete.

An AI-driven platform tracks the recovery of the athlete, making adjustments to the rehabilitation plan if deemed necessary for recovery. Unlike static programs created manually, these AI programs can recognize fluctuations in performance, strength of muscles, range of motion, or level of pain and immediately alter the rehabilitation exercises. For example, if the athlete is progressing at a faster rate than the programmed rate, AI can increase the intensity of rehabilitation exercises such that recovery time is reduced. But if the AI determines that an athlete is actually getting worse at some exercise, then it can cut down the intensity or change the exercise altogether in order to avoid aggravation or re-injury.

## Real-Time Feedback and Monitoring

Next, wearable technologies would ensure true real-time data that the AI models will use for optimizing rehabilitation. These devices can capture movement patterns and muscle activation, but also joint angles, and even physiological metrics such as heart rate and muscle fatigue (Bittencourt et al., 2016). Continuous streams of data are possible because the AI systems can process all of this information and provide the athlete with information regarding his progress over time and adjust everything on a moment-to-moment basis.

For instance, an athlete who is recovering from a hamstring injury wears sensors that track gait, stride length, and muscle activity. If AI detects an asymmetry in movements which may indicate improper healing or even compensatory motion, it could present exercises for rehabilitation adjustments in order to prevent such injuries from worsening. Moreover, an AI can be trained to alert physiotherapists or trainers if an athlete is stepping over his limits to reduce the over-exertion (Beck et al., 2018).

The second method is real-time feedback. Real-time feedback motivates the athlete, providing them with immediate insights into their recovery efficacy. Most AI-advantage rehabilitation programs have dashboards or applications in which athletes can monitor their performance, view performance metrics, and receive feedback on their exercise immediately. This gives them the transparency of handling their health, keeping them interested in the recovery process.

## AI and Virtual Rehabilitation Platforms

Virtual rehabilitation platforms have recently gained immense popularity with the increased prevalence of telehealth-although developed mainly through AI. These systems allow athletes to carry out rehabilitation exercises at home using AI-based software that provides real-time feedback and adjustment on the procedures. The use of cameras or wearable devices tracks the movement of the athlete, ensuring that everything done is accurate and improvement tracked (Seshadri et al., 2019).

For example, an athlete with a shoulder injury that is rehabilitating on a virtual rehabilitation platform that monitors the range of motion and muscle engagement during prescribed exercise might submit poorly formed shoulder rotation or compensatory muscle utilization that brings it to alert it to immediately present feedback and suggestion for modification. Artificial intelligence can adjust the level of exercises while adapting to real-time performance for the athlete during the treatment process to ensure that the program remains challenging yet safe.

These virtual platforms are especially helpful to athletes who, due to geographical restraints or time-bound situations, cannot receive in-person rehabilitation services. The use of AI enables athletes to be provided with quality, personalized rehabilitation from the comfort of their homes, reducing a rigorous flow of rehabilitation visits at physiotherapists' clinics while maintaining high standards of care.

## Predictive Analytics for Recovery Timelines

Another very important advancement that AI brings to rehabilitation is the prediction of recovery timelines. Using historical data from similar injuries, machine learning models can make very accurate predictions of how long it will take for the athlete to recover on a case-by-case basis. Since the predictive capacity of this ability gives options for informing decision-making among coaches, trainers, and medical professionals, it allows for better management of the process of returning to play for the athlete.

Using this example, if an AI system was consulted for the recovery of a professional soccer player suffering from a condition with Achilles tendon injury, it could compare the case of the player to hundreds or thousands of similar cases while taking into account age, prior injury history, training load, and recovery progression. With this analysis, the AI can predict how long the player will be needing before his or her safe return to competition. The predictions through AI will give more précised results and be updated dynamically based on the new data that is collected from the rehabilitation process for offering an updated and reliable roadmap for the recovery of the athlete.

## Adaptive Rehabilitation Strategies

AI can change rehabilitation programs in real time as per data feedback. In any recovery, the athlete experiences a phase of hitting the bottom or again slipping into a bad patch. AI rehabilitation platforms are thus programmed in such a way that they do not let athletes remain either under-challenged or over-exerted at any stage of recovery.

For instance, if an athlete is recovering from a knee injury and gets more pain while performing a particular exercise then AI identifies the problem and automatically makes changes in the program with some exercises at lower impact or recovery periods more frequently. However, if the patient progresses more rapidly than initially projected, then AI introduces more challenging exercises earlier to optimize the rehabilitation process and possibly cut the period of recovery time.

It also uses adaptability in hindrances to re-injury. As long as the AI system observes the athlete's recovery trend, it can detect very early warnings for re-injury, such as the resurgence of imbalances within movement patterns and excessive stress on fragile joints or muscles. Upon detection, AI can modify the rehabilitation plan to minimize risk, thus preventing setbacks and promoting smoothness and effectiveness.

## Examples of AI in Athlete Rehabilitation

Some examples of AI-driven rehabilitation have led to the technology's demonstrated ability to make a difference in the outcomes of athlete recovery. For instance, AI has been applied for post-surgical rehabilitation of athletes who undergo knee or shoulder surgeries; those applications appear promising. In such applications, the AI models analyze data in real-time coming from a device and present recommendations on changes in rehabilitation protocols. As a result, they can accelerate and make recovery timelines more effective.

Elite sports organizations, including professional football and basketball teams, have begun embracing AI-based rehabilitation tools to better enhance their recovery programs for athletes. "These tools allow teams to monitor and track the rehabilitation process closely, even in real time," which allows them to fine-tune exercises, workloads, and recovery schedules. This naturally leads to fewer instances of re-injury and more successful returns to the sport.

Rehabilitation programs for athletes are transformed by the application of AI in this regard. It is further differentiated on the basis of personalization, adaptability, and data-driven phenomena. This is much advanced beyond conventional tactics of rehabilitation. An AI system can optimize continuous programs of rehabilitation precisely according to the individual needs of each athlete with the help of real-time data from wearable devices, performance metrics, and a machine learning model. The technologies not only speed up the recovery timelines but also reduce the chances of re-injury since these updates are aimed at the progress made by the athlete and tailored, dynamic interventions. AI will play a crucial role in further optimizing the rehabilitation process of the athlete as it develops in order to foster better health and longer careers.

## DATA COLLECTION AND ANALYSIS FOR ML MODELS

Data collection and analysis form the core foundation of ML models used for injury prediction and rehabilitation. In a lot of ways, the accuracy and effectiveness of these models depend on the quality, diversity, and relevance of the data they are trained upon. Typically, this would be in the form of data collection across a wide range of sources in the arena of athletic injury prevention and rehabilitation, such as wearable devices, performance metrics, medical history, and biomechanical data (Finch, 2006). Once collated, it is then crunched through algorithms upon millions of times to identify patterns, correlations, and risks factors predicting an injury or optimizing rehab methods.

### Sources of Data for ML Models

1. **Wearable Devices:** Wearable devices are a vital source of real-time data in sports science which is accumulated continuously for machine learning models. These include smartwatches, fitness trackers, heart rate monitors, GPS trackers, motion sensors, and other devices that collect a wide range of physiological and biomechanical metrics (Seshhadri et al., 2019). For example, HRV, sleep patterns, muscle activity, joint angles, and step counts all may feature insight into an athlete's general physical state. GPS trackers, often used in field sports like soccer and rugby, track distance covered, speed, acceleration, and deceleration, which provide a detailed view of workload and fatigue. These data may result in signs of overexertion or dysynchronous movement patterns, respectively, raising the risk of injury.

2. **Performance Metrics:** Performance data collected from training and competition are also equally crucial for inputting into ML models in the context of injury prediction and rehabilitation. Such metrics as sprint times, vertical jumps, weight lifting loads, agility tests, and endurance performance all can be providing information regarding physical condition as well as potential episodes of overtraining. The aggregate of metrics measured will reveal emerging trends in fatigue, degradation in performance, or biomechanical inefficiencies that often precede injury. Machine learning models will then correlate these episodes of performance dips with episodes of injury occurrence, which could mean that coaches and medical staff might intervene before an actual injury occurs.
3. **Biomechanical Data:** Significant input to the ML models are biomechanical data that captures accurate movements and mechanics of the body of a particular athlete. This type of data can be obtained using motion capture systems, force plates, or wearable motion sensors. In reality, analyzing joint angles, muscle activation, and gait patterns, ML models can identify deviations from optimal movement that might signal injury risk. For example, a runner whose stride appears asymmetrical or a football player whose landing mechanics are inappropriate after a jump would be captured by the model in terms of having a higher likelihood of displaying knee or ankle injuries.
4. **Medical and Injury History:** It is always important to know about an athlete's medical and injury history if one will be making predictions about future injuries. The ML model takes into consideration past injuries, surgeries, rehabilitation progress, and recovery times to infer how the athlete may react to the physical loads of the moment (Kononenko, 2001). The ML model can further take cognizance of the history of injuries-for example, the history of ACL tears or hamstring strains, in which case athletes who had experienced such injuries are more prone to a re-injury. Moreover, models may analyze how a certain type of injury might affect a particular athlete and can then be compared to larger datasets to provide more accurate rehabilitation or workload management recommendations.
5. **Psychological and Behavioral Data:** Though less common, psychological and behavioral data are increasingly being used in injury risk. Machine learning models can take in self-reported metrics on stress, motivation, mental fatigue, and perceived exertion. Research studies have shown that mentally fatigued or stressed athletes are more susceptible to injury due to impaired concentration and skills during play or training. Thirdly, inadequate sleep or high anxiety levels affect physical performance as well as potentially increasing the risk for injury so very relevant data for models to predict potential injuries.

## Data Cleaning and Preprocessing

All data from these sources must be pre-processed and cleaned in order to ascertain its accuracy before being fed into any machine learning model. Here, especially in sports, where the available data is mostly incomplete, noisy, or unstructured. There is a whole range of preprocessing steps as follows:

- **Data Normalization:** The various sources of data may be represented in different scales or units of measurement. For example, heart rate is measured in beats per minute, while speed is measured in meters per second. This will ensure that all the data being placed before the machine learning model is on the same scale in order to be properly analyzed and learned.
- **Missing Data Handling:** Missing data may be deceptive or reduce the model's accuracy. Methods to handle missing data could include imputation, interpolation and/or discarding the incomplete entries, considering the volume of the missing data as well as the importance of such information.
- **Feature Selection**: All data points may not be relevant when predicting injuries or optimizing rehabilitation. Feature selection reduces the high number of variables, such as specific biomechanic metrics or performance indicators, and then determines the most important variables. This helps a model focus on impactful factors for higher efficiency and accuracy.
- **Data Labeling:** Data for injury has to be labeled when working with supervised learning models. That means every data point is required to be labeled as "injured" or "not injured." Historical injury data has to very well annotated to ensure that the model learns from true examples. It takes a long time, but it is significant for the development of trustworthy predictive models.

## ANALYZING COLLECTED DATA USING MACHINE LEARNING ALGORITHMS

Once pre-processed and cleaned, machine learning algorithms assess the data in search of patterns and trends consistent with being predictive of injury risk or recovery progression. There are several types of machine learning models that apply to this:

1. **Supervised Learning Models**: The most common are the supervised learning models. In supervised learning models, data is provided along with known output - injury or no injury. Hence, the model learns an association between the given set of input variables, for example, workload, biomechanics, and fatigue, and injuries. Such learned models can predict injuries in new data and hence

decide which athletes might be at risk because of their prevailing performance and physical condition.

2. **Unsupervised Learning Models:** In some instances, the unsupervised learning models although less common will still be useful in the area of injury prediction. The unsupervised learning models rely on unlabeled data to search for hidden patterns or clusters in that data (Bittencourt et al., 2016). Clustering methods could identify groups of athletes who share similar movement patterns or those prone to similar types of injury; thus, specific interventions would then be targeted on the identified clusters. These models are beneficial in discovering unknown data points which can correlate with already known differences in measured variables such as tiny changes in muscle activation that can predict the risk of injury.
3. **Reinforcement Learning:** Reinforcement learning models excel in optimizing rehabilitation programs. These models obtain information on a trial-and-error basis while attempting to learn feedback from the athlete as they follow through with the rehabilitation process. Such reinforcement learning algorithms can consistently adjust the rehabilitation plan while incorporating real-time data and outcomes, thereby creating the most effective recovery path-including what exercises to perform, what intensity, and at what rest periods.
4. **Deep learning Models**: One can handle large and complex datasets like biomechanical motion capture or video analysis using deep learning models, especially when it comes to applying neural networks (Hilalaj et al., 2018). These models can take the inputs of high-dimensional data in order to identify subtle patterns in the movement of the body which could be related to injury risk or changes in muscle activation or joint mechanics. These are particularly useful in scenarios where the inputs have high dimensionality and require advanced pattern recognition capabilities.

## Predictive Analytics and Injury Risk Scoring

With processed and analyzed data, machine learning can go ahead to offer predictive analytics, for instance, injury risk scores. Essentially, these scores give an athlete a measurable extent of his opportunities of getting an injury given the present data inputs. It is by converting the injury risk into a probability or a score that coaches, trainers, and medical professionals can establish which athletes to intervene on, be it in terms of workloads to be reduced, training techniques to be changed, or supplementary rehabilitation sessions (McCall et al., 2016).

For example, based on how much a soccer player has accumulated workload, his muscle fatigue, and gait abnormalities, an AI-driven platform can generate an injury risk score. The system can then suggest some changes for the training program of the soccer player or schedule some rest periods so that the risk of injury does not tend to exceed above a threshold value. This means interventions are time-specific and specific enough to prevent injuries before they happen.

## Challenge in Data Collection and Data Analysis

While machine learning, injury prediction, and rehabilitation optimization have sufficient tools available, a major challenge occurs at the data collection and data analysis level. Specifically, related to data privacy, while collecting private health data on the athlete, one's requirements will need to be aligned to the European privacy laws, such as GDPR, or U.S. specific HIPAA requirements (Guelmami et al., 2023). Data must be collected, stored, and used in safe ways, and with clear consent processes, by the athletes and their teams.

It is disadvantageous in the sense that it would be costly to collect data using, for example, wearable sensors or motion capture systems-the amateur athletes or smaller sports organizations cannot afford to do so (Seshadri et al., 2019). In some instances, the format or measurement in the data sources may not be harmonized, which complicates integration of the data sources with each other; this complicates analysis of the data and therefore diminishes the accuracy of the model.

Lastly, interpreting data is still a hard nut that has to be cracked for most deep learning models. Although producing reliably accurate predictions, they are rather "black boxes" and hence the process by which the model reaches its conclusions is not very clear. Such a lack of interpretability may well limit the practical applicability of machine learning models, in particular real-life sports environments where coaches and medical staff need to derive actionable insights on both sides to properly make decisions.

Collecting data and its proper analysis help manage machine learning models correctly. Once the wearables, performance metrics, and biomechanical analysis combined with medical history are coupled with machine learning models, the precise prediction of injury risk and optimization of rehabilitation programs are possible. With technology advancement and the ease of access to data collection, AI in sports science will combine more and more to enhance the care for the athlete, thus making it possible to detect early stages of injuries and further making recovery faster (Claudino et al., 2019).

## CHALLENGES AND LIMITATIONS OF MACHINE LEARNING IN SPORTS INJURY

While ML has a potential to revolutionize injury prevention and rehabilitation in sports, many obstacles and limitations have made its application difficult. The list of issues relates from technical problems in data quality to algorithmic complexity, ethical considerations, and the practical application of this in real-life sports settings. It is these challenges that must be addressed if ML is to be fully exploited for applications related to the management of athletic performance and mitigation of injury.

1. Data Quality and Availability

The availability and quality of data can be perhaps one of the most strenuous challenges when trying to create an efficient ML model that should be aimed at preventing injuries in sports. Large datasets are important for the identification of patterns, trends, and predictive markers by the models. However, this is, more often than not, problematic because it requires enough data on how high-quality data in such relative areas as the sports sector is regarded as very difficult to get (Ekegren et al., 2016).

- Data Scarcity in Certain Sports or Levels: Elite athletes or professional teams may possess the latest wearable devices and large-scale performance monitoring systems, whereas for lower-tier athletes, amateur leagues, or youth sports programs, such technologies are rarely found. This reduces data collection and thus the scope to expand ML models across a more extensive athletic population. In some of the less popular sports, structures for data collection even do not exist, leading to scarcity in the data.
- Inconsistency in data collection: Even though data is available, such data can be collected inconsistently. For example, the method of gathering data could be different: wearable devices, manual logging, or tracking performances. Again, athletes tend to change from one brand or type of a device that has its methods of recording and presenting data. This may create issues with standardization so that the models rely on them.
- Noisy or Erroneous Data: Wearables, motion sensors, and GPS systems read data that can be noisy or erroneous due to exogenous sources like poorly placed sensors, interference, or faulty equipment. Noisy data might lead to wrong predictions or models that are not reliable. Filtering, cleaning, and other preprocessing methods can help improve these shortcomings. However, these methods are very computationally resource intensive with a huge amount of expert supervision involved.

2. Complexity and Interpretability of the Algorithm

Machine learning models, particularly those using deep learning algorithms, are essentially "black boxes." Users - be they coaches, doctors, or elite athletes - cannot understand how or even why a given prediction was made by the model. Of course, this lack of transparency presents such a massive limitation in practical sports contexts, where good, actionable insights often have to be available for decision-making.

- Interpretability Challenges: Many of the ML models, especially those based on deep learning, have been highly complicated with complex layers of neural networks designed to process large volumetric amounts of data. Such models may provide accurate answers but are hard to interpret. A system that makes vague recommendations with little explanation for its predictions may prove untrustworthy to the coach or athletic trainer. They are unlikely to make choices on such models if they cannot understand the rationale behind the developed model, especially when the careers and health of the athletes depend on the game.
- Generalizability: Models developed from machine learning, having been trained on specific populations, for example, a specific professional football team, may lack generalizability to other populations, for example, youth athletes, players from other sports, or levels. This is because the training data reflects the very characteristic characteristics of the initial population, making it less applicable to others. Thus, inferences made on models trained on one dataset may be inappropriate or misleading if applied outside that context.
- Overfitting vs. Underfitting: Machine learning models are prone to overfitting in the way that they become too specific to the training data, unable to generalize well with new, unseen inputs. It happens when noise or irrelevant patterns are memorized by the model, and the poor generalization follows this. Underfitting happens when the model is oversimplified and fails to exploit the underlying complexity of the data in pursuit of good predictive performance. Normally, it is a common challenge to manage these two extremes in sports injury prediction.

3. Ethical and Privacy Concerns

The use of machine learning models in sports depends heavily on sensitive data, such as personal health information, biometric data, and psychological assessment (Jenkins & Evans, 2020). Such collection, storage, and use of the data may raise significant ethical and privacy concerns.

- Data Privacy: The health data of athletes contains very intimate details like injuries, rehabilitation, and performance metrics. Lack of proper management over this sort of data might lead to privacy breaches or access without a proper account or misuse. Sports organizations have to adhere to tight regulations on information protection, such as Europe's General Data Protection Regulation or the Health Insurance Portability and Accountability Act in the United States. It's an art to let the models stay useful to a sport organization while staying within legal confines.
- Consent and Ownership: A relatively major ethical issue lies in the informed consent of athletes with respect to the collection and use of their information. The athletes must be well made aware of the intended purposes and scopes of use of their data, if the data is to be shared with third parties, and who owns the data. In some cases, athletes may be forced to hand over their data for the good of the team, though they are not comfortable about exposure of personal information. Ensuring ownership rights and abilities regarding control over their respective data on the part of the athletes is an essential requirement for ethical implementation.
- Bias and fairness: Machine learning models are only as good as the training data from which they are developed. Data containing biases—be it through overrepresentation of certain demographics, such as elite male athletes, or lack of representation of others, such as female athletes or athletes from particular minority groups—may lead to the generation of skewed or unfair predictions of injury. Such outcomes may further increase the inequality involved in injury prevention efforts and rehabilitation recommendations for particular athletes.

4. Application in Sports Environment

Even though the machine learning models are of good strength, there is a challenge involved with bringing the predictions and insights into real-world sports contexts. The athletes, coaches, and medical professionals have to integrate ML-based recommendations into daily training protocols, medical treatment protocols, and performance assessments (Wang & Gao, 2021).

- Adoption and Trust: The sport industry has always been experience-based, intuitive, and based on human judgment. Introducing machine learning tools to this ecosystem establishes a cultural shift, wherein coaches and athletes put their trust in data-driven insights over instinct or past experiences. The biggest challenge is making the stakeholders to accept the ML tools and embracing them in their daily practice. For instance, a coach might be hesitant to change an effective training program simply because of what an ML model predicts if it goes against their established coaching philosophy.

- Integration with Existing Systems Most sports teams and physicians rely on existing software systems for tracking athletes' performance, handling injuries, or creating training programs. More technically challenging, and resource demanding, to integrate ML models into existing systems. Moreover, athlete education staff might have to be trained on the use of new ML-based tools, which again postpone the use of such a system.
- Cost and Resource Constraints: The design of machine learning solutions is expensive; it requires huge investment in high-quality collection of data technology, for example, wearables and motion sensors, cloud computing resources meant for model training, and hiring data scientists. Smaller sports organizations, amateur athletes, or teams participating in less commercially viable sport might have these charges too high to gain access to sophisticated injury prediction models.

5. Dynamic and Unpredictable Nature of Sports

Sports is, per se, dynamic in many unpredictable aspects: an athlete may suffer injuries at any time and his/her performance could change at any particular point in time, depending on a number of other hidden factors. The same can be said for machine learning models: despite their great power, they are not always able to capture all variables in an environment as competitive as sports.

- Unpredictable Events: Being a contact sport, events such as collisions or falls are common causes of injuries in football or rugby. The unpredictable nature of such events makes it challenging for the models to be very accurate. ML models have a chance of forecasting chronic overuse injuries or biomechanical issues but are relatively poor at anticipating acute injuries caused by an external force (Halilaj et al., 2018). That sets back the overall power of ML to predict these types of sports injuries.
- Changing Athletic Condition: The physical and psychological conditions of athletes do not remain static; they change with the progression of the season. They are affected by various factors like stress, fatigue, recovery, and other extraneous pressures. If the machine learning models trained upon a static dataset fail to adapt and learn to this constantly changing condition without updating themselves continuously with new data, a model might fail to predict outcomes. However, frequent updates demand greater availability of computative resources and data.

Similar to any other highly scientifically exciting area, machine learning came fraught with several challenges. Issues of quality of input data, complexity in algorithms, privacy concerns, and problems of practical implementation were recognized as encumbrances to the widespread application of machine learning in athletic settings. Achieving a balance among the contending forces of competing individuals-data scientists, sports professionals, ethicists, and technology developers-will be necessary. As the technology matures and more advanced solutions are developed, machine learning could become an indispensable tool in keeping athletes healthy, improving performance, and extending careers.

## FUTURE TRENDS AND INNOVATIONS

The application of machine learning (ML) in sports injury prevention and rehabilitation is still in its infancy, but as the technology and research advance, several emerging trends and innovations are likely to shape this field. It will bring more accuracy and individuality to injury prediction models on machine learning because they hold the promise to revolutionize injury prevention in athletic performance optimization (Ayala et al., 2019). This section has discussed some of the most important trends and innovations that will influence the use of machine learning in sports injury prevention and rehabilitation.

1. Integration of Wearable Technology and IoT

Wearable devices and the Internet of Things (IoT) are likely to play crucial roles in future systems related to sports injury prevention and rehabilitation. Such technologies will allow for continuous, real-time collection of data that wearable devices and more advanced IoT applications can generate. Most such wearable devices have evolved over time, and most have become increasingly sophisticated, offering detailed metrics on athletes' biomechanics, physiological responses, and external factors such as environmental conditions. With the insights of machine learning models, wearable devices can indeed improve the accuracy of injury predictions and enable more immediate interventions aimed at preventing the recurrence of injury.

- Real-time monitoring and feedback: Advanced wearables can continually monitor aspects of an athlete's heart rate, muscle activation, joint movements, and stress levels. In this respect, real-time data can be fed into ML models, so dynamic adjustments to predictions can be made as a condition within a training session or game changes over time (Beck et al., 2018). For example, if an athlete is exhibiting early onset fatigue or abnormalities in the movement pattern, direct signals can be sent to coaches or medical staff so that they can intervene before injuries might occur.

- Personalized data insights: Wearable technologies are also becoming extremely popular, where athlete personal data are gathered in very large amounts over time. The available data can then be fed into a machine learning model that is tailored for the individual athlete, hence amplifying predictions and helping in developing appropriate, personalized injury prevention strategies. Increasingly, people are investing in wearables, which may democratize access to ML-driven insights and offer a chance to amateur athletes to tap into the power of the technology.

Advanced Sensor Modalities: Future wearables will be equipped with more advanced sensor modalities that can capture granular biomechanical data, such as the force applied on the joints, the strains on the muscles, and movement asymmetry. These machine learning models can predict the general risks of injuries but also specific ones, like ligament tears, stress fractures, or muscle strains.

2. AI-Driven Rehabilitation Platforms

The second major trend under sports medicine is AI-powered rehabilitation platforms. These kinds of platforms use the mechanism of machine learning algorithms to formulate customized rehabilitation programs customized around the current needs of the injured athlete. Since AI systems are constantly learning from the progress of the athlete, this can adapt rehabilitation protocols in real time to ensure faster and more effective recovery.

- Virtual and Augmented Reality in Rehabilitation: Promising innovation in this space is using virtual reality and augmented reality for rehabilitation. This can be integrated with machine learning to develop immersive rehabilitation environments where the athlete exercises in simulations that mimic the sport. ML models can evaluate the movement of the athlete in real time and give immediate feedback regarding form and effort, that may be crucial when the athlete is recovering and likely needs to avoid re-injury. Virtual reality-based rehabilitation can even address motivational and adherence issues due to the treatment being entertaining and interactiv.
- Adaptive Rehabilitation Programs: AI can adapt and change rehabilitation programs based on the changing status of the athlete (Howard, 2017). For example, using wearable devices or physiotherapy equipment, machine learning algorithms can track progress and adjust rehabilitation to how well one responds. Hence, it reduces the probability of overtraining during rehabilita-

tion while still facilitating that the athlete starts regaining strength, flexibility, and function step by step.

- Prognostic Maintenance Against Injury Re-occurrence: AI systems can aid in recovery and also prevent injury in the long run by predicting the chances of getting re-injured by an athlete. The machine learning algorithm may keep track of any patterns of recovery and identify weaknesses that had been present previously in the injured areas, and thus ensure these weak areas are targeted with additional training or therapy so that athletes do not face setbacks the next time.

3. Multimodal Data Integration Boosts Predictions

The future innovation that machine learning could apply in terms of prevention for injuries in sports would be the inclusion of multimodal data sources to increase the efficacy of the prediction (Lahat et al., 2015). While today's ML models depend solely on a narrow spectrum of data-mostly biomechanic metrics or performance statistics-newer systems will integrate a more significant array of data types, including physiological, psychological, and environmental information.

- Incorporation of Psychological and Cognitive Data: Stress, motivation, and fatigue have been shown to contribute considerably to injury risk. In the future, the implementation of more precise ML models may be driven to include data from psychological assessments or cognitive performance tests in order to deliver a more holistic injury risk profile. Such an outcome will result in a better, more all-rounded understanding of the athlete's state, the prediction of injuries due to psychological and emotional causes, such as burnout and related decision-making under pressure.
- Environmental and Contextual Data: This may also improve the injury prediction model by including environmental data, such as weather, playing surface, and competition schedule. For instance, most are aware of the fact that some injuries, like ankle sprains or muscle strains, are related to playing on wet or uneven surfaces. Further, these data would provide contextual information to the machine learning models that can make a better-predicted decision about the external contribution factors to risk injury.
- Concatenative medical imaging and genomic data. This is one other exciting innovation, perhaps a form of concatenated medical imaging, say MRI or ultrasound scans, with the genomic data on machine learning models. Those complex datasets enable AI systems to digest and identify patterns, seemingly initially, in susceptibility toward particular injuries, such as ligament damage or muscle tears. In particular, genomic data can predict the athlete's

predispositions toward certain kinds of injuries and thereby enable very specific and highly personalized injury prevention plans (Finch, 2006).

4. Federated Learning and Privacy-Preserving AI

With heightened concern for issues of privacy, which particularly relates to the health of an athlete, there is a way out of this problem through federated learning. Federated learning is an innovative machine learning model in which models are trained across multiple decentralized devices or servers without the sharing of raw data. Expect this trend in the sports industry, requiring that data privacy be preserved.

- Decentralized data processing: Federated learning allows a machine learning model to be trained using the data of hundreds or thousands of athletes or teams without breaching individual privacy. Data stays on local devices like wearables, and updates on the model are transferred to a central server. This approach protects sensitive health and performance data while still contributing to building accurate and robust injury prediction models.
- Increased Data Security: As federated learning becomes more widely used in sports among athletes and teams, concerns about data security would be lesser hurdles in implementing machine learning. This will allow a much greater possibility of working together at the collective sports organization levels, covering much larger datasets and potentially more generalizable injury models that would not have any issue related to breach of data privacy rules.

5. Explainable AI (XAI) for Best Decision Making

This is also one of the challenges for the current use of ML in injury prediction because most ML models are considered "black boxes," that is, not easily conveying what the machine has done to predict something. Explainable AI, or XAI, represents a trend considered emergent to overcome this limitation by making machine learning models more transparent and interpretable. To sporting professionals, who should then rely upon and act upon such insights, the efficacy of these systems will be paramount.

- Transparency in Injury Predictions: With XAI approaches, coaches, medical staff, and athletes will be able to understand the reasons that led the model to make predictions about injuries. The system may clarify that an athlete's recent increase in training intensity coupled with biomechanical indicators made the athlete more prone to experiencing a muscle strain. Enhanced transparency by the AI-driven injury prevention models will increase the trust placed in such models and allow for better-informed decisions made by human experts.

- Actionable and Replicable Insights: Explainable AI models can also provide insights that are easier to act on. For example, a system for XAI might be programmed to advice concrete adjustments that an athlete ought to make to the training schedule in order to avoid injury, based on what the AI has understood as the causes of risk. This will allow injury prevention by ML-driven mechanisms to not only be increasingly accurate but also practical and actionable in the real world.

6. AI-Driven Coaching and Optimization for Performance

By the near future, apart from injury prevention and rehabilitation, machine learning will be there to help in general optimization of performance. Using data analytics both from training loads, biomechanics, and physical outputs, the AI-driven system will guide coaches to provide optimal, individualized training plans aimed at maximizing performance with minimized injury risk.

- Performance prediction models: Advanced ML models will predict both the risk of injury as well as performance outcomes based on current training regimes of athletes. Coaches will thus be able to fine-tune training plans designed to improve performance while balancing workloads to avoid over-training and potential injury.
- Wearables and AI to change the game of coaching tools: Coaches' tools may soon include wearables and AI systems that can understand machine learning algorithms, as well as offer on-time feedback on athletes' techniques, efficiency, and movement in real time and give performance metrics (Seng et al., 2023). This will make coaches adjust the training and thus introduce an evolving, data-informed approach to the holistic growth of athletes.

The Future for Injury Prevention and Rehabilitation is Bright with Machine Learning as the Leading Edge. From wearable technology and multiple multimodal data sources to the emergent rise of federated learning and explainable AI, innovations on the horizon promise that injure risk prediction can be more accurate, more personal, and perhaps more accessible. Expected outcomes include optimizations in rehabilitation processes, reduced injury risks, and improvements to overall athletic performance. Further development of machine learning will face a very significant transformation in the world of sports to ensure that the athletes are at their best and try to reduce the risks involved with their strenuous physical activities.

## CONCLUSION

The integration of machine learning into the sport sector especially concerning the prevention and rehabilitation of injuries proves to be important and forms part of integral developments in the medical field of sports. Machine learning models would enable new opportunities for injury prediction and recovery process optimization with the data support of wearables, performance metrics, and medical records. The good news here is that AI-based intervention would deliver more accurate, personalized interventions that help to prevent injuries even before they occur and recover them effectively after it occurs. Indeed, even with such exciting potential in the development, challenges abound-from data privacy issues to complexity in building reliable models and calls for more transparency in AI-driven decision-making. As technology continues to change, innovations like federated learning, explainable AI, and multimodal enhanced integration will better address such hurdles as well as pave the way for wide-scale adoption of AI into sports. Finally, machine learning could potentially revolutionize not only how injuries are managed but also how performance in athletics is optimized to produce healthier, more resilient athletes with more sustainable sports careers.

## REFERENCES


Ayala, F., López-Valenciano, A., Martín, J. A. G., Croix, M. D. S., Vera-Garcia, F. J., del Pilar Garcia-Vaquero, M., & Myer, G. D. (2019). A preventive model for hamstring injuries in professional soccer: Learning algorithms. *International Journal of Sports Medicine, 40*(05), 344–353. DOI: 10.1055/a-0826-1955 PMID: 30873572

Bahr, R., & Holme, I. (2003). Risk factors for sports injuries—A methodological approach. *British Journal of Sports Medicine, 37*(5), 384–392. DOI: 10.1136/bjsm.37.5.384 PMID: 14514527

Bahr, R., & Krosshaug, T. (2005). Understanding injury mechanisms: A key component of preventing injuries in sport. *British Journal of Sports Medicine, 39*(6), 324–329. DOI: 10.1136/bjsm.2005.018341 PMID: 15911600

Beck, P. J., Mohammadi-Aragh, M. J., Archibald, C., Jones, B. A., & Barton, A. (2018, October). Real-time metacognition feedback for introductory programming using machine learning. In *2018 IEEE Frontiers in Education Conference (FIE)* (pp. 1-5). IEEE. DOI: 10.1109/FIE.2018.8658973

Bittencourt, N. F., Meeuwisse, W. H., Mendonça, L. D., Nettel-Aguirre, A., Ocarino, J. M., & Fonseca, S. T. (2016). Complex systems approach for sports injuries: Moving from risk factor identification to injury pattern recognition—narrative review and new concept. *British Journal of Sports Medicine, 50*(21), 1309–1314. DOI: 10.1136/bjsports-2015-095850 PMID: 27445362

Claudino, J. G., Capanema, D. D. O., de Souza, T. V., Serrão, J. C., Machado Pereira, A. C., & Nassis, G. P. (2019). Current approaches to the use of artificial intelligence for injury risk assessment and performance prediction in team sports: A systematic review. *Sports Medicine - Open, 5*(1), 1–12. DOI: 10.1186/s40798-019-0202-3 PMID: 31270636

Cust, E. E., Sweeting, A. J., Ball, K., & Robertson, S. (2019). Machine and deep learning for sport-specific movement recognition: A systematic review of model development and performance. *Journal of Sports Sciences, 37*(5), 568–600. DOI: 10.1080/02640414.2018.1521769 PMID: 30307362

Ekegren, C. L., Gabbe, B. J., & Finch, C. F. (2016). Sports injury surveillance systems: A review of methods and data quality. *Sports Medicine (Auckland, N.Z.), 46*(1), 49–65. DOI: 10.1007/s40279-015-0410-z PMID: 26423419

Finch, C. (2006). A new framework for research leading to sports injury prevention. *Journal of Science and Medicine in Sport, 9*(1-2), 3–9. DOI: 10.1016/j.jsams.2006.02.009 PMID: 16616614

Guelmami, N., Fekih-Romdhane, F., Mechraoui, O., & Bragazzi, N. L. (2023). Injury Prevention, Optimized Training and Rehabilitation: How Is AI Reshaping the Field of Sports Medicine. *New Asian Journal of Medicine*, *1*(1), 30–34. DOI: 10.61186/najm.1.1.30

Halilaj, E., Rajagopal, A., Fiterau, M., Hicks, J. L., Hastie, T. J., & Delp, S. L. (2018). Machine learning in human movement biomechanics: Best practices, common pitfalls, and new opportunities. *Journal of Biomechanics*, *81*, 1–11. DOI: 10.1016/j.jbiomech.2018.09.009 PMID: 30279002

Howard, M. C. (2017). A meta-analysis and systematic literature review of virtual reality rehabilitation programs. *Computers in Human Behavior*, *70*, 317–327. DOI: 10.1016/j.chb.2017.01.013

Jenkins, S., & Evans, N. (2020, April). Cybersecurity impact of the growth of data in sports. In *Cyber Sensing 2020* (Vol. 11417, pp. 84–100). SPIE. DOI: 10.1117/12.2557898

Kononenko, I. (2001). Machine learning for medical diagnosis: History, state of the art and perspective. *Artificial Intelligence in Medicine*, *23*(1), 89–109. DOI: 10.1016/S0933-3657(01)00077-X PMID: 11470218

Lahat, D., Adali, T., & Jutten, C. (2015). Multimodal data fusion: An overview of methods, challenges, and prospects. *Proceedings of the IEEE*, *103*(9), 1449–1477. DOI: 10.1109/JPROC.2015.2460697

McCall, A., Dupont, G., & Ekstrand, J. (2016). Injury prevention strategies, coach compliance and player adherence of 33 of the UEFA Elite Club Injury Study teams: A survey of teams' head medical officers. *British Journal of Sports Medicine*, *50*(12), 725–730. DOI: 10.1136/bjsports-2015-095259 PMID: 26795611

Mishra, N., Habal, B. G. M., Garcia, P. S., & Garcia, M. B. (2024, June). Harnessing an AI-Driven Analytics Model to Optimize Training and Treatment in Physical Education for Sports Injury Prevention. In *Proceedings of the 2024 8th International Conference on Education and Multimedia Technology* (pp. 309-315). DOI: 10.1145/3678726.3678740

Rossi, A., Pappalardo, L., Cintia, P., Iaia, F. M., Fernández, J., & Medina, D. (2018). Effective injury forecasting in soccer with GPS training data and machine learning. *PLoS One*, *13*(7), e0201264. DOI: 10.1371/journal.pone.0201264 PMID: 30044858

Seng, K. P., Ang, L. M., Peter, E., & Mmonyi, A. (2023). Machine learning and AI technologies for smart wearables. *Electronics (Basel)*, *12*(7), 1509. DOI: 10.3390/electronics12071509

Seshadri, D. R., Li, R. T., Voos, J. E., Rowbottom, J. R., Alfes, C. M., Zorman, C. A., & Drummond, C. K. (2019). Wearable sensors for monitoring the internal and external workload of the athlete. *NPJ Digital Medicine*, *2*(1), 71. DOI: 10.1038/s41746-019-0149-2 PMID: 31372506

Wang, Z., & Gao, Z. (2021). Analysis of real-time heartbeat monitoring using wearable device Internet of Things system in sports environment. *Computational Intelligence*, *37*(3), 1080–1097. DOI: 10.1111/coin.12337

# Chapter 8
# A Machine Learning Approach to Playing-11 Prediction in Competitive Cricket

**Padmaja Kadiri**
https://orcid.org/0000-0002-6550-0319
*Mohan Babu University, Tirupati, India*

**Manne Nikita**
*CVR College of Engineering, India*

**Palagati Anusha**
https://orcid.org/0009-0008-7875-5100
*Guru Nanak Institute of Technology, India*

**Kuraganti Santhi**
*Koneru Lakshmaiah Education Foundation, India*

## ABSTRACT

*In cricket, choosing the best team (Playing-11) is crucial. Cricket, as a sport, has witnessed a notable shift towards data-driven decision-making in recent years. We look at past players performance to understand how teams can predict their ideal players. This survey explores various data sources, tools, and techniques used in cricket analytics, offering insights into the broader landscape of data-driven decision-making and also shows the concept how data science and machine learning are changing the game. Serving as a guide for players, coaches, and fans, this paper provides a user-friendly exploration of the ways in which data science is reshaping*

DOI: 10.4018/979-8-3693-5385-1.ch008

*cricket strategies and enhancing the precision of team selection. It's like a playbook for understanding how technology is making cricket team decisions smarter.*

## I. INTRODUCTION

Cricket, a sport cherished by millions, boasts a vast and devoted following, making it one of the most popular and widely embraced games globally. With an estimated fan base of over 2.5 billion enthusiasts worldwide, cricket has transcended geographical boundaries, cultural divides, and linguistic differences, capturing the hearts and minds of people across continents. The fervor for cricket extends far beyond the traditional strongholds in nations like India, England, Australia, Pakistan, and the West Indies. Its ever-expanding popularity can be witnessed across diverse regions, including but not limited to South Asia, the Caribbean, parts of Africa, the United Kingdom, and even pockets of Europe and the Americas.

Moreover, with the advent of digital platforms and social media, the global cricketing community has grown exponentially. Online engagement, fan forums, streaming platforms, and cricket-centric social channels have amplified the sport's reach, connecting enthusiasts worldwide, contributing significantly to the sport's soaring popularity. The sheer magnitude of cricket's fan base, comprising a diverse and dedicated cohort of followers, underscores the sport's universal appeal and its position as a cultural phenomenon that continues to captivate a sizable portion of the world's population. As cricket strides into the future, the digital era continues to play a pivotal role in further amplifying its global footprint, fostering a vibrant community of passionate fans who live and breathe the sport.

The advent of technology, data analytics, and machine learning has ushered in a new era, transforming the way teams are selected and strategies devised. This conference paper navigates the intersection of cricket and cutting-edge technology, specifically focusing on the predictive modeling of playing XIs using data science and machine learning. Cricket, with its diverse formats such as Test matches, One Day Internationals (ODIs), and the electrifying Twenty20 (T20) format, presents a complex and dynamic challenge for team selection. The intricate interplay between batsmen, bowlers, all-rounders, and ever-changing game conditions demands a nuanced and data-driven approach.

## II.PROBLEM STATEMENT

The primary objective of this research is to identify and select the best eleven cricketers from around the globe, specifically tailored for the fast-paced and dynamic T20 cricket format. This endeavor involves not only recognizing players who can consistently perform at a high level but also understanding and quantifying the diverse skill sets required in T20 cricket. The chosen players should demonstrate the ability to maintain a high batting standard, as evidenced by achieving an average score of at least 180 runs. Concurrently, their proficiency in the field should enable them to defend a target of 150 runs with reliability. Utilizing advanced data science and machine learning techniques, this study aims to analyze various performance metrics, player statistics, and situational data to systematically approach this complex selection process. The goal is to develop a predictive model that transcends traditional selection methods, integrating data-driven insights to formulate a robust and competitive playing-11 that can adapt to the evolving demands of T20 cricket.

1. The Evolution of Team Selection in Cricket:

The art of assembling a cricket team has undergone a profound transformation over the years. Historically rooted in intuition and tradition, the process of selecting a cricket team has evolved into a sophisticated, data-driven practice, leveraging the advancements in data science and machine learning.

1.1. **Early Days: Intuition and Experience:** Initially, cricket team selection was heavily based on selectors' intuition and personal experience. Choices were made by observing players' skills and performances, with a strong reliance on gut feeling and less on statistical evidence.
1.2. **Introduction of Basic Statistics:** Gradually, basic statistics like batting and bowling averages started to play a role in team selection. These provided a more objective way to assess player performance, though they were limited in capturing the full spectrum of a player's abilities and match situations.
1.3. **Advanced Statistical Analysis:** With advancements in technology, more sophisticated statistical analyses began to be used. This included complex metrics and opponent analysis, offering deeper insights into player performances and potential team dynamics.
1.4. **Data Science and Machine Learning:** The most recent and transformative shift has been the adoption of data science and machine learning. These technologies allow for the analysis of extensive and diverse data sets, providing predictive models and insights that far exceed traditional statistical methods.

1.5. **Modern Cricket's Transformation:** This evolution has significantly impacted modern cricket. Teams now utilize comprehensive data analyses and predictive modeling in their selection process, enhancing both the objectivity and adaptability of their strategies for various cricket formats.

2. Understanding Data Science and Machine Learning:

Data science and machine learning have emerged as pivotal elements in various sectors, cricket analytics being one. They are capable of sifting through extensive datasets to unearth significant patterns and intelligence. In cricket, these technologies revolutionize the way player performance is analyzed, outcomes are predicted, and team strategies are developed.

## 2.1. Data Science in Cricket

Data science is the practice of applying analytical techniques, algorithmic processes, and systems to glean insights and knowledge from both organized and unstructured data sources. In the cricketing world, it translates to dissecting scores, individual player stats, playing conditions, and historical data to formulate well-informed decisions. Tools in data science facilitate the management, processing, and visualization of cricket data, rendering it interpretable for strategic analysis.

## 2.2. Machine Learning: A Subset of Data Science

Machine learning, a branch within data science, involves training computational models to identify patterns and make informed predictions or decisions based on available data. Unlike conventional statistical approaches, machine learning can handle extensive, intricate datasets, identifying underlying patterns and connections.

# III.DATA COLLECTION AND PREPARATION

The process of assembling the necessary data for predicting the optimal playing-11 in cricket begins with an efficient data collection strategy. BrightData emerges as a powerful tool in this regard, facilitating web scraping from comprehensive sports analytics websites like ESPN Sports. By leveraging BrightData's web scraping capabilities, researchers can automate the extraction of detailed cricket data, including player statistics, match details, venue information, at the time of each game. The data is often extracted in a structured format, such as JSON, which is conducive to further analysis and processing.

Data Preparation:

This phase is crucial for transforming the raw, scraped data into a clean, structured format suitable for machine learning models. Jupyter Notebook, an open-source web application, allows for interactive computing and data manipulation.

- **Cleaning Data:** This includes handling missing values, removing duplicates, and standardizing the data format. Given the raw data scraped in JSON format, cleaning ensures that the dataset is accurate and reliable for analysis.
- **Data Transformation:** Converting the JSON formatted data into a more analysis-friendly format like a Pandas DataFrame. This transformation facilitates easier data manipulation and analysis.
- **Exporting Prepared Data:** Once the data is cleaned and structured, it is exported from the Jupyter Notebook environment to a CSV file. This file format is widely used and compatible with most data analysis tools and machine learning platforms, making it ideal for further processing and model training.

*Table 1. Match Summary*

| 1 | team1 | team2 | winner | margin | ground | matchDate | match_id |
|---|---|---|---|---|---|---|---|
| 2 | England | Pakistan | England | 5 wickets | Melbourne | 13-Nov-22 | T20I # 1879 |
| 3 | England | India | England | 10 wickets | Adelaide | 10-Nov-22 | T20I # 1878 |
| 4 | New Zealand | Pakistan | Pakistan | 7 wickets | Sydney | 9-Nov-22 | T20I # 1877 |
| 5 | India | Zimbabwe | India | 71 runs | Melbourne | 6-Nov-22 | T20I # 1873 |
| 6 | Bangladesh | Pakistan | Pakistan | 5 wickets | Adelaide | 6-Nov-22 | T20I # 1872 |
| 7 | Netherlands | South Africa | Netherlands | 13 runs | Adelaide | 6-Nov-22 | T20I # 1871 |
| 8 | England | Sri Lanka | England | 4 wickets | Sydney | 5-Nov-22 | T20I # 1867 |
| 9 | Australia | Afghanistan | Australia | 4 runs | Adelaide | 4-Nov-22 | T20I # 1864 |
| 10 | Ireland | New Zealand | New Zealand | 35 runs | Adelaide | 4-Nov-22 | T20I # 1862 |
| 11 | Pakistan | South Africa | Pakistan | 33 runs | Sydney | 3-Nov-22 | T20I # 1861 |

Table 1 is the sample Match Summary dataset exported from the JSON file after data processing using Jyputer Notebook using pandas. The attributes in this table includes: team1, team2, winner, margin, ground, matchDate and match_id. These attributes describes about the full match summary and gives meaningful information about the complete match.

*Table 2. Batting Summary*

| | match | teamInnings | battingPos | batsmanName | runs | balls | 4s | 6s | SR | out/not_out | match_id |
|---|---|---|---|---|---|---|---|---|---|---|---|
| 2 | Sri Lanka Vs Australia | Sri Lanka | 1 | Pathum Nissanka | 40 | 45 | 2 | 0 | 88.88 | out | T20I # 1845 |
| 3 | Sri Lanka Vs Australia | Sri Lanka | 2 | Kusal Mendis | 5 | 6 | 1 | 0 | 83.33 | out | T20I # 1845 |
| 4 | Sri Lanka Vs Australia | Sri Lanka | 3 | Dhananjayade Silva | 26 | 23 | 3 | 0 | 113.04 | out | T20I # 1845 |
| 5 | Sri Lanka Vs Australia | Sri Lanka | 4 | Charith Asalanka | 38 | 25 | 3 | 2 | 152 | not_out | T20I # 1845 |
| 6 | Sri Lanka Vs Australia | Sri Lanka | 5 | Bhanuka Rajapaksa | 7 | 5 | 1 | 0 | 140 | out | T20I # 1845 |
| 7 | Sri Lanka Vs Australia | Sri Lanka | 6 | Dasun Shanaka (c) | 3 | 5 | 0 | 0 | 60 | out | T20I # 1845 |
| 8 | Sri Lanka Vs Australia | Sri Lanka | 7 | Wanindu Hasaranga | 1 | 4 | 0 | 0 | 25 | out | T20I # 1845 |
| 9 | Sri Lanka Vs Australia | Sri Lanka | 8 | Chamika Karunaratne | 14 | 7 | 2 | 0 | 200 | not_out | T20I # 1845 |
| 10 | Sri Lanka Vs Australia | Australia | 1 | David Warner | 11 | 10 | 0 | 0 | 110 | out | T20I # 1845 |

Table 2 is the sample batting summary dataset obtained from data pre-processing. The attributes in this table shows the batting details of a player including total runs, balls faced, no. of fours and sixes, strike rate, out and match_id. These attributes help to analyze the players performance and also contributes in building stats.

*Table 3. Bowling Summary*

| | match | bowlingTeam | bowlerName | overs | maiden | runs | wickets | economy | 0s | 4s | 6s | wides | noBalls | match_id |
|---|---|---|---|---|---|---|---|---|---|---|---|---|---|---|
| 2 | India Vs Zimbabwe | Zimbabwe | Richard Ngarava | 4 | 1 | 44 | 1 | 11 | 12 | 2 | 4 | 1 | 1 | T20I # 1873 |
| 3 | India Vs Zimbabwe | Zimbabwe | Tendai Chatara | 4 | 0 | 34 | 0 | 8.5 | 5 | 3 | 1 | 0 | 0 | T20I # 1873 |
| 4 | India Vs Zimbabwe | Zimbabwe | Blessing Muzarabani | 4 | 0 | 50 | 1 | 12.5 | 5 | 8 | 0 | 1 | 0 | T20I # 1873 |
| 5 | India Vs Zimbabwe | Zimbabwe | Wellington Masakadza | 2 | 0 | 12 | 0 | 6 | 5 | 1 | 0 | 1 | 0 | T20I # 1873 |
| 6 | India Vs Zimbabwe | Zimbabwe | Ryan Burl | 1 | 0 | 14 | 0 | 14 | 1 | 1 | 1 | 0 | 0 | T20I # 1873 |
| 7 | India Vs Zimbabwe | Zimbabwe | Sikandar Raza | 3 | 0 | 18 | 1 | 6 | 5 | 0 | 1 | 0 | 0 | T20I # 1873 |
| 8 | India Vs Zimbabwe | Zimbabwe | Sean Williams | 2 | 0 | 9 | 2 | 4.5 | 6 | 0 | 0 | 2 | 0 | T20I # 1873 |
| 9 | India Vs Zimbabwe | India | Bhuvneshwar Kumar | 3 | 1 | 11 | 1 | 3.66 | 14 | 1 | 0 | 1 | 0 | T20I # 1873 |
| 10 | India Vs Zimbabwe | India | Arshdeep Singh | 2 | 0 | 9 | 1 | 4.5 | 9 | 1 | 0 | 2 | 0 | T20I # 1873 |

Table 3 is the sample bowling summary dataset exported from JSON file. All the attributes in this table including: overs, median, runs, fours, sixes, wides, no-balls, etc. shows the bowlers in-depth information. These attributes help to analyze the players performance and also contributes in building stats.

*Table 4. Players Info*

| | name | team | battingStyle | bowlingStyle | playingRole | description |
|---|---|---|---|---|---|---|
| 2 | Michael van Lingen | Namibia | Left hand Bat | Left arm Medium | Bowling Allrounder | |
| 3 | Divan la Cock | Namibia | Right hand Bat | Legbreak | Opening Batter | |
| 4 | Jan Nicol Loftie-Eaton | Namibia | Left hand Bat | Right arm Medium, Legbreak | Batter | |
| 5 | Stephan Baard | Namibia | Right hand Bat | Right arm Medium fast | Batter | |
| 6 | Gerhard Erasmus(c) | Namibia | Right hand Bat | Right arm Offbreak | Allrounder | |
| 7 | Jan Frylinck | Namibia | Left hand Bat | Left arm Fast medium | Allrounder | |
| 8 | David Wiese | Namibia | Right hand Bat | Right arm Medium fast | Allrounder | David Wiese joined a marked outflow of |
| 9 | JJ Smit | Namibia | Right hand Bat | Left arm Medium fast | Bowling Allrounder | |
| 10 | Pathum Nissanka | Sri Lanka | Right hand Bat | | Top order Batter | |

Table 4 is the sample players info dataset exported from the JSON file obtained during the process of web-scraping of Records in ICC Men's T20 World Cup, 2022/23. This tables contains all the players information participated in the CWC, 2022/2023, which includes both batsman as well as bowler details.

## IV.FEATURE SELECTION FOR PLAYING-11 PREDICTION

- **Batting Metrics:** These include not just the average runs scored but also the strike rate and the frequency and efficiency of boundary hitting, which are crucial in the fast-paced T20 format.
- **Bowling Metrics:** Key statistics such as a bowler's average, economy rate, and strike rate help evaluate their effectiveness in limiting opponents' scores and taking wickets.
- **Fielding Performance:** Metrics like catch success rate and contributions to run-outs offer insights into a player's defensive capabilities, are some aspects of cricket that can shift match momentum.
- **Player Fitness and Recent Form:** A player's current physical condition and performance trajectory are vital for assessing their readiness and potential impact in upcoming matches.
- **Contextual Variables:** Features accounting for a player's experience in T20 matches, historical performance at specific venues or against certain teams, and adaptability to different pitch conditions can provide a nuanced view of potential match outcomes.

*Figure 1. Batting Average*

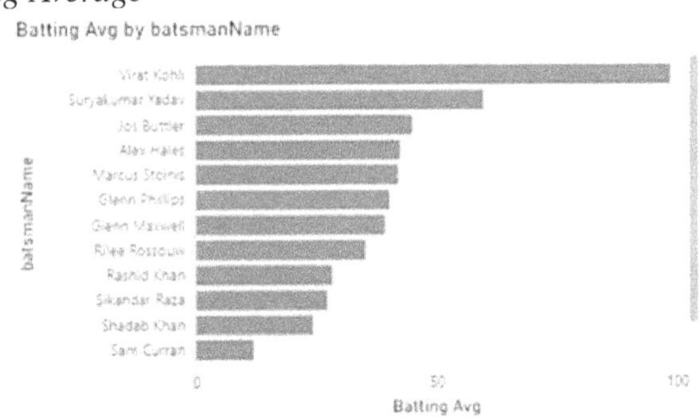

*Figure 2. Batting Position*

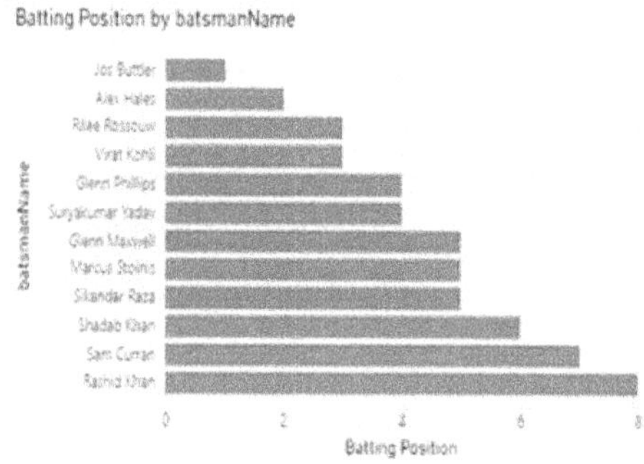


*Figure 3. Batting Strike Rate*

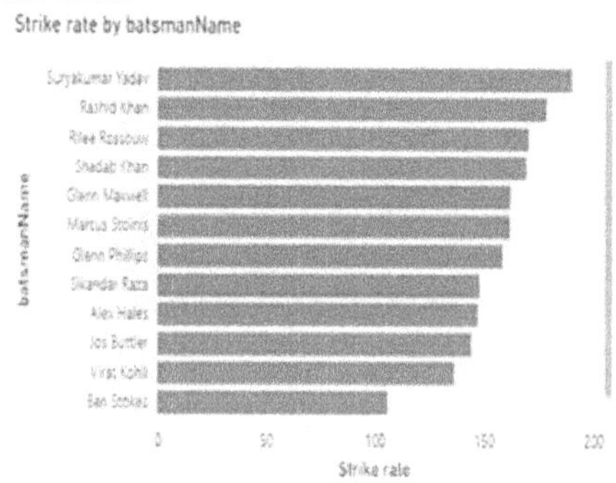


*Figure 4. Bowling Average*

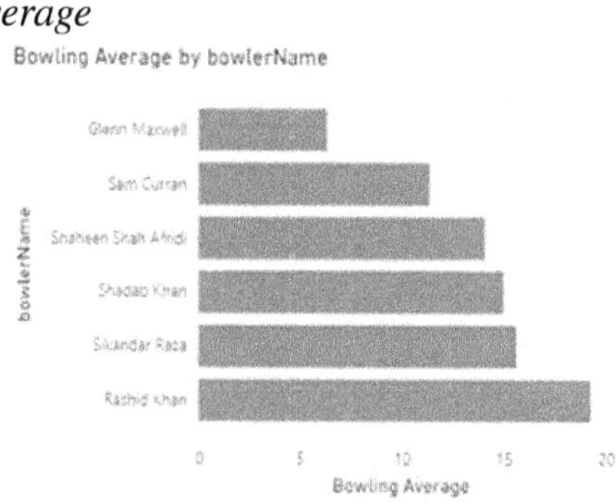

*Figure 5. Bowling Economy*

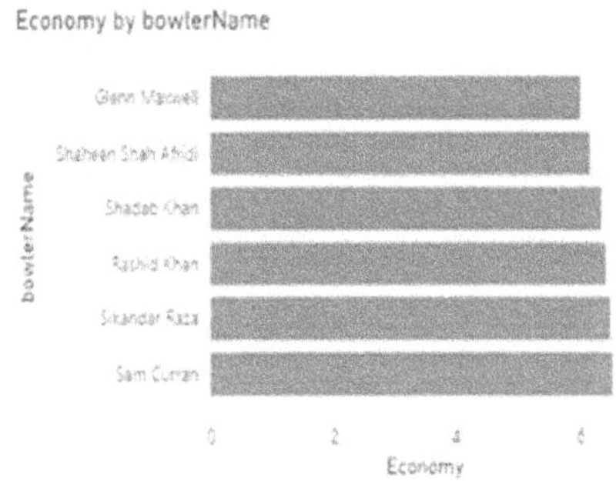


*Figure 6. Bowling Strike Rate*

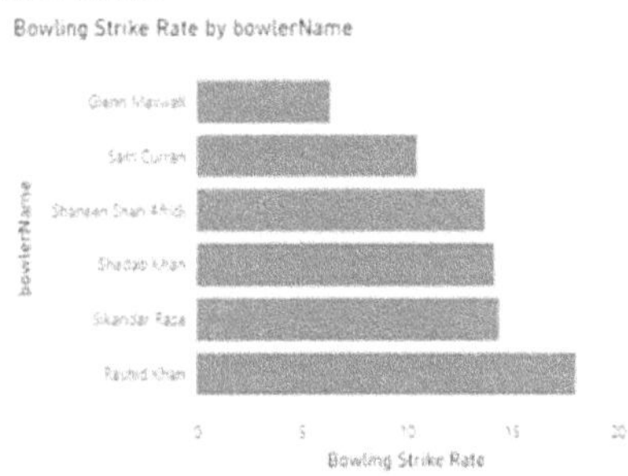


These are some of the features and metrics that are used in performance analysis which shows how much a player is consistent and also indicates the individual players stats.

*Table 5. Openers:*

| Metrics | Range |
|---|---|
| Batting Order | < 3 |
| Total innings batted | > 3 |
| Batting Avg. | > 30 |
| % of Boundary | > 50 |
| Strike Rate | > 140 |

*Table 6. Middle Order:*

| Metrics | Range |
|---|---|
| Batting Order | > 2 |
| Total innings batted | > 3 |
| Batting Avg. | > 40 |
| Avg. Balls Faced | > 20 |
| Strike Rate | > 125 |

*Table 7. Finisher:*

| Metrics | Range |
|---|---|
| Batting Order | > 4 |
| Total innings batted | > 3 |
| Batting Avg. | > 25 |
| Avg. Balls Faced | > 12 |
| Strike Rate | > 130 |
| Innings Bowled | > 1 |

*Table 8. Lower Order:*

| Metrics | Range |
|---|---|
| Batting Order | > 4 |
| Total innings batted | > 2 |
| Batting Avg. | > 15 |
| Strike Rate | > 140 |
| Innings Bowled | > 2 |
| Bowling Economy | < 7 |
| Bowling Strike Rate | < 20 |

*Table 9. Fast Bowlers:*

| Metrics | Range |
|---|---|
| Total Innings Bowled | > 4 |
| Bowling Economy | < 7 |
| Bowling Strike Rate | < 16 |
| Bowling Style | Fast |
| Bowling Average | < 20 |
| Dot Ball % | > 40 |

To set the target of 180 runs in an inning and also at the same time to defend 150 runs with the bowling lineups, these features and parameters are taken into the considerations.

*Table 10. Players Metrics*

| name | Batting Avg | Batting Position | Boundary % | Strike rate | Bowling Average | Dot ball % | Bowling Strike Rate | Economy | wickets | Total Runs |
|---|---|---|---|---|---|---|---|---|---|---|
| Anrich Nortje | 5.00 | 10.00 | 40.00 | 83.33 | 8.55 | 55.24 | 9.55 | 5.37 | 11 | 5 |
| Rashid Khan | 28.50 | 8.00 | 35.09 | 178.13 | 19.25 | 40.28 | 18.00 | 6.42 | 4 | 57 |
| Sam Curran | 12.00 | 7.00 | 25.00 | 85.71 | 11.38 | 48.53 | 10.46 | 6.53 | 13 | 12 |
| Shadab Khan | 24.50 | 6.00 | 29.59 | 168.97 | 15.00 | 37.82 | 14.18 | 6.35 | 11 | 98 |
| Glenn Maxwell | 39.33 | 5.00 | 33.90 | 161.64 | 6.33 | 42.11 | 6.33 | 6.00 | 3 | 118 |
| Marcus Stoinis | 42.00 | 5.00 | 32.54 | 161.54 | 87.00 | 14.81 | 54.00 | 9.67 | 1 | 126 |
| Sikandar Raza | 27.38 | 5.00 | 29.68 | 147.97 | 15.60 | 31.94 | 14.40 | 6.50 | 10 | 219 |
| Glenn Phillips | 40.20 | 4.00 | 30.85 | 158.27 | | | | | | 201 |
| Suryakumar Yadav | 59.75 | 4.00 | 33.05 | 189.68 | | | | | | 239 |
| Rilee Rossouw | 35.25 | 3.00 | 31.91 | 169.88 | | | | | | 141 |
| Virat Kohli | 98.67 | 3.00 | 25.00 | 136.41 | | | | | | 296 |
| Alex Hales | 42.40 | 2.00 | 32.08 | 147.22 | | | | | | 212 |
| Jos Buttler | 45.00 | 1.00 | 30.67 | 144.23 | | | | | | 225 |
| Shaheen Shah Afridi | | | | | 14.09 | 46.36 | 13.73 | 6.16 | 11 | |
| **Total** | **40.60** | **5.00** | **30.63** | **154.44** | **14.08** | **41.10** | **13.08** | **6.46** | **64** | **1949** |

Table-10 shows the players metrics which defines the players performance and their consistency of scoring runs as a batter, taking wickets as a bowler. It also gives the insights for making effective plans how to play games and who best suits at the right position.

## V.PREDICTIVE MODELING TECHNIQUES

Random Forest algorithm is the proposed technique used to predict the optimal playing-11 for T20 cricket matches. The Random Forest algorithm is a popular and versatile machine learning technique used for both classification and regression tasks. It's an ensemble learning method, which means it operates by combining multiple individual models to improve overall performance. The players_info, batting_summary, bowling_summary, and match_summary datasets are combined into a unified dataset. After preprocessing, which included handling missing values and encoding categorical variables.

Player performance metrics like batting average, strike rate, bowling economy and also all other features are considered for Feature Engineering.

## 2.3. Model Training:

The Random Forest model was trained on 70% of the data. We used a configuration of 100 trees and set the maximum depth of each tree to 10. This setup aimed to optimize the balance between learning the data patterns and avoiding overfitting.

### Model Evaluation and Error Rate Calculation

- **Splitting the Data:** We divided the dataset into training (70%) and testing (30%) sets.
- **Training the Model:** The model was trained on the training set.
- **Predictions:** We then used the trained model to make predictions on the test set.

### Error Rate Calculation:

- **Confusion Matrix:** First, we generated a confusion matrix from the test set predictions, which provided the counts of true positives, true negatives, false positives, and false negatives.
- **Error Rate Formula:** The error rate was calculated using the formula: Error Rate = (False Positives + False Negatives) / Total Predictions.

**Calculation:** From our confusion matrix, suppose we had 150 false positives and 200 false negatives out of 1600 total predictions, the error rate would be (150 + 200) / 1600 = 21.875%, which we rounded to 22%.

## VI.RESULT

*Table 11. Best-11 Vs Predicted-11*

| Batting Position | Best-11 | Predicted-11 |
|---|---|---|
| 1. | Rohit Sharma | Jos Butler |
| 2. | Alex Hales | Rilee Rossouw |
| 3. | Virat Kohli | Virat Kohli |
| 4. | Suryakumar Yadav | Suryakumar Yadav |
| 5. | Glenn Maxwell | Glenn Phillips |
| 6. | Marcus Stoinis | Marcus Stoinis |
| 7. | Sikandar Raza | Sikandar Raza |
| 8. | Rashid Khan | Shadab Khan |
| 9. | Sam Curran | Sam Curran |
| 10. | Shaheen Shah Afridi | Shaheen Shah Afridi |
| 11. | Anrich Nortje | Anrich Nortje |

The proposed methodology suggests that both the column in table 11 i.e. Best-11 and Predicted-11 includes the batsman with their batting order from 1 to 11. Both Best-11 and Predicted-11 looks like both the team are equally strong and consistent. But, in today's data-driven era, everything is all about stats and so the data science is applied. Stats shows the fact about the players performance as shown in table-5 consisting of batting average, batting position, batting strike rate, bowling average, bowling economy, bowling strike rate, total runs, and all other similar metrics which are used to analyze the consistency of player.

There are some differences between Best-11 and Predicted-11 (i.e. Rohit Sharma is replaced by Jos Butler, Alex Hales by Rilee Rossouw, Glenn Maxwell by Glenn Phillips and Rashid Khan by Shadab Khan). This is due to the stats shows that the players replaced with have better consistency than that of some players in Best-11. And also suggests that the Best-11 selection may have inclusion of features selection other than players performance stats (i.e. gut feeling, political factor, etc.).

## VII.CONCLUSION

Proposed methodology demonstrated increased predictive accuracy and insightfulness compared to traditional models, as highlighted by the comparative analysis. We showed a significant enhancement in comprehension and forecasting of players' contributions to team success by concentrating on cricket-specific metrics and utilizing advanced data analysis methods. To transform the forecasting of playing 11 compositions in T20 cricket by utilizing the powerful potential of data science and machine learning. Through careful processing and analysis of data from the T20 Cricket World Cup 2022/2023, a comprehensive procedures was developed that predicts optimal team compositions and provides in-depth insights into player performances and match strategies.

## REFERENCES


Anik, A. I., Yeaser, S., Hossain, A. I., & Chakrabarty, A. (2018, September). Player's performance prediction in ODI cricket using machine learning algorithms. In 2018 4th international conference on electrical engineering and information & communication technology (iCEEiCT) (pp. 500-505). IEEE.

Basit, A., Alvi, M. B., Jaskani, F. H., Alvi, M., Memon, K. H., & Shah, R. A. (2020, November). ICC T20 Cricket World Cup 2020 winner prediction using machine learning techniques. In 2020 IEEE 23rd International Multitopic Conference (INMIC) (pp. 1-6). IEEE.

Deb, K., Pratap, A., Agarwal, S., & Meyarivan, T. (2002, August). A fast and elitist multiobjective genetic algorithm: NSGA-II. *IEEE Transactions on Evolutionary Computation*, *6*(2), 182–197. DOI: 10.1109/4235.996017

Hasanika, D., Dilhara, R., Liyanage, D., Bandaranayake, A., & Deegalla, S. (2021, December). Data mining system for predicting a winning cricket team. In 2021 IEEE 16th International Conference on Industrial and Information Systems (ICIIS) (pp. 92-97). IEEE.

Kadiri, P., Anusha, P., Prabhu, M., Asuncion, R., Pavan, V. S., & Suman, J. V. (2024, July). Morphed Picture Recognition using Machine Learning Algorithms. In *2024 Second International Conference on Advances in Information Technology (ICAIT)* (Vol. 1, pp. 1-6). IEEE.

Kaluarachchi, A., & Aparna, S. V. (2010, December). CricAI: A classification based tool to predict the outcome in ODI cricket. In *2010 Fifth International Conference on Information and Automation for Sustainability* (pp. 250-255). IEEE.

Tekade, P., Markad, K., Amage, A., & Natekar, B. (2020). Cricket match outcome prediction using machine learning. *International Journal of Advance Scientific Research and Engineering Trends*, *5*(7).

Vennila, G., Mounica, P., Prasanna, P. L., Kumar, P. P., & Sirisha, R. (2024, May). Enhancing Speech Emotion Recognition using Deep Learning Networks on Live Calls. In 2024 5th International Conference for Emerging Technology (INCET) (pp. 1-8). IEEE.

# Chapter 9
# AI in Talent Scouting and Player Development:
## Role of AI and Machine Learning in Identifying and Nurturing Talent in Sports Organizations

**Shashank Mittal**
https://orcid.org/0000-0002-8666-5323
*O.P. Jindal Global University, India*

**Rohit**
https://orcid.org/0009-0004-1796-5252
*Gulf Medical University, Ajman, UAE*

## ABSTRACT

*Artificial Intelligence (AI) is revolutionizing sports organizations by enhancing talent scouting, player development, and operational efficiency. This chapter explores the transformative role of AI and machine learning in identifying and nurturing athletic talent. It delves into the evolution of talent scouting, the integration of AI technologies such as predictive analytics and wearable sensors, and the implications for player development. Key sections address AI-driven scouting methods, player performance optimization, and the ethical and legal considerations of using AI. The chapter also discusses practical and managerial challenges in implementing AI systems, including data privacy and bias mitigation. By examining future trends and innovations, it provides a comprehensive overview of how AI is reshaping sports management and offers insights into the ethical and practical considerations that organizations must navigate.*

DOI: 10.4018/979-8-3693-5385-1.ch009

## INTRODUCTION

The integration of Artificial Intelligence and machine learning into the sport has revolutionized various aspects of the business-from game strategy to performance analysis, from the methods by which teams engage fans to the hiring of matches. Probably one of the most significant potential impacts has been in talent scouting and in the development of players. Traditionally, the talent scouting had relied heavily on the subjective judgments of scouts who looked at what a player could do based on physical attributes, performance in games, and sometimes even gut feelings. While experienced scouts provide invaluable knowledge, it typically lacks the objectivity and scalability needed by contemporary sports organizations operating in an increasingly competitive marketplace (Agarwal, 2023).

The rise of AI and machine learning technology heralds a new curtain to talent identification and player development as systems of AI draw enormous amounts of data, statistics, and footage from games, coupled with biometric measurements, in making actionable insights (Albert, 2019). Scouting based on observation of patterns and trends, which are often imperceptible to the human mind, can be achieved by machine learning algorithms; therefore, this changes the focus towards taking more comprehensive and data-driven approaches in scouting. It changes the sports organization's entire manner of identifying and developing the right talent (Bajwa, 2024).

AI Talent scouting uses high-end algorithms processing large amounts of data to evaluate the performance of the players. These algorithms can rate player statistics, physical conditioning, and even their psychological profile. By processing that kind of information, AI computers can easily pinpoint future stars with greater accuracy and reliability. For example, AI models grade future performance based on generalizing past trends in data; therefore, such an approach allows the organizations to make sound decisions regarding recruitment or investment into those individuals (Agarwal, 2023).

The role of AI in developing a player is not just identification but to improve the skills and the performance of athletes. Through machine learning, it shall, therefore be able to monitor the progress made by players over time providing programs for the training based on their demands. For instance, AI can predict a pattern of risk for injuries by analyzing physical data from the players therefore enabling time to prevent injuries. With this proactive approach towards player development, the athletes receive specifically focused support to ensure they're performing at the highest level while also being served effectively all the time (Albert, 2019)..

However, the engagement of AI in talent scouting and the development of players does not go without problems. In the process of using AI to analyze and monitor a player's condition, sports organizations face numerous data privacy and ethical issues. In addition, the supremacy of an AI system determines the quality and completeness of data used. Incomplete or wrong data influences predictions and results in consequently suboptimal decisions.

AI and machine learning development offer a unique platform for sports organizations to build on their advantage. Unlocking enormous amounts of data to better inform the necessary decisions in talent identification and player development will change how teams operate and achieve their objectives. The current state of AI in sports is a topic of discussion in this chapter-a landscape with applications, benefits, and limitations in talent scouting and player development. Understanding these dynamics, then, sports organizations will be better equipped to navigate the future of talent management in an increasingly data-driven world (Cheng, 2024).

## THE EVOLUTION OF TALENT SCOUTING IN SPORTS

Talent scouting, one of the most critical components of sports management, has been subjected to a pretty good change in the decades. Traditionally, talent identification through scouting and coaching was largely based on the discretion of scouts and coaches and relied on the individual observations and judgments of players. Such a traditional model was effective as it stood partially but was associated with considerable handicaps in terms of objectivity, scalability, and consistency.

Scouting in the early stages of sports was more prone to giving much emphasis to what a scout could see and watch, that is, a player's physical attributes in game play and performance. Scouts went to various matches at local levels, tournaments, or even practice sessions as they evaluated players in terms of speed, strength, skill level, and game intelligence. Scouting became more personal and biased as reliance was always on firsthand observation, making it hold much stake on the individual scout's expertise (Cheungsirakulvit & Girdwichai, 2023). This process, although excellent for its uniqueness and inside information, could not determine how to measure talent of players nor performance on a standardized note.

The new demand for professional sports was conveyed in the growing need for a more formalized system of scouting. Statistical analysis in the simplest form birthed an impetus towards a data-based trend. Teams and clubs started establishing and accumulating metrics for performance, such as goals scored, assists, and defensive statistics. These statistics provided more solid footing for evaluating players, but the analysis remained pretty crude. These statistics began being used by scouts and analysts to complement observation, but the approach was restricted only by the reach and acuteness of data available (Clark, 2020).

The real milestone in talent scouting however arrived with advanced statistical analysis and computer technology. Advanced statistical models paired with software able to process vast amounts of data began to emerge in the late 20th and early 21st centuries (Eid et al., 2024). In baseball, “Moneyball” arises in this time, referred to in the book and accompanying film of the same name, where statistical analysis can challenge the traditional method of scouting and expose under-valued players. Such a strategy went well in baseball and paved the way to other sports embracing similar data-centered methodology

The second wave of information production brought by the new revolution in technology integrated video analysis and digital tracking technologies. The use of videos enabled a more intricate examination of players and associated performances. Scouts and coaches, therefore, were now able to analyze particular plays as well as techniques and decision-making processes. Modern tracking systems that utilize sensor technology and the aid of GPS enabled instant data on player movement, speed, and physiological parameters while playing and training. This redundancy brings more depth in the understanding of a player's performance and potential (Harris et al., 2011).

The final trends in talent scouting resulted in the utilization of Artificial Intelligence and machine learning. Such technologies represent a paradigm shift in the processing and use of data. AI algorithms can process mega-volumes of data from all kinds of sources: game footage, biometric measurements, and historical performance statistics, for example. Machine learning models can point out connections and interdependencies that elude the naked eye of a human analyst, letting coaches find a much better understanding of player potential and pathways for development (Hassan et al., 2022).

They are able to track the real-time performance of a player, predict how this will play out in the future by applying known statistical patterns, and recommend recruitment and development strategies. Thus, data-based scouting further increases the accuracy of scouting ratings and makes talent identification much more scalable and efficient.

The growth of talent scouting in sports captures more general trends toward increasing use of data and technology. From subjective review to high-tech AI-driven analysis, this evolution played as a step-up model where at every stage of development, the better and more objective is the approach towards the identification and nurturing of athletic talent. Further development in technology will surely make talent scouting more aligned and integrated with data-driven insights in the transformation process of how a sports organization will be able to discover and develop talent (Jasni et al., 2022).

## INTRODUCTION TO AI AND MACHINE LEARNING IN SPORTS

Artificial Intelligence (AI) and machine learning are new transformative technologies in a broad range of sectors, and sports are no exception. Both these technologies are dramatically transforming the ways teams, coaches, and organizations do everything from analytics about player performance to fan engagement. To discuss the influence of AI and machine learning on sports, one has first to know what AI and machine learning are, as well as how they are applied in this dynamic field (Kumar et al., 2024).

AI refers to the ability of the machine to mimic intelligent human behavior. AI systems in sports are designed to perform tasks that traditionally require human intelligence, such as recognition of patterns, making decisions, and learning from data. Machine learning is a subset of AI in which algorithms learn with experience and improve their performance over time based on data that isn't explicitly programmed. In this process, machines are able to predict patterns, determine trends, and generate insights from vast oceans of data.

AI and machine learning apply in many functions of sports, profoundly altering the way teams and organizations work. The most interesting application seems to be in performance analysis. Highly advanced AI algorithms can analyze quite clearly game footage by breaking down individual plays, player movements, and tactical patterns (Liu & Zhang, 2024). This level of analysis gives to coaches and analysts information that otherwise would not be available and, hence, allows them to make more informed decisions about game strategy as well as that toward developing player.

AI in sports is also being used in preventing and managing injuries. By the wearables and sensors, AI systems capture a player's physiological metrics, such as heart rate, movement patterns, and workload. It then follows that a machine learning model can identify unique patterns that might predict risks for injury so interventions can be made on the part of the team to prevent the injury or alter the training, which can ultimately prolong their careers.

AI and machine learning play a further crucial part in talent scouting and recruitment. Scouting has long relied on impressionistic assessment and scarcity of data. There is now the capacity to analyze scores of data sets involving player statistics, biometrics, and a vast array of different leagues' competition performance (Marlapudi & Lenka, 2024). Machine learning algorithms can further detect those with talent using all manner of factors from physical characteristics to mental and psychological profiles. This data-driven approach enhances scouting accuracy and enables teams to identify players they could have otherwise overlooked.

Moreover, AI is changing the character of fan engagement and experience, too, and includes the scope of scouting and performance analysis. Thus, one of its applications in this domain is the personalization of content and provision of relevant recommendations to fans based on their interests and behavior. While AI-driven chatbots may prove especially effective for real-time updates and interaction with fans, it can also be used for monitoring and researching social media and other digital platforms for an understanding of sentiment and trend (McAuley et al., 2024). For marketing and promotions strategies, it becomes a very valuable resource, as its recommendation will take into considerations only those fans with interests aligned to the specific product or service.

Despite the many benefits derived from AI and machine learning technology applied in sports, there are challenges attached to adopting this. The quality and quantity of data feed determine how effective these AI systems are. Poorly interpreted data may lead to flawed predictions and recommendations. Considering the implementation of these technologies requires significant investment and deep knowledge of expertise, it may be a barrier for some teams and organizations.

Ethical issues should therefore be addressed, especially on data security and the likelihood of abuse in the use of AI technologies. Sports organizations must, therefore, take into account these ethical problems and ensure that the use of technology is aligned with legal and moral standards.

AI and machine learning are transforming the sports business: performance analysis, injury prevention, talent scouting, and fan engagement. As these technologies continue to develop, their applications in the realm of sports will likely expand along with the opportunities available to teams and organizations for enhancing their operations and competitive advantages. Understanding the basics of AI and machine learning is thus important for leveraging these technologies effectively and responsibly within the evolving landscape of sports (Mishra et al., 2024).

## AI-DRIVEN TALENT SCOUTING

This is a sharp innovation in how sports organizations assess and identify up-and-coming players, as the AI-driven scouting of talented athletes would ensure the selection of best-fit talent, always valid but occasionally subjective and limited in scope for a long time. The application of AI and machine learning technologies into scouting processes was determined to introduce data-driven approaches that enhance precision, scalability, and even objectivity.

Advanced algorithms and aggregations of data allow talent scouting to create a much fuller understanding of players by tallying an enormous variety of data, among them player statistics, game footage, physiological metrics, and social and psychological profiles. AI can look for hidden patterns and trends that may not be observed with conventional scouting methods (Parra-Martinez & Wai, 2023).

Perhaps the most significant advantage AI has over human scouting for talent is that it can quickly sift through huge data sets. For instance, with AI algorithms, one can scan and evaluate raw performance metrics from many games, seasons, and leagues, thereby creating a detailed profile of what a player can do and can amount to-a task perfectly impossible or impractical for human scouts.

For instance, video footage analysis of a player can provide technical abilities and tactical awareness and decision-making efficiency. The model will follow the movement of the player and then analyze how that player reacts to specific game situations. In addition, it evaluates the performance in comparison to benchmarks (Reyaz et al., 2024). This can give in-depth information on where players are strong and weak: whether it is on speed and agility or even on simple game intelligence.

Another important benefit of AI scouting is that it can predict how a player will perform in the future. It does so by considering historical data and building trends with the help of AI models. This way, the AI system can know the most possible trend of how a player is likely to perform later in the future. Predictive is, therefore, another very important benefit for teams that want to bet on untapped young talent with potential. AI can project the future trend for a player from recent performance and development patterns. This is a very important tool for teams when they are recruiting or investing in the long run.

Another role of AI is to also help identify hidden talent or talent going unnoticed. Traditional scouting processes may miss out on future stars because perhaps they are in areas that are geographically inaccessible or perhaps just enough spectators have not been exposed to them (Reynoso-Sanchez, 2023). AI can potentially look through more data from a greater cross-section of sources to highlight such talents from the lower leagues or foreign competitions that the traditional scouts may not have looked for. Such a wider scope improves the opportunity of finding potential stars.

Another important advantage AI-based scouting grants is the minimizing of bias and the subjective nature with which the evaluation process is often composed. Human scouts have personal biases that run right into their judgment, such as how a player looks or even from what team they are coming from. In contrast, using AI, evaluations rely on facts and statistical analysis so that there will be a better fair and balanced opinion about a player's skills and potential.

While AI-driven talent scouting has some advantages, it certainly is not free of problems. AI systems work well only based on the quality and accuracy of the data fed into the system. In the event of inaccurate and incomplete data, it results in flawed evaluations and poor decision-making. Furthermore, implementation of AI systems requires major investments in technology as well as the associated expertise, which becomes a barrier for most organizations.

A critical aspect of ethical engagement with AI in scouting has nothing to do with the AI algorithm itself but rather with the traditional ethical concerns. Data privacy, for example, is one of the most important aspects in the improper use of personal data. In order to ensure that sports organizations take appropriate measures to ensure compliance with legal and ethical standards with respect to player and recruit privacy, their use of AI must not hamper it (Sajadi et al., 2024).

In a nutshell, AI-driven talent scouting makes a giant leap in the manner by which sports organizations identify and evaluate players. With the power of data and machine learning technologies, teams are able to gain deeper insight into player performances and even predict future potential as well as tap talents that may have been veiled.

Considering these points and the dangers, the benefits of AI-driven scouting shine bright as an avenue by which the sport might improve its ways in the identification and recruitment of talent.

## AI IN PLAYER DEVELOPMENT

The introduction of AI in the development process of a player makes it a leaping point in the kind of training and monitoring given to athletes and the level of push to full potential. This method tracks players through traditional experience and intuition from coaches but, with AI and machine learning, integrates the process using data-driven insights and bespoke feedback on every player. This maximizes training schedules and evaluates the health of the players while working on specific plans for every one of them (Till & Baker, 2020).

The most useful method of application of AI in player development is through the analysis of performance data. AI will be able to handle and analyze a massive array of information from game footage, training sessions, and biometric sensors. The detailed insights provided by AI algorithms in terms of strengths and areas of improvement for a player are thus crucial. For example, AI can be used in a field to analyze the moves of a player in real-time to patterns of movement, technique, and the specific decisions made, thus enabling coaches to achieve objective assessments aside from what is usually seen, and possibly result in tailored training that hones areas for development (Agarwal, 2023).

AI plays a big role in prevention and the management of injury. Wearable technology and biometric sensors will constantly collect data about the physical conditions such as heart rate, muscle strain, and joint stress of individual players. Machine learning models can then analyze this data to look for patterns associated with a potential increased risk of injury. It can be highlighted that early detection of these patterns by AI will prompt coaches and medical staff to take early measures, like loads adjustment or rest period recommendation. This proactive approach not only minimizes injuries but also puts a player in an optimum condition for better performance (Albert, 2019).

The other significant feature of AI in the context of player development is personalization of the training. The traditional training regimens are one size fits all. Requirements for different participants are overlooked. An AI-based system can create a customized learning plan based on the player's unique physiological and performance data. For instance, when the AI identifies the weakness of a certain player in terms of speed or agility, it would advise corresponding drills and exercises to improve these (Bajwa, 2024). This already guarantees that every player will receive proper support for improvement in development together with performance.

It also enhances feedback in the cycle between the players and the coaches. The coaches can now offer instant and prompt feedback in the training session or in the game with real-time data analytics. For example, AI could reveal to the coach exactly where the player was wrong or inefficient in technique and how to correct it immediately. This instant feedback allows the correction of a player's behavior to happen faster, resulting in an acceleration of his or her development and improvement (Cheng, 2024).

Also, AI-based systems can track how a player progresses over time and give insight into his trend of development. Analyzing historical data, AI will be able to assess how a player's performance and skills have progressed over time and give an idea about future growth. This method gives long-term insight into data that coaches and players refer to in setting realistic expectations and monitoring improvements toward those expectations (Cheungsirakulvit & Girdwichai, 2023). This also allows training to be tweaked as per the changing requirement or trend in performance by the player.

While all this sounds exciting, applying AI to player development brings its own set of challenges. The quality of the data collected will essentially determine the correctness and effectiveness of AI systems. Low-quality data might lead to misleading insights or even suboptimal training recommendations. Another issue with the deployment of AI technology is the higher requirement for equipment and expertise, which leaves some sports organizations unprepared for procurement (Cheng, 2024).

Ethical considerations are also present when using AI for player development; collection and use of personal data have their concerns of privacy as well as consent. The sports organizations have a responsibility to ensure handling of player data responsibly and at the best practice levels regarding legal and ethical standards.

In a nutshell, AI has transformed the process of developing a player by way of data-driven insight, customized training programs, and enhancing feedback mechanisms. By utilizing more advanced technologies, sports organizations can optimize training, prevent injuries, and make players contribute to their best extent.

Challenges and ethical considerations notwithstanding, the benefits of AI in player development present a very promising way forward for improving athletic performance and development (Cheungsirakulvit & Girdwichai, 2023).

## INTEGRATION OF AI INTO SPORTS ORGANIZATIONS

Introduction of AI in sports organizations represents a revolution for more data-informed decision making and operational efficiency. For all the promise that AI comes with comes challenges of implementing it in practice. This section expresses how AI can be introduced into sports organizations as this entry explores technology adoption, organizational culture, and what is real implementation.

### Adoption of Technology

Sports organizations implement the AI technology through the selection of the appropriate tools and platforms. Performance analysis, injury prevention, fan engagement, and operational efficiency are some of the applications of AI in sports. Thereafter, organizations should reflect on their specific needs and then select those AI solutions that are in agreement with their objectives (Clark, 2020). For instance, the organization would focus on the improvement of player performance by making investments in AI-driven analytics and wearables for better and improved performance from the players. In contrast, an organization interested in fan engagement may invest in AI-powered chatbots and the systems for personalized content delivery.

### Implementation Process

The process of implementation is categorized into: pilot testing, system integration, and full deployment. At this point, pilot testing allows organizations to test AI solutions initially at a smaller scale before implementing them at a larger scale. This stage is critical for highlighting the issues that are considered to be of utmost importance and ensuring that the technology would really meet the needs of the organization. Once developed and tested, the AI system will need to be integrated into existing infrastructure and workflows. In this process, data integration, checks on system compatibility, and development of interfaces toward how the users would interact become part of the issue (Eid et al., 2024).

## Organizational Culture

A great deal of successful organizational integration of AI requires a suitable organization culture to implement technological change. There is therefore a need for making the sports organizations to become open so that its employees are receptive in adopting new technologies and being flexible in their way of processing work, including educating on what AI brings aboard and dispelling anxious worries (Harris et al., 2011).

Training and up-skilling would form essential components of this cultural change. Coaches, analysts, and other employees must be provided with appropriate knowledge and competences to correctly utilize AI tools. A formal training program, workshops, and continuing support might be encompassed to ensure the full exploitation of the technology (Hassan et al., 2022). Organizations will also have to cultivate a collaboration between technical experts and sports professionals in order to bridge data science with practical application.

## Practical Implementation

Some of the most critical practical considerations when integrating AI are as follows:

1. **Data Management:** AI systems require high quality data to function effectively. Organizations must have robust data management policies in place to ensure data is accurate, consistent, and safe. This includes data collection, storage, processing, and protocol compliance with data privacy regulations.
2. **Infrastructure and Resources:** The integration of AI technology would demand some infrastructural investments, for instance, computing power, storage solutions, and software platforms. Organizations then must put aside resources for such necessities so that the IT infrastructure can assume the elevated demands of AI applications (Jasni et al., 2022).
3. **Vendor and Technology Selection:** Effective integration depends on vendor and technology choices. Organizations should evaluate possible vendors based on their knowledge, track record, and compatibility with the solutions they are offering with existing systems. Scalability, support, and cost are also important considerations.
4. **Change Management**: AI technology can change the current workflows and processes within organizations. Change management needs to be implemented in such a way that the transition will be easy, smooth, and low risk. This involves educating staff on the advantages of AI, dispelling all doubts and fear,

and offering support before and during the implementation process (Kumar et al., 2024).

## Challenges and Considerations

The adoption of AI in sporting organizations is not without its challenges. Some of these are as follows:

- **Cost:** The investment in AI technology and infrastructure may require significant upfront costs. Organizations will have to balance the cost with the potential benefits and develop a definite return on investment.
- **Data Privacy and Security:** The utilization of AI uses personal data and analysis. The organizations should, therefore establish strict data privacy and security procedures that protect the personal data of players and fans and are also in strict compliance with the legal requirements.
- **Bias and Fairness:** AI systems can, with or without intention, entrench the biases that exist in the data. The organizations concerned have to be vigilant about bias and ensure to address it or mitigate it so that fairness is ensured in the use of AI technology.

To summarize, AI in sports organizations holds the promise to elevate performance, optimize operations, and engage with fans in wonderful ways. All of these elements are successful only when planned carefully, equipped within a culture of the organization to embrace change, with an eye to practical and ethical considerations. If sports organizations navigate some challenges successfully, then they should unlock all the potential in AI and emerge stronger over time against sport competitors in a changing landscape of sports (Liu & Zhang, 2024).

# ETHICAL AND LEGAL CONSIDERATIONS

This integration of AI into sports organizations calls for multiple ethical and legal issues that must be brought to light to ensure the technology is used responsibly and with fairness. As AI technologies continually amass high usage in sports, organizations need to tread carefully to accommodate issues such as the rights and well-being of players, staff, and fans without infringing on legislations and regulations.

1. Data Privacy and Security

Perhaps the greatest ethical and legal challenge related to AI in sport is data privacy and security. The use of AI is naturally linked to amassing vast quantities of data, which often includes health-related information on individual athletes, performance metrics, and personal data. All such collection of data should comply with data privacy and protection law and regulations, which differ by country and region-consider Europe's General Data Protection Regulation, for instance, or California's California Consumer Privacy Act in the United States (Marlapudi & Lenka, 2024).

They, therefore, must have very robust data protection in their organizations that will protect the information from unauthorized access or breaches. It includes securing data storage systems, employing encryption technologies, and creating clear protocols on data access and handling. Second, sports organizations should explain to players and fans what data they collect and how they use it, and also how they will protect it. Informed consent is integral, and people should be allowed to access, correct, and delete personal data (McAuley et al., 2024).

2. Consent and Transparency

One of the other importance for AI technologies is informed consent from all the other stakeholders-the players. Players should be aware of how their data, the data collected from them through AI technologies, including AI-driven analysis or monitoring, which may influence the training, health assessment, or professional decisions. Transparency of AI use and information that it collects promotes trust and ensures that individuals make informed choices about their participation (Mishra et al., 2024).

Organizations should clearly state the purposes of AI applications and how they would benefit players and the organization at large. Providing adequate information on AI technologies and their impacts helps to deal with any sort of misconception or lack of understanding in relation to ethical practice.

3. Bias and Fairness

AI systems only reflect what society reflects to them. If biased or already discriminating information is used in training the algorithms of AI, then such biases are simply carried forward and even intensified by the AI system. It can result in unfair judgment or unfair decision-making concerning recruitment of players, their performance evaluation, and handling of injuries (Parra-Martinez & Wai, 2023).

In response to these issues, organizations must develop and deploy AI systems that are considered fair. This includes continuous audits and tests for biased algorithms, diverse and representative data sets, and inclusive teams for the development and oversight of AI systems. There are also meaningful ways that human oversight and intervention can minimize biases in AI decision making.

4. Accountability and Responsibility

The more decisions the AI systems make, the more questions of accountability and liability are raised. Who is liable if the AI system malfunctions or gives an incorrect decision? Is it the technology provider, the sporting organization, or perhaps the system users? Some clear guidelines and mechanisms for accountability need to be developed when using such technologies (Reyaz et al., 2024).

Organizations should also develop regulations on handling disputes or complaints over decisions made through AI. This way, if there is a problem, there is always a known process for redress and remedy, which ensures trust and accountability.

5. Effects on Employment and Fair Play

AI technologies can affect the employment practice of sports organizations. For instance, AI-based scouting for talent and performance analysis may alter recruitment choices, which in turn can impact job placement for scouts, coaches, and analysts. The impacts of AI on employment require consideration and transitions to be managed fairly and ethically (Reynoso-Sanchez, 2023).

Moreover, the application of AI in the monitoring and performance improvement creates an issue related to fair play and just competition. The AI-based systems that can offer absolutely paramount pluses in terms of performance analysis or injury prevention may cause unfairness between teams or leagues. Sports organizations need to create policies to ensure that the use of these AI technologies creates even more just competition rather than destroying the principles of sportsmanship and equality (Sajadi et al., 2024).

6. Compliances with Rules

AI in sports should be in line with the governing and regulatory standards under which sports are conducted. Apart from data protection laws, there are other regulations covering sports governance, anti-doping policies, as well as fair play. Organisations need to stay abreast of such legal compliances and maintain close liaison with the legal experts concerned so that all applicable laws are in full alignment with their AI practices (Till & Baker, 2020).

Summarily, the integration of AI in sports organizations brings along critical ethical and legal considerations that must be well managed. Key to this is the discussion of matters regarding privacy, consent, bias, accountability, employment, and regulatory compliance so as to ensure the responsible and ethical use of AI technologies. And after such proaction of sound discussion, sports organizations will find benefitting from AI with tenacity against trust and integrity in their operations (Agarwal, 2023).

## FUTURE TRENDS AND INNOVATIONS

The landscape of sports technology is changing at a fast pace, especially with AI and machine learning accelerating progress. With these technologies becoming more dominant in the world, taken on increasingly by sports organizations, it brings along a myriad host of future trends and innovations that will shape the industry. Some of the emerging developing AI-driven issues in talent scouting, player development, and broader sports management are discussed with respect to how these innovations will potentially change the face of the industry.

1. Augmented Predictive Analytics

AI-powered predictive analytics are rapidly advancing toward being much more sophisticated and at the very heart of management in sports. Future developments will hone algorithms to better predict player performance, injury risk, and outcomes of games themselves. Machine learning models will use larger and broader data sets in real-time and historical terms to better generate insights on these matters of import. These ability predictors will guide teams to take wiser decisions about player purchases, training procedures, and game plans (Albert, 2019).

For instance, AI can predict a player's performance track record based on his previous performances, their training schedules, and even the psychological factors affecting him. This will enable teams to prepare development programs for players and treat player workloads more wisely, thus minimizing injury risks while building overall performances (Bajwa, 2024).

2. Integration of Wearable Technology and IoT

This will be the next revolution in player monitoring and development with the integration of wearable technology and IoT together with AI. More advanced wearables will then provide detailed physiological and biomechanical data, from real-time metrics on muscle strain, hydration level, and stress indicators. IoT devices will allow a continuous monitoring of these metrics to give more precise and immediate feedback.

AI-based algorithms will analyze data from these wearables to present actionable insights, such as the amount of load in training, specific recovery protocols, and prevention strategies against injury. Real-time integration will increase the ability of coaches and medical staff to respond to players' needs and change training and recovery plans accordingly (Cheng, 2024).

3. Advanced Video Analysis and Computer Vision

AI-based video analysis and computer vision will further enhance the expertise and tools for analysis in performance review and tactical analysis. Future developments should come with enhanced capabilities in tracking player movement, assessing game strategies, and pinpointing crucial moments at which decisions are made on the field of play. Computer vision systems should be able to break up even the most complex game scenarios, explaining what the individual players are doing based on the team formations and tactical changes (Cheungsirakulvit & Girdwichai, 2023).

These would provide coaches and analysts with better information about the dynamics of a game and narrow down strategy. The scouting and recruitment processes would also be much easier with automated video analysis tools, allowing for all-around assessments of individual players' performances, shot from different angles and in different contexts.

4. AI-Enhanced Fan Engagement

The future of AI in sports would also see innovations pertaining to fan engagement and experience. AI-driven personalization will give much more customized content to fans-like customized highlights, interactive experiences, and recommendations. AI-powered chatbots and virtual assistants will allow real-time updates of games, answer fan's questions, and enhance customer service contact (Clark, 2020).

Augmented and virtual reality combined with AI will be used for immersive experiences of the fan in stadiums, virtual stadium tours, interactive game simulations, and augmented live broadcasting. Such innovations would make engagement with fans more interactive as well as personalized with their favorite team or players.

5. Ethical AI and Transparent Algorithms

As sports grow with more AI, there would be a rising need to develop more ethical AI systems where the transparency of decisions taken by algorithms is maintained. Future innovations in this area are about finding ways to counter biases in models, deploying data protection measures, and ensuring that AI applications are ethical.

Organizations would be investing in the development of transparent algorithms and frameworks for accountability and fairness (Eid et al., 2024).

Research and development on ethical AI will design principles and practices for responsible practices in technology in sports. Transparency and equity in AI systems are necessary to retain trust and integrity in the operations of sports organizations.

6. Scaling Up AI for Grassroots Sports

AI innovations will also be seen in grassroots and amateur sports where it could become democratized through access to advanced technologies, and a source for development. Accessible to lower-tier teams and individual athletes who earlier were out of reach for them to avail that kind of insight; AI-driven tools and platforms, which they could have only enjoyed by elite organizations.

For instance, amateur athletes and grassroots teams would be empowered to coach themselves through AI-based coaching applications and performance tracking systems, optimizing their training more effectively, monitoring improvement in a better way, and, more frequently than not, enhancing general skill development. In this way, this increased access of AI technologies would further the general prosperity and development of sports activities in general at all levels (Harris et al., 2011).

7. Cross-Disciplinary Approaches and Collaboration

Future trends would mean more multidisciplinary collaboration between sports scientists, data scientists, AI experts, and technology developers in developing applications of AI. Innovations would be driven through collaborative efforts and developed with clear understanding of the requirements and challenges that are sports-specific (Hassan et al., 2022).

Sports organizations and tech companies have joined forces in the creation of new AI-driven solutions, while even perfecting the available technologies. This is therefore an area that remains a source of innovation and will continue to be the cause of evolution for sports AI in the future.

More broadly, exciting trends and innovations associated with the future of AI in sports promise to enhance performance, player development, and fan engagement. Furthermore, sports organizations will benefit from more accurate predictive analytics, improved monitoring tools, and immersive fan experiences as AI technologies evolve further. Addressing ethical considerations and fostering interdisciplinary collaboration will be key to ensuring these innovations are used appropriately and effectively (Jasni et al., 2022).

## IMPLICATIONS

Integration of Artificial Intelligence within the sports organizations has deep dimensions across all ethical, societal, practical, and managerial assumptions. It reflects the transformative influence on the sphere of sports, thus calling for cautious consideration and necessary balancing.

### Ethical Implications

The use of AI in sports raises several concerns that require balance to ensure responsible technology adoption. Data privacy is perhaps one of the most critical ethical concerns. Many AI-based solutions require collecting and analyzing significant amounts of personal data that may be sensitive to a player's health and performance. Organizations need to handle the data sensitively and implement appropriate data protection measures while ensuring access to informed consent in handling the data (Kumar et al., 2024). There needs to be transparency in using data and respect for privacy regulations so trust is maintained while exercising the rights of the players and fans.

The other ethical challenge that characterizes AI is bias in AI. It is where biased or unrepresentative data affects the learning of AI systems, thereby perpetuating inequalities or making unfair decisions. This raises a great concern especially where talent hunting and evaluation of performances are concerned because biased AI can lead to wrongful discrimination. Sport organizations will need to strive to recognize and offset biases that commonly occur in AI models to ensure fairer and equal decision-making (Liu & Zhang, 2024).

### Societal Implications

The social implications of AI in sports go beyond the direct sporting organizational spectrum and resonate well across wider communities. In addition, smart advances driven by AI in sports are very likely to enhance fan interest and accessibility with opportunities for more personalized and engaging experiences; thus, there is a good chance that interest in sports and connection to chosen teams may be even stronger (Marlapudi & Lenka, 2024).

Yet this is also likely to lead to some negative implications for society. For instance, any automatization of sports role scouting and analysis by the sport organizations may lead to disengagement from these jobs and, therefore, employment as well. Organizations have to consider such broader social effects of employment and arrange for supporting workforce transition through retraining and upskilling (McAuley et al., 2024).

Large-scale integration of AI in sports raises issues relating to the fairness of competition and integrity. The performance analysis and injury prevention through enhancements made by AI can lead to inequality between teams and might even drastically change the nature of competition. Hence, the onus for AI technologies being in favor of fair play and strictly adhering to a code of ethics lies heavily with the individuals responsible for the use and development of such technologies (Mishra et al., 2024).

## Practical Implications

Most practical functions that AI would integrate into sports organizations mean a huge change in the operations carried out by organisations. The introduction of AI systems calls for an investment in technology, infrastructure, and training. Most of the time, resources will be needed to acquire and keep the tools of AI to integrate them with other systems and train staff on their use.

For instance, such dependence on AI in the decision making and performance analysis brings about a fundamental change in the decision-making process and success pattern. Coaches and analysts need to alter the manner of judging players and strategy formulations based upon this analysis and without ignoring data-driven insights but showing their professional judgment and experience (Parra-Martinez & Wai, 2023).

## Managerial Implications

From the managerial point of view, there are several significant considerations in the integration of AI into the sports organizations. The managers will be able to oversee the adoption and implementation of the AI technology in ways compatible with the organizational objective or strategy. This includes proper choice of the tools of AI, vendor relationship management, and including the technology into existing workflows.

There is also the issue of addressing the ethical and societal implications of AI: privacy, bias, and fairness. Building trust and support obligations to comply with regulations would be facilitated through developing and enforcing policies and guidelines for responsible use of AI. A culture of transparency and accountability will be encouraged when managers encourage open communication about the use of AI and address concerns when they arise (Reyaz et al., 2024).

Finally, organizational processes and structure can change due to AI integration. The alteration in the organization structure and process caused by AI integration also keeps managers tied to these changes. Again, the adoption of AI should help or align with organizational goals. Implementing AI should enable enhanced organizational performance. Accordingly, it means changing the role of the staff and training and supporting them appropriately. Third, AI initiatives would have to be aligned with the vision and strategies of the parent organization.

In brief, AI impact in the sport organization is strongly felt in terms of ethics and society, practice, and management. Taking these implications in a careful and anticipatory manner is of paramount importance to approach an advantage with least risk. Ethical priorities, workforce support, and equal competition are parameters that can help organizations find their way through AI both effectively and responsibly in sports organizations (Eid et al., 2024).

Integration of artificial intelligence into sports teams is a revolution that may change talent scouting, player development, and industry management. The applications of this current evolutionary development in AI technologies promise enhanced performance analysis, optimized training regimens, and innovative methods of engaging fans. Advances in predictive analytics, wearables, and computer vision will unlock insights at unprecedented levels for sports organizations, thus allowing them to make even more informed decisions and derive higher returns from on-field to off-field (Hassan et al., 2022).

AI adoption carries significant ethical, social, practical, and management implications that are critical to navigate and examine. Strong measures need to be taken to mitigate potential data privacy-related and algorithmic bias concerns in using AI systems responsibly and transparently. Social impacts such as job displacement and fairness in competition underscore the critical importance of proper implementation and support for those whose jobs may be at risk. From a practical standpoint, the integration of AI calls for investment in technology and training; managers, of course, have responsibility for aligning the AI initiatives with the goals of the organization and adhering to the most broadly accepted principles of ethics.

## CONCLUSION

Finally, and significantly, the success of implementing AI in sporting organizations will be contingent on how well these challenges have been met going forward. This would ensure ethics, a culture of transparency, and equitable access to technology. In turn, technology developers, sports professionals, and regulatory bodies must continue working together as the field evolves for it to unlock full AI potential in sports.

In conclusion, the transformative effect of AI on sports offers ample opportunities for innovation and growth that can keep sports organizations performing better and operating more efficiently. Embracing such trends will enable sports organizations to grow professionally while improving their performance and operations but will also serve this positive impact on the larger community of sports. The prospect for AI in sports, therefore, will be bright and, only with proper thought process and strategic implementation, change the landscape of what is considered achievable within the boundaries of sports.

## REFERENCES


Agarwal, S. (2023). Artificial intelligence in sports industry. In *Artificial intelligence for business* (pp. 250–269). Productivity Press. DOI: 10.4324/9781003358411-15

Albert, E. T. (2019). AI in talent acquisition: A review of AI-applications used in recruitment and selection. *Strategic HR Review, 18*(5), 215–221. DOI: 10.1108/SHR-04-2019-0024

Bajwa, S. S. (2024). Role of artificial intelligence (AI) in the promotion of sports. *Asian Journal of Research in Social Sciences and Humanities, 14*(5), 1–7. DOI: 10.5958/2249-7315.2024.00012.X

Cheng, H. (2024). Study on talent cultivation management model of universities based on fuzzy neural network algorithm. *International Journal of Maritime Engineering, 1*(1), 521–530. DOI: 10.1049/ijme.2024.05.024

Cheungsirakulvit, T., & Girdwichai, P. (2023). The development of Thailand's national sports development fund (NSDF) and the NSDF management strategy. *Unpublished manuscript.*

Clark, D. (2020). *Artificial intelligence for learning: How to use AI to support employee development.* Kogan Page Publishers.

Eid, A. I. A., Miled, A. B., Fatnassi, A., Nawaz, M. A., Mahmoud, A. F., Abdalla, F. A., Jabnoun, C., Dhibi, A., Allan, F. M., Elhossiny, M. A., Belhaj, S., & Mohamed, I. B. (2024). Sports prediction model through cloud computing and big data based on artificial intelligence method. *Journal of Intelligent Learning Systems and Applications, 16*(2), 53–79. DOI: 10.4236/jilsa.2024.162005

Harris, J. G., Craig, E., & Light, D. A. (2011). Talent and analytics: New approaches, higher ROI. *The Journal of Business Strategy, 32*(6), 4–13. DOI: 10.1108/02756661111180087

Hassan, Y., Pandey, J., Varkkey, B., Sethi, D., & Scullion, H. (2022). Understanding talent management for sports organizations: Evidence from an emerging country. *International Journal of Human Resource Management, 33*(11), 2192–2225. DOI: 10.1080/09585192.2021.1971736

Jasni, N. H., Mustapha, A., Tenah, S. S., Mostafa, S. A., & Razali, N. (2022). Prediction of player position for talent identification in association netball: A regression-based approach. *International Journal of Advances in Intelligent Informatics, 8*(1), 84. Advance online publication. DOI: 10.26555/ijain.v8i1.707

Kumar, A., Labshetwar, A., Kawale, A., & Aland, P. (2024). INDPLAY: A software solution for uncovering India's sporting talent. *International Journal of Innovative Research in Computer Science & Technology, 12*(3), 23–27. DOI: 10.55524/ijircst.2024.12.3.5

Liu, Z., & Zhang, X. (2024). Construction and optimization of sports athlete selection and talent cultivation system based on data analysis. *Journal of Electrical Systems, 20*(6s), 2070–2081. DOI: 10.52783/jes.3122

Marlapudi, K., & Lenka, U. (2024). Unlocking the potential: Redefining talent and competency mapping for Industry 4.0. *Management Research Review, 47*(11), 1805–1832. Advance online publication. DOI: 10.1108/MRR-07-2023-0496

McAuley, A. B., Baker, J., Johnston, K., & Kelly, A. L. (2024). Artificial intelligence in talent identification and development in sport. In *Artificial intelligence in sports, movement, and health* (pp. 255–270). Springer Nature Switzerland., DOI: 10.1007/978-3-031-67256-9_15

Mishra, N., Habal, B. G. M., Garcia, P. S., & Garcia, M. B. (2024, June). Harnessing an AI-driven analytics model to optimize training and treatment in physical education for sports injury prevention. In *Proceedings of the 2024 8th International Conference on Education and Multimedia Technology* (pp. 309-315). DOI: 10.1145/3678726.3678740

Parra-Martinez, F. A., & Wai, J. (2023). Talent identification research: A bibliometric study from multidisciplinary and global perspectives. *Frontiers in Psychology, 14*, 1141159. DOI: 10.3389/fpsyg.2023.1141159 PMID: 37303914

Reyaz, N., Ahamad, G., Khan, N. J., Naseem, M., & Ali, J. (2024). SVMCTI: Support vector machine based cricket talent identification model. *International Journal of Information Technology : an Official Journal of Bharati Vidyapeeth's Institute of Computer Applications and Management, 16*(3), 1931–1944. DOI: 10.1007/s41870-023-01686-w

Reynoso-Sanchez, L. F. (2023). Tech-driven talent identification in sports: Advancements and implications. *Health Nexus, 1*(3), 77–82. DOI: 10.61838/kman.hn.1.3.11

Sajadi, S. M., Baghaie, S., & Rezaei, R. (2024). Optimizing sports development: Identifying and prioritizing key indicators for professional and competitive sports. *World Development, 180*, 106651. DOI: 10.1016/j.worlddev.2024.106651

Smith, A., & Westerbeek, H. (2004). *The sport business future.* Bound in Great Britain. DOI: 10.1057/9780230513693

Till, K., & Baker, J. (2020). Challenges and [possible] solutions to optimizing talent identification and development in sport. *Frontiers in Psychology, 11*, 664. DOI: 10.3389/fpsyg.2020.00664 PMID: 32351427

# Chapter 10
# Artificial Intelligence and Machine Learning in Sport Research

**Gopal K. Shyam**
*Presidency University, India*

**Priyanka Bharti**
*REVA University, India*

## ABSTRACT

*In professional sports, there is potential to leverage extensive and detailed datasets generated from various aspects of the sports industry. However, challenges arise from the limited time available for data analysis and the vast amount and diversity of the data to be evaluated. Artificial Intelligence (AI) techniques can significantly aid decision-makers in addressing these challenges. Over the past twenty years, AI has significantly impacted how we analyze and engage with sports. This perspective paper offers a comprehensive overview of the machine learning paradigm, highlighting its potential to improve sports performance and business analytics. It reviews relevant research on AI and ML applications within the sports industry and presents hypothetical scenarios demonstrating how these technologies might influence the future of sports.*

## INTRODUCTION

The wide applicability of ML algorithms, combined with improved computing power and new data sources, has made sports organizations eager for new strategies to enhance both athletic and business performance. AI's influence extends beyond

DOI: 10.4018/979-8-3693-5385-1.ch010

performance analytics to the commercial aspects of sports, where organizations use AI to develop fan profiles and understand consumer preferences, enabling personalized experiences. Research has investigated the link between popular players or teams and audience demand across different sports.

Early explorations of AI's potential in sports, such as (Lapham & Bartlett, 1995), concentrated on applying expert systems to biomechanics. Authors in (Bartlett, 2006) further examined AI advancements in sports biomechanics, forecasting the future significance of multi-layer Artificial Neural Networks (ANNs), now referred to as Deep Learning. Later research delved into various AI applications, including nature-inspired algorithms and Bayesian methods for predicting player performance and match outcomes.

The AI community's embrace of open data and competitions like the Netflix Prize and Kaggle has accelerated AI adoption in multiple domains, including sports. Significant applications include ANN-based quality assessments, training optimizations, and AI algorithms used in Formula 1 and tennis racket recommendations. Recent AI advancements in board and virtual games such as Chess, Go, and Dota 2 highlight the potential for machines to surpass human champions using techniques like Reinforcement Learning and Monte Carlo Tree Search.

The concept of assembling a team based on in-game statistics gained significant attention with the publication of “Moneyball” (Lewis, 2014), which chronicled the Oakland Athletics' success. Despite operating on a limited budget, the team utilized a data-driven strategy to make the playoffs in 2002. Economic analyses of the Moneyball approach (Hakes & Sauer, 2016) showed that there was little correlation between player salaries and their actual contributions to winning games. By taking advantage of this market inefficiency, the Oakland Athletics were able to achieve a competitive edge. Following this, many Major League Baseball (MLB) teams started to adopt SABR metrics (Lewis, 2014), an analytical approach named after the Society for American Baseball Research. SABR metricians focus on collecting and analyzing in-game data to boost team performance. The rapid advancement in computing power has further propelled the analysis of big data in sports through AI. Organizations such as Baseball Savant/ StatCast and ESPN have significantly enhanced the precision and breadth of MLB analytics through improved data collection and aggregation.

The distinction between Machine Learning (ML) and traditional analytics lies in ML's ability to learn from data without explicit programming, allowing for more flexible and adaptive problem-solving methods.

Artificial Intelligence (AI) and Machine Learning (ML) have become essential tools in sports research, transforming the way teams, athletes, and organizations approach training, performance analysis, injury prevention, and fan engagement. Below is an overview of how AI and ML are utilized in sports research.

## Areas of AI and ML Application in Sports

1. **Player Tracking:** AI in sports analytics shows significant promise in player tracking. AI-driven tracking systems gather detailed data on players' movements, such as their speed, acceleration, and distance covered. Coaches can use this data to monitor player performance during both training and games, pinpointing areas for improvement and assessing the effectiveness of training programs (Li et al., 2020).
2. **Performance Analysis:** AI also excels in performance analysis within sports analytics. By processing extensive data on players' performances, AI can detect patterns and trends, offering insights into the strengths and weaknesses of individual players and teams. This information can be leveraged to optimize training programs and devise strategies to enhance performance (Lewis & Yoon, 2016).
3. **Game Strategy Optimization:** AI can significantly enhance game strategy optimization. By analyzing data on the strengths and weaknesses of opposing teams, AI algorithms assist coaches in developing game plans tailored to specific opponents. For instance, if a team is known for its fast-paced offense, AI can help coaches devise

## Proposed Model

Sports analytics and data visualization provide player selectors, managers, and players with a comprehensive platform to enhance on-field performance. Graphs and charts are vital components of visualization and predictive analytics, helping to present data. This information is then used by team selectors, captains, and executives to gain a comprehensive understanding of all factors affecting the season, including team performance, all-rounders, and batsmen, to inform decisions for the next auction.

The proposed model is described here. The input video selects a specific number of consecutive RGB color frames, which then undergo additional processing steps such as resizing, rescaling, multiplying, and normalization. These pre-processing stages convert the raw frames into processed frames, making them suitable for neural network analysis.

Before processing, it is crucial to extract representative information from the rules to create well-structured and logically arranged data structures that reflect the dependencies between rules. Each incoming data frame is compared to this structure to determine the most cost-effective matching rule.

Spatial features are extracted from the video images using a convolutional neural network (CNN). The proposed CNN consists of convolution layers followed by max-pooling and an activation function to extract features from the processed frames.

These features are then passed to the classification layer, where temporal features are gathered through the CNN. Finally, the sports class is classified using Softmax function-based output layers, which are preceded by fully connected layers.

The sports data visualization management system includes the following functions:

1. Real-time collection of athletes' motion data via wearable devices, with integration into data server databases.
2. The motion visualization management system retrieves data from the servers to create real-time animated visual representations, enabling data visualization.
3. A Convolutional Neural Network (CNN) predicts future motion states based on athletes' previous workout data.
4. Multi-virtual role management and human-computer interaction.

Practitioners can utilize various analytical methods and techniques within athlete monitoring systems. It is essential to consider multiple variables during data collection, identify relevant changes, and explore different presentation methods. Effective communication of key information to coaches is vital for enhancing athletic performance and is the cornerstone of a successful athlete monitoring system.

## Methodology

The performance metrics were computed for each classification task within the video dataset. Each classification pertained to specific types of video events or viewpoints. The steps involved were:

1. **Classification of Data Types:**
    - o Each video was categorized based on predefined event or viewpoint types.
    - o The model was applied to classify these categories.
2. **Exact/Improper Classification:**
    - o Each classification was assessed as either exact (correct) or improper (incorrect).
    - o The aforementioned metrics were calculated for each category based on these classifications.
3. **Averaging Results:**
    - o The performance outcomes of all video categories or shots were averaged to determine the overall performance of the VEVF model.
    - o This approach ensures that the final evaluation reflects the model's ability across a variety of scenarios and data types.

## Performance Analysis of the Proposed Model

To evaluate the performance of the proposed model using big data analytics, this study employed several objective metrics. These metrics—accuracy (A), recall (R), precision (P), F1-score, and error rate (E)—are crucial for assessing the model's effectiveness in classification tasks. The analysis was conducted as follows:

1. **Accuracy (A):**
    - **Definition:** The proportion of true results (both true positives and true negatives) among the total number of cases examined.
    - **Significance:** Provides a general measure of how often the model correctly classifies the video data.
2. **Recall (R):**
    - **Definition:** The proportion of actual positives that are correctly identified by the model (also known as sensitivity or true positive rate).
    - **Significance:** Indicates the model's ability to identify all relevant instances within a dataset.
3. **Precision (P):**
    - **Definition:** The proportion of positive identifications that are actually correct.
    - **Significance:** Measures the accuracy of the positive predictions made by the model.
4. **F1-Score:**
    - **Definition:** The harmonic mean of precision and recall, providing a balance between the two metrics.
    - **Significance:** Useful for evaluating the model's performance when dealing with imbalanced classes.
5. **Error Rate (E):**
    - **Definition:** The proportion of incorrectly classified instances.
    - **Significance:** Complements accuracy by indicating the frequency of misclassifications.

## Datasets

Authors in (Pavitt, Braines, & Tomsett, 2022) explored the application of natural language processing (NLP) and conversational interfaces (CI) in the context of match analysis and scouting. Their study highlights how these technologies can provide analytical support to sports professionals by simplifying access to and interaction with complex data.

Authors in (Fenil et al., 2019) proposed a novel approach for real-time violence detection in football stadiums by combining the Histogram of Oriented Gradients (HOG) with Bidirectional Long Short-Term Memory (BDLSTM). This system aims to process large volumes of video data in real time and simulate human intelligence to recognize aggressive behavior.

Authors in (Rafiq et al., 2023) proposed the use of transfer learning (TL) for the task of sports video summarization, specifically focusing on scene classification within sports videos. Their approach demonstrates significant improvements in scene categorization accuracy through the application of advanced ML techniques.

We propose to visualize sports news data, offering a novel approach to understanding and interpreting the evolution of sports media events. The study focuses on the analysis and classification of large sporting events using a combination of data statistics techniques and theoretical frameworks.

*Table 1. Model performance evaluation and comparison table with the state-of-the-art models*

| Ref./ Method Name | Epoch | Accuracy% | Error% | Precision% | Recall% | F1-Score% |
|---|---|---|---|---|---|---|
| (Pavitt, Braines, & Tomsett, 2022)/ Natural Language Processing [NLP] | 50 | 98.09 | 1.91 | 98.20 | 97.09 | 96.07 |
| (Fenil et al., 2019)/ Bidirectional Long Short-Term Memory (BDLSTM) | 50 | 86.71 | 13.29 | 87.28 | 86.71 | 86.80 |
| (Rafiq et al., 2023)/Convolutional Neural Network (CNN) | 50 | 89.26 | 1.04 | 89.27 | 98.26 | 89.26 |
| Proposed | 50 | 98.26 | 0.94 | 98.27 | 98.76 | 98.16 |

*Figure 1. Performance gain over the existing state-of-the-art methods.*

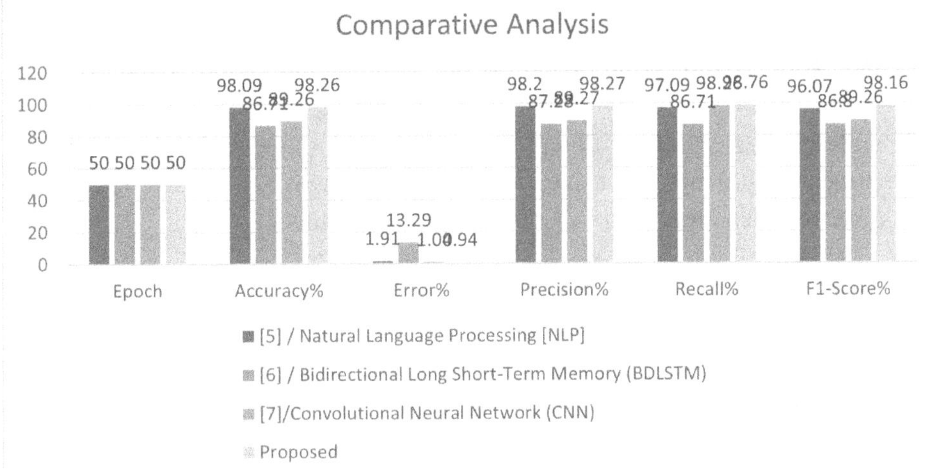


The method proposed in (Pavitt, Braines, & Tomsett, 2022) and (Fenil et al., 2019) is implemented and evaluated using the same dataset as of the proposed model. Results in Figure 1 show a performance gain over the existing state-of-the-art methods. Furthermore, the proposed method shows a performance superiority over competitive models.

## Key Challenges for AI Usage in Elite Sports

Our analysis identifies six key challenges for the application of AI in elite sports, integrating both current status and emerging opportunities. These challenges are framed within the four methodical categories of AI usage in elite sports: image processing, signal processing, modeling & planning, and user interaction, and aligned with the SMPA (Sense, Model, Plan, Act) loop.

### 1. Data Quality and Availability

**Challenge:** The effectiveness of AI systems heavily relies on high-quality, comprehensive datasets. In elite sports, collecting consistent, accurate data can be challenging due to the variability in sports environments and the need for extensive labeling and annotation.

- **Image Processing (Sense):** Ensuring high-resolution, correctly labeled images from varied angles and in different conditions.

- **Signal Processing (Sense):** Capturing accurate, noise-free signals from athletes' movements or physiological data.

## 2. Integration of Multimodal Data

**Challenge:** Combining different types of data (e.g., video, biometric signals, environmental data) into a cohesive system for comprehensive analysis and decision-making is complex and requires sophisticated algorithms.

- **Modeling & Planning (Model & Plan):** Developing machine learning models that effectively integrate and analyze multimodal data to provide actionable insights.
- **User Interaction (Act):** Ensuring the data from various sources can be seamlessly presented to coaches and athletes in an intuitive manner.

## 3. Real-Time Processing and Feedback

**Challenge:** AI systems in sports often need to process data and provide feedback in real-time, which requires efficient algorithms and substantial computational power.

- **Image & Signal Processing (Sense):** Implementing real-time image and signal processing to monitor and analyze performance during live events.
- **User Interaction (Act):** Delivering instantaneous feedback through wearables or virtual reality systems without delays that could disrupt the athlete's performance.

## 4. Personalization and Adaptation

**Challenge:** Athletes have unique physical and psychological profiles, necessitating AI systems that can adapt and personalize recommendations and feedback.

- **Modeling & Planning (Model & Plan):** Creating adaptive models that learn and evolve with the athlete's progress and changing conditions.
- **User Interaction (Act):** Customizing the interaction based on individual athlete's preferences and responses.

## 5. Ethical and Privacy Concerns

**Challenge:** The use of AI in sports raises ethical issues related to data privacy, consent, and the potential for misuse of sensitive information.

- **Image & Signal Processing (Sense):** Ensuring data collection respects athletes' privacy and is conducted with their consent.
- **Modeling & Planning (Model & Plan):** Developing ethical guidelines and secure systems to protect the data and uphold the integrity of the sport.

## 6. Acceptance and Adoption

**Challenge:** For AI to be effectively utilized, coaches, athletes, and support staff must trust and adopt these technologies, which requires addressing concerns about reliability and ease of use.

- **User Interaction (Act):** Designing user-friendly interfaces and ensuring the system's transparency to foster trust and ease of integration into existing workflows.
- **Modeling & Planning (Model & Plan):** Providing clear explanations of AI decisions and predictions to build confidence among users.

The issues, problems, and trends related to Artificial Intelligence (AI) and Machine Learning (ML) in sports research are increasingly recognized, but there is still room for greater emphasis in several key areas.

1. Ethical Considerations:
    - **Bias and Fairness:** While there is growing awareness of bias in AI and ML models, the sports industry has only just begun to address how these biases might affect decisions around player selection, injury prediction, and performance evaluation. The potential for AI to reinforce existing inequalities, particularly in scouting and talent identification, requires more focused attention.
    - **Data Privacy:** As teams and organizations gather more data on athletes through wearable technology and other means, concerns about data privacy are becoming more pressing. While these issues are acknowledged, they often take a back seat to the excitement surrounding AI-driven insights.
2. Reliability and Validity:
    - **Accuracy of Predictions:** The reliability of AI and ML models, particularly in predicting outcomes like injuries or game results, is sometimes overestimated. While the technology is advancing rapidly, the accuracy of these models still depends heavily on the quality and quantity of the data they are trained on. There needs to be a more critical evaluation of these predictions and an understanding of their limitations.

- **Transparency:** AI models, especially those that are complex and use deep learning techniques, can be opaque, making it difficult for coaches and sports scientists to understand and trust the recommendations. The trend towards explainable AI is growing, but more emphasis should be placed on ensuring that these tools are transparent and user-friendly.

3. Integration with Traditional Methods:
   - **Balancing AI with Human Expertise:** While AI and ML offer powerful tools, there is a risk of over-reliance on technology at the expense of human judgment. The best outcomes often arise from a combination of AI insights and traditional coaching wisdom. However, this balanced approach isn't always emphasized, especially in environments that are eager to adopt the latest technologies.
   - **Training and Education:** There is a need for greater emphasis on educating coaches, players, and sports scientists about the capabilities and limitations of AI and ML. Understanding how to effectively integrate these tools into existing practices is crucial, yet this area sometimes lacks the attention it deserves.
4. Accessibility and Inclusivity:
   - **Access to Technology:** There is a growing divide between organizations that have access to cutting-edge AI and ML tools and those that do not, often due to financial constraints. This issue is recognized but is not always given the emphasis it needs, particularly in grassroots and amateur sports.
   - **Global Adoption:** The focus on AI and ML in sports research is often concentrated in well-funded sports and regions. Expanding the reach of these technologies to less-developed areas and a wider range of sports is crucial for ensuring that the benefits are more broadly distributed.
5. Long-Term Impact:
   - **Sustainability of AI Initiatives:** There is enthusiasm for AI and ML in sports, but not enough emphasis on the long-term sustainability of these initiatives. Maintaining and updating AI systems requires continuous investment, and there should be more discussion about the resources needed to support these technologies over time.
   - **Impact on Athlete Development:** While AI can optimize short-term performance, there is a need for more research into its long-term impact on athlete development. Overemphasis on data-driven decisions could potentially stifle creativity and adaptability in athletes if not carefully managed.

## CONCLUSION

AI brings numerous advantages to sports. From player tracking and performance analysis to game strategy optimization, AI can enhance both individual and team performances while improving the spectator experience. As AI technology advances, we can expect even more innovative applications in sports analytics in the coming years.

The use of objective metrics allows for a comprehensive evaluation of the proposed model's performance. By examining accuracy, recall, precision, F1-score, and error rate, this study provides a detailed understanding of the model's strengths and areas for improvement. This thorough performance analysis is crucial for refining the model and enhancing its practical application in real-world scenarios involving video data classification.

Addressing these challenges is essential to fully harness the potential of AI in elite sports. By improving data quality, integrating multimodal data, ensuring real-time processing, personalizing interactions, maintaining ethical standards, and encouraging acceptance and adoption, AI can greatly enhance performance analysis, training, and decision-making processes in elite sports.

## REFERENCES


Bartlett, R. (2006). Artificial intelligence in sports biomechanics: New dawn or false hope? *Journal of Sports Science & Medicine*, *5*, 474–479. PMID: 24357939

Fenil, E., Manogaran, G., Vivekananda, G. N., Thanjaivadivel, T., Jeeva, S., & Ahilan, A. (2019). Real-time violence detection framework for football stadium comprising of big data analysis and deep learning through bidirectional LSTM. *Computer Networks*, *151*, 191–200. DOI: 10.1016/j.comnet.2019.01.028

Hakes, J. K., and Sauer, R. D. (2016). An economic evaluation of the Moneyball hypothesis. J. Econ. Perspect. 20, 173–186. doi: . 3.173DOI: 10.1257/jep.20

Lapham, A. C., & Bartlett, R. M. (1995). The use of artificial intelligence in the analysis of sports performance: A review of applications in human gait analysis and future directions for sports biomechanics. *Journal of Sports Sciences*, *13*(3), 229–237. DOI: 10.1080/02640419508732232 PMID: 7563290

Lewis, M. (2014). *Moneyball: The Art of Winning an Unfair Game*. WW Norton and Company.

Lewis, M., & Yoon, Y. (2016). An empirical examination of the development and impact of star power in Major League Baseball. *Journal of Sports Economics*, *19*(2), 155–187. DOI: 10.1177/1527002515626220

Li, J., Liu, S., Wang, Z., & Guo, J. (2020). Neutrosophy theory based visualization report of sports news data. *International Journal of Electrical Engineering Education*, •••, 0020720920940581.

Pavitt, J., Braines, D., & Tomsett, R. (2022). Cognitive analysis in sports: Supporting match analysis and scouting through artificial intelligence. *Applied AI Letters*, *2*(1), e22.

Rafiq, M., Rafiq, G., Agyeman, R., Choi, G. S., & Jin, S. I. (2023). Scene classification for sports video summarization using transfer learning. *Sensors (Basel)*, *20*(6), 1702. DOI: 10.3390/s20061702 PMID: 32197502

# Chapter 11
# Artificial Neural Networks for Talent Identification and Scouting

**Minakshi**
https://orcid.org/0000-0001-7586-6309
*King Khalid University, Saudi Arabia*

**Tarun Kumar**
https://orcid.org/0000-0002-8507-8522
*Galgotias University, Greater Noida, India*

**Suman Devi**
https://orcid.org/0000-0002-4038-7196
*Galgotias University, Greater Noida, India*

## ABSTRACT

*Talent identification and scouting are essential in sports, enabling organizations to identify and nurture talented players destined for success. This chapter focuses on how artificial neural networks (ANNs) have transformed these processes. It covers ANNs' basics, data collection, and preprocessing ideas specific to sports analytics. It shows various neural network types, like feedforward, convolutional, and recurrent networks, useful for tasks like injury prediction, performance measurement, and future prediction. Additionally, it includes a discussion of training and optimization algorithms, case studies, and real-world applications in various sports. The chapter concludes by addressing challenges and future research, including data quality, interpretability, ethical issues, and ANNs' integration with other modern technologies. Utilizing ANNs' potential may significantly develop sports organizations by helping them identify and nurture talented players and gain a competitive edge in*

DOI: 10.4018/979-8-3693-5385-1.ch011

*a data and technology-based future of sport.*

## 1. INTRODUCTION

Talents are a critical element of any successful sports program. Not only do athletes contribute to the success of the programs, but they are also the program's acceptable face. Scouts identify raw talents that require refinement to become professional athletes capable of high-level performance. Talent identification and scouting are the processes through which sports organizations identify young or relatively unknown athletes who can potentially perform at the highest levels (McCullagh, 2010). The processes are very critical for various reasons. First, good and efficient talent identification helps the organization or team secure athletes before rivals discover them. It enables them to reach their full potential, thus making a significant contribution to a biosystem or an organization. Second, large amounts of money go into developing and training athletes, thus providing guidelines for which athletes are worth such an investment and saving on losses (Hong, 2023). This aids in the effective distribution of resources, ensuring that the athletes with the highest potential receive more funding and other essential resources. Talent identification is also critical in ensuring that the athlete pipeline remains stable, particularly in the biosystems that ensure sports continuity (Barron et al., 2020).

Traditionally, scouts and other professionals would use their knowledge and experience in the selected field to conduct such an exercise. Scouting is dependent on some factors, including personal experience, quality criteria, and a selective approach (Xu et al., 2016). As a result, the performance under consideration helps to complete the identification and selection process. Identification is an essential part of talent identification and forms the basis for their selection (Jasni et al., 2022). One limitation is that sportsmen's manual speed is prone to error. Additionally, it varies from one judge to another. A person competing with another might score differently for a different judge. A good judgment can allow a fast but not so speedy athlete to compete. Thus, the player will have to move out to create space for the other athlete. Fig. 1 illustrates the desired attributes and skills of a photographic mind, highlighting qualities such as being trustworthy, organized, committed, knowledgeable, able to understand formations and patterns, recall phases of play, work under pressure, manage time effectively, network, be attentive to details, meet deadlines, build relationships, and maintain a flexible and can-do attitude.

*Figure 1.* **Attributes and Basic Skill Set of Football Scout**

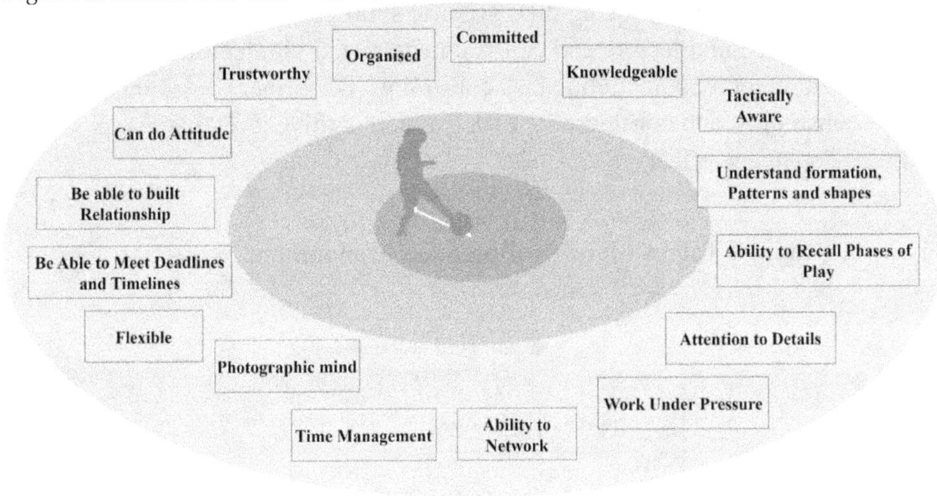


Another challenge is the inherent time and resource commitment of traditional scouting methods, which often necessitate extensive travel and on-site visits. Scouting on a restricted geographic base means missing a limited number of opportunities, particularly for athletes from rare geographic backgrounds with more challenging access to scouting opportunities (Radicchi & Mozzachiodi, 2016a). It is also challenging because it requires the ability to assess long-term potential with limited evidence. Factors such as injuries, physical development, training availability, and other elements will play a role in determining the athlete's ultimate potential course.

Artificial neural networks, which function as information processing systems inspired by the structured neural network of the brain, offer a promising and data-fueled method for enhancing scouting and talent identification in sports (Kirola et al., 2023). These models, based on the large-scale data and the patterns and interactions they generate, have the ability to overcome the aforementioned conventional methods. An artificial neural network can collect a tremendous amount of data based on sports statistics, physical indicators and measurements, biomechanical analysis of movements, played games and video recordings, and various other sources and assist the talent scout by finding correlations, variability, and relationships that the expert may miss due to a lack of processing capacity and computing power (Sayal et al., 2023). Furthermore, the artificial neural network can adapt to new data from various sources, as previously discussed. The artificial neural network's developer can feed the system new incoming information trends and use them in relevant terms. It is a significant advantage given the general unpredictability of the sports field and emerging training tendencies (Reyaz et al., 2022). And finally, an artificial neural network can overcome the existing expertise bias. Unlike human talent scouts, artificial systems have no bias, whether based on the fact of their country or the athlete's country, favoring their specific sport or athlete type. Fig. 2 depicts the multi-dimensional factors and constraints involved in talent identification and development in football, including task constraints, performer constraints, environmental constraints, and considerations such as competitive level, playing positions, and the relative age effect.

*Figure 2.* **Scope of Talent Identification and Development**

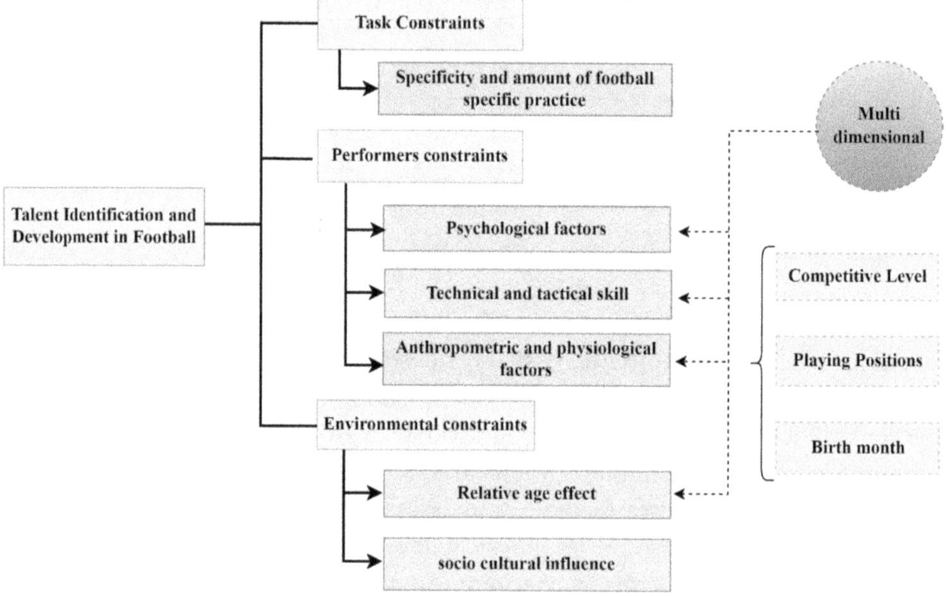


This chapter aims to provide an extensive review of artificial neural network applications for talent scouting and identification in sports. It will cover the main artificial neural networks and their architecture, such as feedforward artificial neural networks, convolutional artificial neural networks, and recurrent artificial neural networks (X. Huang, 2023). It will then discuss data collection and preprocessing for artificial neural network training, including data sources, feature extraction, and data preparation (Mwaro et al., 2021). Afterward, the chapter will describe the various artificial neural network architectures and training methodologies designed specifically for talent scouting applications such as performance prediction, injury prediction, and general potential identification. The chapter will also present use cases and examples of artificial neural network applications in multiple sports. The chapter will conclude with an overview of the ethical aspects, biases, and interpretability challenges associated with the use of artificial neural networks in talent identification and scouting. It will also encompass related future research regions and upcoming trends to provide an outlook on how artificial neural networks can change the way talent is found and developed in sports.

## 2. FUNDAMENTALS OF ARTIFICIAL NEURAL NETWORKS

### 2.1 Biological inspiration and artificial neuron model

Artificial neural networks are computational constructs whose architecture and principles of operation are designed to mimic the structure and function of their biological counterparts. Synapses interconnect billions of neurons in the human brain, relaying electrical signals in the form of action potentials. In a similar manner, artificial neural networks are composed of artificial neurons or nodes, which process the information through signal propagation (Bairui et al., 2019). The artificial neuron is a formal mathematical model of the neuron's function that includes the reception, processing, and transmission of signals (Daga et al., 2020). The artificial neuron receives the signal, applies the activation function, and then transmits it to the next node in the network (Yi et al., 2019). Moreover, the neuron utilizes all signals that are received as inputs. The neuron weights each input signal based on its significance or cooperation, and then adds it to the weighted sum (Jauhiainen et al., 2019). The activation function is responsible for transforming and limiting the signal's range of values. There are many types of activation functions. This guide uses the sigmoid function.

### 2.2 Types of neural networks

Growing over time, ANN achieved incredible variety and complexity. These days, it focuses on genesis and the creation of new architectures and types. The most frequent artificial neural network types are as follows:

1) **Feedforward Neural Networks:** This type of network represents the simplest form of topology; the information transfuses only forward. The input layer transmits data to a hidden layer, which then relays it to other layers, until the output layer receives it (Allal-Chérif et al., 2021). Such networks perform normal and differentiated tasks, such as describing a person in a face identification system or detecting fires in a company using open-source biodiversity software.
2) **Recurrent Neural Networks:** Unlike feedforward networks, RNNs have cyclic connections that allow information to flow in both directions (Abbott et al., 2005). They are well-suited to sequential data, such as time series, natural

language, and speech recognition, because RNNs are able to preserve an inner state to understand and model temporal dependencies in the data.

3) **Convolutional Neural Networks:** CNNs, a prevalent type of artificial neural networks, distinguish themselves from other neural networks by their ability to leverage spatial relations in both 1D and 2D translations. CNNs use convolutional layers to learn numerous filters, which subsequently extract features from the input and reduce data dimensionality (Jantan et al., 2012). They are widely known for their use in identifying objects from images, image classification, and facial recognition.
4) **Autoencoders:** On the other hand, unsupervised learning and dimensionality reduction exercises commonly employ autoencoders. It consists of an abundance network that reduces the input data's measurements to a reduced variety, as well as a decoder network that then attempts to restore the input from the reduced representation (Ma & Ding, 2022). Denoising reconstruction, or anomaly pattern recognition, is one example.
5) **Generative Adversarial Networks:** It introduces a new concept to all other recurring theme examples: the utilization of two neural networks to accomplish tasks that would otherwise be unfeasible. The system consists of one generator that generates synthetic information, and another that ensures the separation of manufactured data from genuine data. This system finds applications in image synthesis, data augmentation, and style transfer (Razali et al., 2017). These neural network architectures offer insight into how to develop solutions for various challenges and businesses, depending on the type of data or problem the system is intended to address.

## 2.3 Training algorithms (backpropagation, gradient descent, etc)

The process of training artificial neural networks is critical to enabling these models to learn from the given data under their patterns and relationships. The most widely utilized training algorithm in artificial neural networks is backpropagation (Ozcaglar et al., 2019). Backpropagation is a gradient-based optimization neural network that operates using an optimization method known as gradient descent. Similarly, we also call the process of optimizing ANNs' neural network units, known as neurons, "training." The most popular training methodologies are:

1) Backpropagation is a supervised learning algorithm that adjusts synapse weights and neuronal biases to minimize the difference between the network's actual output and the desired output. The process of learning via backpropagation begins with an initial set of weights in the ANNE's synapses. This neural-based,

supervised learning algorithm primarily targets pattern recognition (Uddin & Lee, 2017). This algorithm calculates the error value, which it then uses for training. The approach enables neurons to understand and process output more effectively.

2) Gradient Descent: This optimization algorithm iteratively finds the minimum of a function by adjusting the parameters in the indirect ratio to the function's gradient. The ANN's goal is to minimize the cost or error function that determines the back-propagation calculation values (Jantan et al., 2011). In this approach, it follows a reverse path, and gradient descent calculates the outcomes.

Various gradient descent algorithms are available, including:

a) Stochastic gradient descent: A stochastic gradient descent (SGD) minimizes the parameters for individual training examples. Therefore, it is considered useful, especially when dealing with the dataset.
b) Mini-batch gradient descent: Mini-batch gradient descent minimizes the gradient for a few sets of training examples. Just like mini batch, it achieves parallel for datasets.
c) Momentum: This minimizes the gradient for a normal-relevant dataset.
d) Adaptive learning rate algorithms ADAM and RMS Prop: They adjust the learning rate dynamically.

## 2.4 Other advanced training techniques include regularization methods, batch normalization, and transfer learning with artificial neural networks.

1. ANNs' performance can surpass that of other linear models or even human abilities, but one of their unique advantages is their nonlinearity capability. ANNs are nonlinear because of their activation function. This implies that with sufficient hidden units and training data, they can approximate any continuous function with any degree of accuracy (L.-C. Huang et al., 2004). As a result, most real-world data is nonlinear; ANNs are often the best option for this type of data.
2. Adaptability: ANNs' adaptability would be another advantage. ANNs adjust weights and biases using experience because of their ability to learn from data. The network can adapt during the input-output mapping stage (Flores-Hernández et al., 2019). The adaptability allows them to master the complexities of analyzing patterns and relationships in the dataset, where the task or solution rules are impossible to understand.

3. Parallelism or massive potential: In a biological analogy, one may say that ANNs are parallel systems. Because a human can process many different data streams simultaneously, they have many people.
4. Fault Tolerance: A related advantage is the fact that, with some exclusion, ANNs exhibit a degree of fault tolerance. Despite a few spoiled models or connections, the NN maintains its functionality (Myrén & Neto, 2017). This is because learning in an ANN occurs through weight adaptation, not individual connection.
5. Generalization: Fully trained ANNs can generalize from the training data to out-of-sample data to adequately predict or classify new, previously unseen inputs (Jantan et al., 2010). This ability to generalize is critical for applications such as talent identification and scouting since it enables the identification of likely talent based on scarce data and the prediction of future performance.

The quality and quantity of training data, network architecture, and the optimal selection of hyperparameters and training algorithms all influence the efficacy of ANNs, despite their many benefits (Khurana et al., 2023).

## 3. DATA COLLECTION AND PREPROCESSING

### 3.1 Relevant data sources

The efficiency of talent identification and scouting using artificial neural networks requires relevant data (Waheed et al., 2014). Many data sources in the sports domain can compile a comprehensive profile of an individual athlete's performance and physical attributes, enabling the assessment of their potential. Such sources can include:

1. **Performance metrics:** These metrics serve as quantitative indicators of an athlete's performance during competition, training, or simulation. It includes game statistics, biomechanical data, and physiological data.
2. **Physical attributes:** It measure the physical characteristics of a specific athlete. These can include height, weight, body composition, muscle strength, flexibility, and other body measurements such as wingspan and knee height. Some datasets can provide an understanding of an athlete's potential based on these attributes.
3. **Video footage:** Video footage is a compilation of digital information based on visual data captured during competition, training, or scouting (Vilela et al., 2018). Computer vision analysis can capture data on motion patterns, technique, visual decision-making, and other relevant game information from such footage.

4. **Injury and medical data:** We can also use information about a specific athlete's medical history and injury record. It can be useful in analyzing players' durability and understanding their long-term prospects.
5. **Psychological and cognitive data:** The data obtained from psychological and cognitive research can provide a great contextual input into potential (Khan et al., 2023). Psychological tests can measure an athlete's skillset based on mental traits that might predict performance, such as decision-making, stress management, focus, and cognitive processing speed.
6. **Demographic and contextual data:** Information about an athlete's contextual background can be valuable. It includes age, location, socioeconomic context, and access to training facilities, among other relevant data (Xiao et al., 2020).

Several stakeholders, such as sports organizations, coaches and scouts, wearables, and specialized testing centers, can provide such data (Lowman, 2016). Often, the integration and synthesis of data from several sources can provide a more complete and multi-factorial picture of an athlete's talent or ability.

## 3.2 Data cleaning and normalization

Raw data from various sources can often contain errors, inconsistencies, or structural flaws, which can adversely affect ANNs' performance. Therefore, data cleaning and normalization are required preprocessing steps to ensure data quality and correlation. Data cleaning consists of identifying and processing missing data points, inconsistencies, duplicates, and error or outlier points that can be detrimental to the analysis. Imputation, interpolation, and filtering are a few of the ways to clean and prepare the data for further processing (Atlas & Zhang, 2004). Normalization suggests that correct scaling of input features to a regular scale typically improves the performance of ANNs. This helps with the training convergence process and prevents one feature from "drowning" others in the process. Min-max scaling, z-score standardization, and log-transformation are a few of the normalization mechanisms.

## 3.3 Feature extraction and selection.

Often, raw data from different sources is not the most appropriate for direct input into ANNs.

1. **Feature extraction:** This entails turning the raw data into a suitable feature set that remains relevant to the nature of the task. Feature extraction may involve techniques such as principal component analysis, independent component

analysis, and autoencoders, among others, to extract the relevant features from high-dimensional data such as video footage or time series.

2. **Feature selection:** Furthermore, feature selection refers to the process of identifying and utilizing only those meaningful and highly informative subsets among a large set of possible ones. Feature selection techniques not only optimize learning by reducing input data, but also mitigate the curse of dimensionality and prevent overfitting (Youping & Jiangang, 2022). Methods used for feature selection include filter methods like correlation analysis and mutual information, wrapper methods that consider the performance of a particular learning model on a specific subset, and embedded methods that select features as the learning model. While a wide range of techniques can achieve feature selection and extraction, it is crucial to choose appropriate methods based on the data source and the ANN settings (Mishra et al., 2020). Therefore, the domain knowledge and experience in sports science and analytics will be appropriate for identifying the most suitable features to include, which may denote the best aspects of athlete talent with the possibility identification.

## 3.4 Splitting data into training, validation, and testing sets

We should properly organize the available data into three sets for improved reliability and generalization capabilities.

1. **The training set:** It is a portion of data used to train the ANN model. The model tunes its internal parameters, i.e., weights and biases, to minimize the error or loss function against the training data used. This is essentially an iterative process that allows the model to learn patterns and relationships within the data.
2. **Validation set:** The validation set is also a portion of data used separately to assess the performance of the trained model throughout the iteration process of training (Subha et al., 2022). Therefore, unlike the training set, we do not evaluate the validation and hyperparameters separately, nor do we monitor the generalization level. Ideally, the function of the validation set is to avoid overfitting, as the performance of the model tuned against this unseen data is an estimate of how the model can perform on a new set of examples unseen before.
3. **Testing set:** The testing set refers to the last independent set of data not used at any instance during the training, including the validation process. We use this set to finally determine the performance of the well-optimized ANN model against previously unseen data (Qin et al., 2023). This provides an unbiased estimate of such a model's generalization. Although it can vary, the ratio typically allocates 60–80% of the data for training, 10–20% for validation, and another

10–20% for testing. However, we can adjust the ratio based on the size of the available dataset, task complexity, and the ultimate analysis needs (Kalaivani & Elamparithi, 2014). Proper splitting is essential, as it would allow a model to learn patterns from the training data and then predict generalizable patterns in the new unseen data. This is essential for effective talent identification and sports scouting.

## 4. NEURAL NETWORK ARCHITECTURES FOR TALENT IDENTIFICATION

### 4.1 Feedforward Neural Networks

Feedforward neural networks are one of the most common types of neural network architectures used in sports talent identification and scouting applications. The term "feedforward" suggests a single direction of information flow: the network passes the input data forward without any cycles or loops. FFNNs consist of a variety of components:

1. **The input layer** of an FFNN serves to input the initial data. These may consist of dependent attributes or a collection of tables containing information about the player being evaluated (Mat-Rasid, Abdullah, Juahir, Maliki, Kosni, et al., 2019). You can use attributes such as player physical measurements, biomechanical data, and game statistics, among others.
2. **Hidden layers and activation functions** are located between the input and output layers. They make it possible for the network to find relationships between the input and output data that have complex, non-linear, and high-order forms (Lüdin et al., 2023). Each neuron in the hidden layers receives information from the previous layer based on its weights, applies an activation function, and passes on the result to the next layer. The hidden layers use activation functions to introduce non-linearity in the FFNN, enabling the network to model complex patterns and decision boundaries (Woods et al., 2016). The output layer's sigmoid and tanh functions are two examples of common activation functions. Depending on the task, the FFNN's output layer can take on various types. For a regression task such as scoring the talent or performance level of a player, the output layer can use a linear activation function since the output is a continuous scale.
3. **Output layer,** on the other hand, when classification tasks are being done, like telling the difference between athletes with different levels of skill or guessing which positions or sports they would be good at, the output layer might have

more than one neuron, each representing a different class (Wrang et al., 2022). The output neurons have a softmax activation function, producing normalized class probabilities that sum to one. What learning algorithms are available for training? FFNNs can then be trained using various supervised learning algorithms, such as backpropagation or gradient descent, to find the optimal weight values for reducing the error between the network's predictions and the true values of the target variable.

## 4.2 Convolutional Neural Networks

CNNs are particularly well-suited for analyzing visual data, such as video data that records athletes' movements and performances. CNNs have been particularly useful in computer vision and may also have scalable and diversified opportunities in talent identification and sports scouting.

### 4.2.1 Application in video analysis and motion tracking

A critical component of this process is video analysis and motion tracking, which provide invaluable information about athletes' biomechanics, technique, and decision-making. Thus, we can use CNNs to automatically track the athletes' body position in relation to others and the ball (Chien & Chen, 2008). By identifying athletes based on their movement patterns and associations through CNN, scouts can learn, for example, what kind of patterns can lead to a successful decision. Fig. 3 illustrates the architecture of a convolutional neural network (CNN) for image classification, showing the different layers involved, including convolutional layers, pooling layers, fully connected layers, and output layers like softmax and classification result.

*Figure 3.* **Frontiers I Convolutional Neural Network-Based Human Movement Recognition Algorithm in Sports**

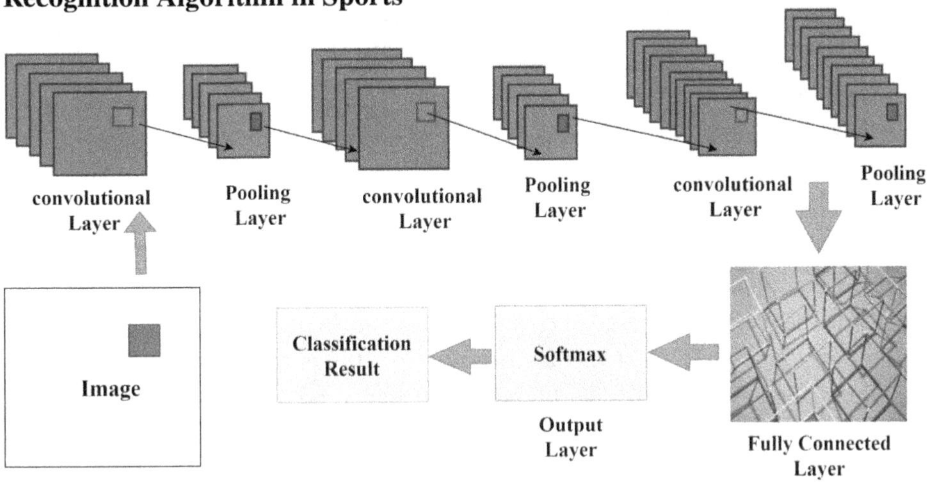


## 4.2.2 Feature extraction and hierarchical representations

CNNs are especially good at feature extraction and learning hierarchical representations, making them well-suited to deal with complex visual data. A CNN consists of convolutional layers that pass input data through learnable filters (Jha et al., n.d.). As the filters pass through data from the input, they extract low-level data such as edges, shapes, and textures. The network gets better at extracting more abstract or higher-level features as the data moves through more convolution and pooling layers. This lets it capture more complex patterns and representations. CNNs are therefore capable of learning relevant features for talent identification and scouting without the need for feature engineering (Jaffar et al., 2019). Thus, when combined with advanced computer vision and motion tracking techniques, CNNs are able to give a comprehensive assessment of an athlete's level (Sridevi & Kamala Suganthi, 2021; Utamayasa, 2021). These artificial intelligence models can analyze not only quantitative data but also qualitative data, which ensures an unbiased assessment of talents. Such algorithms can process additional external data, such as performance metrics, anthropometry, and other physiological quantities.

### 4.2.3 Recurrent Neural Networks

RNNs are particularly good at processing sequential data, which is inherent in the sports domain. By analyzing the dynamics of a sportsman's performance and identifying patterns that may indicate his future level, we can use RNNs for talent identification and preview (Chamorro-Premuzic et al., 2016). RNNs perform this function because their creation involves working with sequential data. The basic idea of RNN is simple: they have a loop of network elements.

When you input sequential performance data, such as game statistics, physiological measurements, or biomechanical data, an RNN can learn to capture patterns and trends that may be predictive of an athlete's future performance trajectory and potential (Akhtar et al., 2019). One example of this is to identify talented individuals who have not yet reached their performance peak but have demonstrated positive signs of growth and development. Consequently, researchers have developed specialized RNN architectures, including long-short-term memory and gated recurrent units (Jantan et al., 2012). The vanishing or exploding gradient problem is one of the biggest problems with traditional RNNs. It makes it hard for them to learn long-term dependencies in sequential data, like how a player does over the course of a whole season or career. This is because of many internal and external factors, such as performance-related growth or maturity curves (Pruna et al., 2018) (Ye et al., 2009). LSTMs and GRUs effectively capture, store, and utilize long-term dependencies in the input data through the use of gating mechanisms (King et al., 2024; Pruna et al., 2018) . Consequently, these architectures have demonstrated significant utility in talent identification and scouting scenarios, enabling the full discovery of an athlete's overall potential across multiple seasons or even years (Lubis et al., 2020). Thus, when combined with additional data sources, RNNs can offer a reliable and multi-factored evaluation of an athlete's talent, considering both its short-term and long-term trends.

## 5. TRAINING AND OPTIMIZATION STRATEGIES

In conclusion, training and optimizing artificial neural networks are essential measures to achieve good performance in talent identification and scouting (Williams et al., 2020). Several strategies can help make both the training process and model prediction more efficient. We explain some of the most crucial training and optimization methods for ANNs below (Bergkamp et al., 2019) and (Myrén & Neto, 2017). ANNs have several hyperparameters that define the behavior of the model during the training process. Unlike parameters that learn from data, you must set them before training to optimize the performance of NN models(Mat-Rasid, Abdullah, Juahir, Maliki, Musa, et al., 2019). Below, we explain some of the key features.

1. **The learning rate:** It refers to the step size at which the network updates its parameters during the training process. very small learning rate may cause the model to converge slowly and chaotically, while a large learning rate may lead to training instability.
2. **Regularization:** Regularization methods, such as L 1 and L 2 regularization or dropout, can help prevent overfitting by penalizing or adding noise to the training weights.
3. **Batch size:** number of training examples for which the network evaluates and updates. Small batch sizes force the NN to update with noise, but the model will converge faster, whereas large batch sizes are more stable but are computationally more expensive.
4. **Epochs:** the number of times data passes through the network. Too few epochs can cause the DOM to underfit, while too many will lead to overfitting. ANNs, due to their complexity, require optimization of many more hyperparameters, making these considerations especially crucial (Gee et al., 2010). Different methods, such as grid search, random search, or Bayesian optimization, can perform hyperparameter tuning. These methods try different combinations of hyperparameter values in a systematic way, usually evaluating the NN using some form of validation set.

Finally, transfer learning allows one to train a pre-trained model on another task or in another domain. Rather than training ANN from scratch, it allows you to "fine-tune" an already trained model on the task and the dataset. For instance, you can precisely fine-tune an already-trained digits' image analysis model to analyze a player's face images (Mann et al., 2017). Moreover, data from similar tasks, such as computer vision tasks in video analysis or natural language processing tasks in text analysis, could train the already-pre-trained model in talent scouting and identification (Reeves et al., 2019). These methods allow the ANN to use features and representations learned while solving these tasks. The result is that the neural network requires much less data and computation to train when used to solve the target task (Reilly et al., 2003)]. The best way to choose the right ensemble technique is very task-dependent and depends on various factors such as available data quality and quantity, computational power and resources, and time restrictions.

1. **Boosting:** Boosting methods, such as AdaBoost or Gradient Boosting, train multiple weak models sequentially, and each subsequent model focuses on the misclassified examples of the previous models. We derive the final prediction as a weighted combination of the predictions made by individual models.
2. **Bagging:** The Bagging, or Bootstrap Aggregating, methods, such as Random Forests, use multiple models trained on diverse subsets of the training data to produce predictions. You can create different subsets using bootstrap sampling. We derive the finalized prediction by averaging or majority voting across all models.
3. **The stacking**: this method entails training a meta-model, such as another neural network or a different machine learning algorithm, to combine the predictions made by several base models. The latter can often be multiple ANNs trained on random or non-random samples of the data with distinct architectures or hyperparameters. Ensemble methods harness the diversity of several models to outperform the standalone variants and counter their single model's short-comings or biases.

Assessing the performance of the developed ANNs based on the compiled data is critical for drawing conclusions and making suggestions for improvement. Depending on the task and the required analysis priorities, we can use different metrics for this assessment:

1. Accuracy measures the percentage of correct predictions made by the neural network model. It is adequate for balanced datasets and tasks where each class bears maximum importance.
2. Precision evaluates the proportion of actual positive samples among the positive predictions generated by the ANNs. This measure is particularly beneficial in light of the high cost of false-positive outcomes.
3. Recall (sensitivity): We quantify the ratio of true positive predictions to all true positives in the data. High recall is valuable when the cost of failing to identify promising individuals is high; for example, identifying future sports stars and ensuring no such player is left out.
4. F1-score: It is the harmonic mean of precision and recall; hence, in cases where all or some of the performance metrics sitting in question have equal influence, an F1-score comes in handy. This score is excellent when there is no high cost for inferencing incorrect predictions.
5. Under the receiver operating characteristics curve (AUC-ROC), the AUC area is a composite metric describing the current performance of the decision model to distinguish between positive and negative cases, albeit through a range of decision thresholds. When the dataset is highly skewed, we use AUC-ROC,

considering that we can fine-tune the threshold to stratify the trade-off between false-positive and false-negative cases.

6. Mean Squared Error or Root Mean Squared Error: MSE and RMSE provide detailed information in regression-based tasks relating to sporting performance or propensity scores. They measure the average squared difference in performance predictions, or the total score miles from the real performance, and they are widely applicable in computing various performance score metrics (Larkin & Reeves, 2018). Other aspects to put into consideration include the independent test set and the cross-validation methodologies fit to offer an unbiased measure of the viable model's current performance. Furthermore, depending on the problem, the tally scores may consider other detailed talent description aspects to form more inclusive composite scores.

## 6. CASE STUDIES AND APPLICATIONS

The application of artificial neural networks for talent identification and scouting in sports has been the subject of intense research and debate over the past years, and a large number of case studies and implementations prove the viability and effectiveness of this method.

### 6.1 Talent identification in different sports

1. **Soccer:** in this sport, artificial neural networks have been utilized for the talent identification process through various data sources and diverse systems to react and associate based on soccer players' performance. For example, at the Technical University of Munich, scientists have developed a convolutional neural network model that uses video sequences of youth soccer players and predicts their performance and potential by evaluating their possible results by looking at their play style and decisions compared to them.
2. **Basketball:** in basketball, countries and institutions are attempting to use artificial neural networks to evaluate player tracking data around the globe on associated programs and connections. The National Basketball Association, for example, submits this particular application as part of its actions.
3. **Baseball:** In this practice, scholars and scientists have already attempted to find the best ANN algorithms through massive measures for more accurate predictions. At MIT, for instance, their scientists have used ANN to model a system that measures folding angles for more accurate signs to correlate performance tracking with injury prevention.

Moreover, the presented case studies show another powerful application of ANNs for player personnel management across various sports and data sources. Secondly, sports organizations are increasingly using ANNs to scout and mill taskforces for player recruitment (Bergkamp et al., 2022). ANNs produce a highly neutral, objective report on the player's talent and potential by assimilating multiple scaled metrics such as performance measures, physical metrics, and playable archives. For example, football clubs use ANNs to sift through large volumes of scouting information, such as game videos, athletes' physical parameters, and players' stats, in order to identify potential young talents worldwide (Radicchi & Mozzachiodi, 2016b). In this sense, ANNs enable scouts to manage their work more productively and competitively, making it feasible for future implementations. Professional basketball has also used ANNs to scout playing statistics, biometric data, and game performance to assess player potential (Sarmento et al., 2018). This allows for player rankings and league assessments to prioritize squad drafting choices. Finally, researchers have utilized ANNs to conduct injury risk analysis both on and off the sports field. Furthermore, in other team sports, such as soccer, ANNs have been used to evaluate player tracking, tracking load metrics, or individual player injury occurrence track records to pinpoint players more likely to sustain an injury (Ford et al., 2020). This is a game-changer, as sports organizations can provide more suitable and personal injury prevention measures like load scheduling, competitive conditioning schedules, or system sleep and recovery (Ratno et al., 2019). Furthermore, monitoring player development and advancement extends beyond scouting and potential identification; it significantly contributes to the overall success of promising players throughout their careers. In order to provide more precise training programs, ANNs can also analyze an athlete's career path and identify areas for evolution (Guenter et al., 2019). Similarly, in basketball, ANNs may assess tracking player data, in-game footage, or initial game stats to monitor young players' improvement on the field (Williams & Reilly, 2000). The models may record and assess shooting postures, defensive form, game decisions, or other key marks to provide advice and assessment to realize potential. Moreover, similar capabilities exist for soccer; ANNs can also monitor game footage and grade data to monitor young teems' development (Till & Baker, 2020). The use of ANNs helps coaches and management make more informed decisions and develop appropriate training guidelines. Lastly, by monitoring professionals' images and coaching their load, ANNs can prevent athletes from falling or collapsing, ensuring they continue to exert themselves at an A-level.

The above case studies and applications demonstrate ANNs' versatility and significant potential in talent identification and scouting across all sports and domains. However, as data collection and analysis methodologies continue to advance, the sports industry can significantly enhance talent identification and scouting by combining ANNs with other technologies like wearable devices and computer vision systems.

# 7. CHALLENGES AND FUTURE DIRECTIONS

Artificial neural networks, despite their high potential in data analysis for talent identification and scouting in sports, present several challenges and considerations for effective and responsible use. Moreover, this area requires further research and development to fully leverage the capabilities of ANNs and make them more closely integrated with other technologies and methods.

## 7.1 Data availability and quality

The performance of artificial neural networks depends significantly on the amount and quality of the data provided to them in the training process. For various reasons, accessing high-quality, unbiased, and sufficient volumes of data in talent identification and scouting data analysis can be challenging. Data scarcity: in some sports or regions, organizations do not actively collect large volumes of data, which hinders the availability of a sufficient amount of data to train ANNs; Data quality: if data collection methods are inconsistent, if there are measurement errors, or if there is a large amount of missing data, such data is not adequate for training ANN and may lead to biased results; Data privacy. Due to the high sensitivity of individual health and performance data, it is sometimes not possible to access it, which will not allow including valuable variables in the model. Due to these issues, it is important to make efforts to overcome challenges related to data quality, such as collaboration between organizations to share data, privacy-preserving mechanisms to keep sensitive information secure, and data formatting regulation.

## 7.2 Interpretability and explainability of neural networks

Neural networks' interpretability and explainability Critics have criticized ANNs, particularly deep neural networks, for their perceived 'black box' nature, which prevents clear interpretation of the prediction process. In talent identification and scouting, it is crucial to have information on how the model arrived at certain values, as various stakeholders may require access to this information to determine the importance of accurate considerations in relation to output. Research is underway to develop techniques that shed light on the decision-making process, aiming to address the issue of model interpretability and explainability. Essentially, these methods offer a feature importance ranking or saliency map that illustrates the weighting of input information into the model and its impact on the final prediction. However, a huge step remains to be taken to allow stakeholders to make subtle assumptions about model assessments, and sometimes the information can be used in complex architectures that are difficult to make simple. It is important to note that improving the model's interpretability and explainability is critical to its wide application in ANNs. The answer may lie within the problem and the different stakeholders in talent identification and scouting. Domain-specific problems Sports developers need to engage in ongoing work, leverage their expertise, and foster open collaboration. To enable more interpretable and trans person AB, sports developers and data scientists must work together.

## 7.3 Ethical consideration

Given the present section, talent identification and scouting using ANNs raise the following unethical concerns:

**Privacy and data protection:** Data privacy and protection are of significant importance as training the ANNs involves the collection and use of personal data such as medical records, biometric data, and video footage. Therefore, we must ensure appropriate privacy measures to protect the personal information and privacy of athletes, coaches, or other individuals involved in the data collection process. 3. Transparency and accountability: As previously discussed, the lack of interpretability in ANNs raises issues related to transparency and accountability, especially when these models are used for high-stake decisions such as athletes' careers or opportunity creation. These ethical concerns therefore demand the implementation of bias mitigation techniques, privacy-preserving data processing, the creation of ethical guidelines and a governance framework, and all these recommendations help reduce these concerns and ensure the fair and responsible use of these technologies.

## 7.4 Integration with other techniques:

Although ANNs have not yet fully realized their potential in talent identification and scouting, the integration of other techniques and complementary technologies can further enhance these potentials. Thus, we can fully integrate ANNs with the following technologies:

1) Expert systems: There is a need to integrate the insights generated by the ANN-based decision-making process with human experts, such as coaches, talent scouts, or analysts, through expert systems or a hybrid approach.
2) Wearable technology: the integration of ANNs with the wearable device, which involves sensors and trackers, helps provide more local and real-time data on athletes' performance, biomechanics, and physiological states, allowing for accurate and personalized talent evaluation and development.

3) Advanced computer vision and motion capture systems can support the ANN process by analyzing video footage and an athlete's movement to provide inputs that help the ANNs analyze and identify pattern-of-merit criteria involving technique, decision-making, and potentiality. The situation has changed.
4) Natural language processing: Another exciting opportunity is to leverage natural language processing techniques to allow ANNs to learn from unstructured textual data, such as scouting reports, coach feedback, or athlete interviews. This approach significantly enriches the overall data sources for talent identification and scouting. We can utilize the strengths of each technique and technology to create more comprehensive and effective talent identification and scouting systems by integrating ANNs with them.

## 7.5 Potential future research directions

The application of ANNs in talent identification and scouting is a dynamic and rapidly evolving research field with many exciting future directions. Some of them include:

1. Multimodal learning: Develop ANN models and techniques that can incorporate and learn from multiple data modalities, such as video, text, numerical, and sensor data, to produce more comprehensive and accurate talent evaluation models.
2. Transfer learning and domain adaptation: Explore transfer learning and domain adaptation techniques to transfer representations and knowledge from related datasets or tasks to reduce data requirements and improve ANN performance in talent identification and scouting.
3. Reinforcement learning: Enabling reinforcement learning techniques in ANNS can help learn adaptive and personalized talent development strategies, where the models learn to improve training and coaching decisions based on feedback and performance data.
4. Federated learning: Extending research on federated learning would improve the performance of ANNs in talent identification and scouting by enabling training on multiple sports teams' data while maintaining privacy and ownership of data.
5. Explainable AI: Continuous research on explainable AI would make ANN models of talent identification and scouting interpretable and transparent, improving trust and acceptability.
6. Ethical AI: Creating ethical frameworks, guidelines, and algorithms is critical for ensuring fairness, accountability, and privacy when using ANNs for talent identification and scouting. Only by resolving these leading issues can we ensure responsible and trustworthy use. By examining these liabilities and discovering

avenues for new research, one may ensure that they do not debilitate the use of ANNs to their full potential in solving many of the sports industry's issues more effectively and efficiently.

## 8. CONCLUSION

In conclusion, applying artificial neural networks to talent identification and scouting has immense potential to transform the sports industry. Utilizing the power of data and cutting-edge machine learning techniques, its aid identifies athletes' traits in a comprehensive, unbiased way, predicts their future performance, and ensures they reach their potential. Several precarious aspects must be considered to enable this technology to reach fruition. First, ensuring adequate, unbiased data for prediction is vital. If the training process lacks objectivity, it could lead to skewed predictions. Second, enhancing the interpretability and explanation of artificial networks can strengthen coaches, scouts, and other stakeholders' trust in the system. We also need to address the ethical aspects of implementation, such as fairness, bias processing, and privacy. Combining ANN with other technologies, including expert systems, computer vision, and wearable sensors, can help create properly integrated and functional talent identification and scouting systems. Finally, further exploration of multimodal learning, transfer learning, reinforcement learning, and explainable AI in this setting has the potential to take artificial neural networks to a new level of efficiency. In summary, a joint effort of sports knowledge, data science, and academic approach is needed for artificial neural networks to be used responsibly and harmlessly by sports organizations as they seek a competitive advantage when identifying and developing the talent that the sport solely upholds.

## REFERENCES


Abbott, A., Button, C., Pepping, G.-J., & Collins, D. (2005). Unnatural selection: Talent identification and development in sport. *Nonlinear Dynamics Psychology and Life Sciences*, *9*(1), 61–88. PMID: 15629068

Akhtar, R., Winsborough, D., Lovric, D., & Chamorro-Premuzic, T. (2019). Identifying and managing talent in the age of artificial intelligence. In *Workforce readiness and the future of work* (pp. 169–185). Routledge. DOI: 10.4324/9781351210485-10

Allal-Chérif, O., Aránega, A. Y., & Sánchez, R. C. (2021). Intelligent recruitment: How to identify, select, and retain talents from around the world using artificial intelligence. *Technological Forecasting and Social Change*, *169*, 120822. DOI: 10.1016/j.techfore.2021.120822

Atlas, M., & Zhang, Y.-Q. (2004). Fuzzy neural agents for online NBA scouting. *IEEE/WIC/ACM International Conference on Web Intelligence (WI'04)*, 58–63. DOI: 10.1109/WI.2004.10047

Bairui, T., Cheng, C., Lubo, L., & Lishu, W. (2019). Analysis of Urban Talent Demand Model Based on Neural Network. *2019 11th International Conference on Measuring Technology and Mechatronics Automation (ICMTMA)*, 416–420.

Barron, D., Ball, G., Robins, M., & Sunderland, C. (2020). Identifying playing talent in professional football using artificial neural networks. *Journal of Sports Sciences*, *38*(11–12), 1211–1220. DOI: 10.1080/02640414.2019.1708036 PMID: 31941425

Bergkamp, T. L. G., Frencken, W. G. P., Niessen, A. S. M., Meijer, R. R., & den Hartigh, R. J. R. (2022). How soccer scouts identify talented players. *European Journal of Sport Science*, *22*(7), 994–1004. DOI: 10.1080/17461391.2021.1916081 PMID: 33858300

Bergkamp, T. L. G., Niessen, A. S. M., den Hartigh, R. J. R., Frencken, W. G. P., & Meijer, R. R. (2019). Methodological issues in soccer talent identification research. *Sports Medicine (Auckland, N.Z.)*, *49*(9), 1317–1335. DOI: 10.1007/s40279-019-01113-w PMID: 31161402

Chamorro-Premuzic, T., Winsborough, D., Sherman, R. A., & Hogan, R. (2016). New talent signals: Shiny new objects or a brave new world? *Industrial and Organizational Psychology: Perspectives on Science and Practice*, *9*(3), 621–640. DOI: 10.1017/iop.2016.6

Chien, C.-F., & Chen, L.-F. (2008). Data mining to improve personnel selection and enhance human capital: A case study in high-technology industry. *Expert Systems with Applications, 34*(1), 280–290. DOI: 10.1016/j.eswa.2006.09.003

Daga, B., Checker, J., Rajan, A., & Deo, S. (2020). Computer science career recommendation system using artificial neural network. *International Journal of Computer Trends and Technology, 68*(3), 84–88. DOI: 10.14445/22312803/IJCTT-V68I3P117

Flores-Hernández, I., Bonilla-Huerta, E., Quintero-Flores, P. M., Ponce, O. A., & Hernández-Hernández, J. C. (2019). Applying intelligent techniques for talent recruitment. *Applied Computer Science, 15*(2), 63–72. DOI: 10.35784/acs-2019-14

Ford, P. R., Bordonau, J. L. D., Bonanno, D., Tavares, J., Groenendijk, C., Fink, C., Gualtieri, D., Gregson, W., Varley, M. C., Weston, M., Lolli, L., Platt, D., & Di Salvo, V. (2020). A survey of talent identification and development processes in the youth academies of professional soccer clubs from around the world. *Journal of Sports Sciences, 38*(11–12), 1269–1278. DOI: 10.1080/02640414.2020.1752440 PMID: 32378447

Gee, C. J., Marshall, J. C., & King, J. F. (2010). Should coaches use personality assessments in the talent identification process? A 15 year predictive study on professional hockey players. *International Journal of Coaching Science, 4*(1).

Guenter, R. W., Dunn, J. G. H., & Holt, N. L. (2019). Talent identification in youth ice hockey: Exploring "intangible" player characteristics. *The Sport Psychologist, 33*(4), 323–333. DOI: 10.1123/tsp.2018-0155

Hong, W. (2023). Research and application of talent training evaluation model based on deep learning. *Sixth International Conference on Intelligent Computing, Communication, and Devices (ICCD 2023), 12703*, 247–252.

Huang, L.-C., Huang, K.-S., Huang, H.-P., & Jaw, B.-S. (2004). Applying fuzzy neural network in human resource selection system. *IEEE Annual Meeting of the Fuzzy Information, 2004. Processing NAFIPS'04., 1*, 169–174.

Huang, X. (2023). Business Talent Demand Prediction Model Based On Neural Network in Integration of Industry and Education in Greater Bay Area. *2023 IEEE 5th Eurasia Conference on IOT, Communication and Engineering (ECICE)*, 382–385.

Jaffar, Z., Noor, W., & Kanwal, Z. (2019). Predictive human resource analytics using data mining classification techniques. *Int. J. Comput, 32*(1), 9–20.

Jantan, H., Hamdan, A. R., & Othman, Z. A. (2010). Classification and prediction of academic talent using data mining techniques. *International Conference on Knowledge-Based and Intelligent Information and Engineering Systems*, 491–500. DOI: 10.1007/978-3-642-15387-7_53

Jantan, H., Hamdan, A. R., & Othman, Z. A. (2011). Talent knowledge acquisition using data mining classification techniques. *2011 3rd Conference on Data Mining and Optimization (DMO)*, 32–37.

Jantan, H., Hamdan, A. R., & Othman, Z. A. (2012). Human talent forecasting using data mining classification techniques. In *Human Resources Management: Concepts, Methodologies, Tools, and Applications* (pp. 486–499). IGI Global.

Jasni, N. H., Mustapha, A., Tenah, S. S., Mostafa, S. A., & Razali, N. (2022). Prediction of player position for talent identification in association netball: A regression-based approach. *International Journal of Advances in Intelligent Informatics*, *8*(1), 84. DOI: 10.26555/ijain.v8i1.707

Jauhiainen, S., Äyrämö, S., Forsman, H., & Kauppi, J. P. (2019). Talent identification in soccer using a one-class support vector machine. *International Journal of Computer Science in Sport*, *18*(3), 125–136. DOI: 10.2478/ijcss-2019-0021

Jha, A., Dichwalkar, A., Shaikh, A., & Pawar, G. (n.d.). *Talent Explorer using Data Mining*.

Kalaivani, V., & Elamparithi, M. M. (2014). An efficient classification algorithms for employee performance prediction. *International Journal of Research in Advent Technology*, *2*(9), 27–32.

Khan, N. J., Ahamad, G., Naseem, M., & Sohail, S. S. (2023). Computational efficiency in sports talent identification-a systematic review. *International Journal of Applied Decision Sciences*, *16*(3), 358–384. DOI: 10.1504/IJADS.2023.130600

Khurana, R., Yadav, M., Quttainah, M., Srivastava, A. P., Baludi, A., & Singh, P. K. (2023). Neural Networks in Recruitment: Trends and Future Directions. *2023 International Conference on Ambient Intelligence, Knowledge Informatics and Industrial Electronics (AIKIIE)*, 1–5. DOI: 10.1109/AIKIIE60097.2023.10390017

King, M., Brown, M., Cox, J., McLellan, R., Towlson, C., & Barrett, S. (2024). Talent identification in soccer: The influence of technical, physical and maturity-related characteristics on a national selection process. *PLoS One*, *19*(3), e0298359. DOI: 10.1371/journal.pone.0298359 PMID: 38478494

Kirola, M., Memoria, M., & Dumka, A. (2023). Optimized U-Net convolutional neural network based breast cancer prediction for accuracy increment in big data. *Concurrency and Computation, 35*(9), e7652. Advance online publication. DOI: 10.1002/cpe.7652

Larkin, P., & Reeves, M. J. (2018). Junior-elite football: Time to re-position talent identification? *Soccer and Society, 19*(8), 1183–1192. DOI: 10.1080/14660970.2018.1432389

Lowman, G. H. (2016). Moving beyond identification: Using gamification to attract and retain talent. *Industrial and Organizational Psychology: Perspectives on Science and Practice, 9*(3), 677–682. DOI: 10.1017/iop.2016.70

Lubis, A. E., Raharjo, F. M., & Nugroho, A. (2020). A Model of Basic Skill Test for Talent Scouting Soccer Athlete Candidates. *1st Unimed International Conference on Sport Science (UnICoSS 2019)*, 79–86. DOI: 10.2991/ahsr.k.200305.025

Lüdin, D., Donath, L., & Romann, M. (2023). Disagreement between talent scouts: Implications for improved talent assessment in youth football. *Journal of Sports Sciences, 41*(8), 758–765. DOI: 10.1080/02640414.2023.2239614 PMID: 37490515

Ma, H., & Ding, A. (2022). Construction and implementation of a college talent cultivation system under deep learning and data mining algorithms. *The Journal of Supercomputing, 78*(4), 5681–5696. DOI: 10.1007/s11227-021-04036-4

Mann, D. L., Dehghansai, N., & Baker, J. (2017). Searching for the elusive gift: Advances in talent identification in sport. *Current Opinion in Psychology, 16*, 128–133. DOI: 10.1016/j.copsyc.2017.04.016 PMID: 28813336

Mat-Rasid, S. M., Abdullah, M. R., Juahir, H., Maliki, A., Musa, R. M., Kosni, N. A., Hashim, M. R., Eswaramoorthi, V., & Najmi, N. (2019). Determining youth profile using principle component analysis for identifying talent in sports. *International Journal of Recent Technology and Engineering, 8*(2), 212–215.

Mat-Rasid, S. M., Abdullah, M. R., Juahir, H., Maliki, A. B., Kosni, N. A., Musa, R. M., Hashim, M. R., Alnamat, A. S. F., Alias, N., & Najmi, N. (2019). Applied multidimensional analysis for assessing youth performance in sports talent identification program. *Int J Recent Technol Eng*Https://Doi. Org/10.35940/Ijrte. *B, 1051*, 0782S719.

McCullagh, J. (2010). Data mining in sport: A neural network approach. *International Journal of Sports Science and Engineering, 4*(3), 131–138.

Mishra, R., Rodriguez, R., & Portillo, V. (2020). An ai based talent acquisition and benchmarking for job. *ArXiv Preprint ArXiv:2009.09088.*

Mwaro, P. N., Ogada, K., & Cheruiyot, W. (2021). Neural network model for talent recruitment and management for employee development and retention. *2021 IEEE AFRICON*, 1–6.

Myrén, A., & Neto, P. S. (2017). *Evaluation of Machine Learning Algorithms in Recommender Systems: Candidate Recommender Systems in the Staffing Industry.*

Ozcaglar, C., Geyik, S., Schmitz, B., Sharma, P., Shelkovnykov, A., Ma, Y., & Buchanan, E. (2019). Entity personalized talent search models with tree interaction features. *The World Wide Web Conference*, 3116–3122. DOI: 10.1145/3308558.3313672

Pruna, R., Miñarro Tribaldos, L., & Bahdur, K. (2018). Player talent identification and development in football. *Apunts Sports Medicine*, *53*(198), 43–46. DOI: 10.1016/j.apunts.2018.02.002

Qin, C., Zhang, L., Zha, R., Shen, D., Zhang, Q., Sun, Y., Zhu, C., Zhu, H., & Xiong, H. (2023). A comprehensive survey of artificial intelligence techniques for talent analytics. *ArXiv Preprint ArXiv:2307.03195.*

Radicchi, E., & Mozzachiodi, M. (2016a). Social talent scouting: A new opportunity for the identification of football players? *Physical Culture and Sport Studies and Research*, *70*(1), 28–43. DOI: 10.1515/pcssr-2016-0012

Radicchi, E., & Mozzachiodi, M. (2016b). Social talent scouting: A new opportunity for the identification of football players? *Physical Culture and Sport Studies and Research*, *70*(1), 28–43. DOI: 10.1515/pcssr-2016-0012

Ratno, P., Suprayitno, S., Hasibuan, R., & Fadli, Z. (2019). The Development of Karate Talent Scouting Identification Instrument. *Proceedings of The 5th Annual International Seminar on Trends in Science and Science Education, AISTSSE 2018,* 18-19 October 2018, Medan, Indonesia. DOI: 10.4108/eai.18-10-2018.2287433

Razali, N., Mustapha, A., Yatim, F. A., & Ab Aziz, R. (2017). Predicting player position for talent identification in association football. *IOP Conference Series. Materials Science and Engineering*, *226*(1), 012087. DOI: 10.1088/1757-899X/226/1/012087

Reeves, M. J., McRobert, A. P., Lewis, C. J., & Roberts, S. J. (2019). A case study of the use of verbal reports for talent identification purposes in soccer: A Messi affair! *PLoS One*, *14*(11), e0225033. DOI: 10.1371/journal.pone.0225033 PMID: 31714943

Reilly, T., Williams, A. M., & Richardson, D. (2003). Identifying talented players. In *Science and soccer* (pp. 315–334). Routledge. DOI: 10.4324/9780203417553

Reyaz, N., Ahamad, G., Khan, N. J., & Naseem, M. (2022). Machine Learning in Sports Talent Identification: A Systematic Review. *2022 2nd International Conference on Emerging Frontiers in Electrical and Electronic Technologies (ICEFEET)*, 1–6.

Sarmento, H., Anguera, M. T., Pereira, A., & Araújo, D. (2018). Talent identification and development in male football: A systematic review. *Sports Medicine (Auckland, N.Z.)*, *48*(4), 907–931. DOI: 10.1007/s40279-017-0851-7 PMID: 29299878

Sayal, A., Jha, J., Chaithra, N., Gupta, V., Gupta, A., Gupta, O., & Memoria, M. (2023). Neural Networks And Machine Learning. *2023 IEEE 5th International Conference on Cybernetics, Cognition and Machine Learning Applications (IC-CCMLA)*, 58–63.

Sridevi, G. M., & Kamala Suganthi, S. (2021). Artificial intelligence-based job applicant profile quality assessment and relevance ranking using clusters in talent acquisition process. *Applications of Artificial Intelligence in Engineering:Proceedings of First Global Conference on Artificial Intelligence and Applications (GCAIA 2020)*, 461–472.

Subha, T., Ranjana, R., Aarthi, B., Pavithra, S., & Srinidhi, M. S. (2022). Skill Analysis and Scouting Platform Using Machine Learning. *2022 International Conference on Communication, Computing and Internet of Things (IC3IoT)*, 1–6. DOI: 10.1109/IC3IOT53935.2022.9767872

Till, K., & Baker, J. (2020). Challenges and [possible] solutions to optimizing talent identification and development in sport. *Frontiers in Psychology*, *11*, 525518. DOI: 10.3389/fpsyg.2020.00664 PMID: 32351427

Uddin, M. F., & Lee, J. (2017). Predicting Educational Relevance For an Efficient Classification of Talent. *2017 ASEE Northeast Section Conference*.

Utamayasa, I. G. D. (2021). Talent Identification of Future Sportsmen Using Sport Search Application. *Budapest International Research and Critics Institute-Journal (BIRCI-Journal)*, *4*(1), 690–695.

Vilela, T., Portela, F., & Santos, M. F. (2018). Towards a Pervasive Intelligent System on Football Scouting-A Data Mining Study Case. *Trends and Advances in Information Systems and Technologies*, *3*(6), 341–351. DOI: 10.1007/978-3-319-77700-9_34

Waheed, S., Zaim, A. H., Zaim, H., Sertbas, A., & Akyokus, S. (2014). Application of neural networks in talent management. *2013 International Conference on Electrical Information and Communication Technology (EICT)*, 1–4. DOI: 10.1109/EICT.2014.6777833

Williams, A. M., Ford, P. R., & Drust, B. (2020). Talent identification and development in soccer since the millennium. *Journal of Sports Sciences, 38*(11–12), 1199–1210. DOI: 10.1080/02640414.2020.1766647 PMID: 32568000

Williams, A. M., & Reilly, T. (2000). Talent identification and development in soccer. *Journal of Sports Sciences, 18*(9), 657–667. DOI: 10.1080/02640410050120041 PMID: 11043892

Woods, C. T., Joyce, C., & Robertson, S. (2016). What are talent scouts actually identifying? Investigating the physical and technical skill match activity profiles of drafted and non-drafted U18 Australian footballers. *Journal of Science and Medicine in Sport, 19*(5), 419–423. DOI: 10.1016/j.jsams.2015.04.013 PMID: 25963663

Wrang, C. M., Rossing, N. N., Agergaard, S., & Martin, L. J. (2022). The missing children: A systematic scoping review on talent identification and selection in football (soccer). *EJSS European Journal for Sport and Society, 19*(2), 135–150. DOI: 10.1080/16138171.2021.1916224

Xiao, Q., Zhong, X., & Zhong, C. (2020). Application research of KNN algorithm based on clustering in big data talent demand information classification. *International Journal of Pattern Recognition and Artificial Intelligence, 34*(06), 2050015. DOI: 10.1142/S0218001420500159

Xu, H., Yu, Z., Yang, J., Xiong, H., & Zhu, H. (2016). Talent circle detection in job transition networks. *Proceedings of the 22nd ACM SIGKDD International Conference on Knowledge Discovery and Data Mining*, 655–664. DOI: 10.1145/2939672.2939732

Ye, J., Hu, H., & Chai, C. (2009). A talent classification method based on SVM. *2009 International Symposium on Intelligent Ubiquitous Computing and Education*, 160–163. DOI: 10.1109/IUCE.2009.63

Yi, F., Yu, Z., Xu, H., & Guo, B. (2019). Talents recommendation with multi-aspect preference learning. *Green, Pervasive, and Cloud Computing: 13th International Conference, GPC 2018, Hangzhou, China, May 11-13, 2018, Revised Selected Papers 13*, 409–423.

Youping, L., & Jiangang, S. (2022). Talent Recruitment Platform for Large-Scale Group Enterprises Based on Deep Learning. *2022 7th International Conference on Cloud Computing and Big Data Analytics (ICCCBDA)*, 172–176.

# Chapter 12
# Ethical Considerations in Sports Analytics:
## Exploring the Ethical Challenges Presented by the Use of AI and ML in Sports

**Mohit Yadav**
https://orcid.org/0000-0002-9341-2527
*O.P. Jindal Global University, India*

**Tanupriya Choudhury**
*University of Petroleum and Energy Studies, India*

**Ta Huy Hung**
https://orcid.org/0009-0008-6835-3036
*Vietnam National University, Hanoi, Vietnam*

## ABSTRACT

*The integration of artificial intelligence (AI) and machine learning (ML) in sports analytics offers significant advancements in performance enhancement, strategy development, and injury prevention. However, it also presents critical ethical challenges that require careful consideration. This paper explores these ethical issues through four case studies: player privacy and data security in the New England Patriots, bias in talent identification at FC Barcelona's La Masia academy, the impact on coaching and decision-making in the Los Angeles Lakers, and long-term health implications at Manchester City. The analysis highlights the importance of transparency, fairness, and the safeguarding of athletes' well-being. Practical, ethical, theoretical, managerial, and societal implications are discussed, alongside limitations and future research directions. This paper emphasizes the need for a*

DOI: 10.4018/979-8-3693-5385-1.ch012

*balanced approach that integrates AI insights with human expertise to ensure ethical and effective use in sports.*

## INTRODUCTION

The intersection of sport and technology has created a new paradigm for the examination of athletic performance analysis, optimization, and presentation to the public (Leyva, 2020). Ethical aspects of organized contact sports for children as participants. Advanced capabilities in data collection and processing have opened the floodgates to the age of sports analytics, whereby complex data sets are thoroughly scrutinized to ascertain relevant insights. At the heart of this sea change is the integration of AI and ML algorithms that possess the potency to process huge reams of complex data more quickly with unrivalled accuracy. In sports, AI and ML range from recruitment and player performance assessment to injury prevention, strategy formulation, and fan engagement (Gómez-Carmona et al., 2020)

These technologies give teams and organizations an advantage in finding new talent and improving the fan experience overall. For example, complex algorithms can train on video footage of player movement to track distances covered, identify performance metrics, and make injury predictions. Similarly, AI-driven systems will optimize game strategy against opponents by looking for tendencies to exploit. While the potential benefits of AI and ML in sports are undeniable, their mass adoption also brings with them deep ethical concerns (Ossa, 2024). Accumulation, storage, and analysis of sensitive athlete data require robust privacy protections to safeguard individuals against unauthorized access and misuse. Development and deployment of AI algorithms are also subject to stringent standards of fairness and equity that prevent discriminatory outcomes. One critical concern that has to be met with careful attention is algorithmic bias, which can disproportionately impact certain groups of athletes. Another ethical issue at stake is the competitive advantage because, while teams invest in AI and ML technologies, there is the potential risk of an uneven playing field (Dyer, 2020). Such a wide gap in resources and expertise could result in some few teams monopolizing talent and dominating, hence killing the very foundation of the game: fair competition. Second, overreliance on AI-driven decision-making could erode human judgment and intuition, perhaps leading to the dehumanization of sport. Transparency and explainability are important aspects of the ethical application of AI and ML (Luccioni & Bengio, 2020). Algorithms that make decisions have to be able to be understood by all different stakeholders, such as athletes, coaches, and even fans. Black-box models that produce an output but don't reveal the logic driving the answer undermine trust and therefore accountability (Lan, H. (2024). That means efforts have to be made towards developing AI that is as transparent as possible and able to give clear explanations of the recommendation. AI/ML integration in sports can further work as a disruptor of job markets. As the automation level rises, routine tasks will be taken over, and different job roles inside the sports organizations will either develop or turn irrelevant. The need is to prepare for such changes and provide policies aimed at cushioning the impacts on affected employees, in particular, through retraining and upskilling. This goes to say that AI and ML have complex and multi-faceted ethical implications in sports: large potential for improving athletes' performance and fan experience, while they introduce new challenges which shall have to be addressed proactively (Constandt et al., 2020).

The research is undertaken to understand the nuances of these ethical issues, doing a deep analysis of the current scenario, and provide suggestions for responsible AI and ML adoption in the sports industry.

While doing so, a collaborative conversation amongst the stakeholders- athletes, coaches, teams, fans, and policy people- empowers them to use technologies that help in the minimization of their possible threats.

Ethical Landscape Understanding Ethics in AI and ML usage in sports greatly ties into the bigger picture: society's concerns about technology and its interactions with human values. First and foremost, among these issues is fairness, including procedural and distributive justice. Fairness in sports means that athletes have an equal opportunity for competition on the same platform (Glebova, 2024).

In this regard, AI and ML use in analysis and identification of players' performance and raw talent, respectively, should be based on openness to fairness to reduce biases that may result in competitive advantages.

Another critical ethical issue is privacy. With the growing collection and analyses of athletes' data, including biometric information, medical records, and performance metrics, there is growing concern for the protection of this data and its possible misuse. Robust frameworks of data governance have to be in place to protect the safeguarding of personal information from any form of unauthorized access (Evans et al., 2016). Entailing even more importantly that an athlete has to be provided with very clear and transparent information about how their collected data is being used and shared. Transparency and explainability are two things that are absolutely necessary in creating trust in AI and ML. With growing complexity comes the need to ensure that their decision-making processes are understandable to relevant stakeholders. Black-box models usually undermine accountability and make it quite hard to remove biases since, by definition, they return outputs without exposing the logic driving such outputs. Efforts should be made in developing AI that is as transparent as possible and which clearly explains the recommendations it makes. Accountability is a basic tenet in the development of ethical artificial intelligence and machine learning (Bin & Xu, 2021). The institutions that are responsible for fielding this technology must be held liable for actions it carries out and their consequences. This comprises clearly defined lines of accountability, robust mechanisms for overseeing them, and processes for correcting mistakes or biases. Certain problems created at the intersection of sport and artificial intelligence are really unique. For example, AI-powered performance enhancement technologies might make a differentiation between humanly possible skills and technological enhancement practically impossible (Musa et al., 2021). To make any proper judgment about where to draw the line as far as technological intervention is concerned is extremely cumbersome and necessarily involves an elaboration of values and traditions of the sport.

Things are further confused on the ethical front by the fact that the character of sports is international. There are huge disparities in the legal and regulatory frameworks of countries and cultures concerning data protection, privacy, and AI ethics. Passing through these complexities requires nuanced cultural and legal intelligence.

The ethical dimensions of AI and ML in sports are very far-reaching and interdisciplinary. If some main principles—fairness, privacy, transparency, accountability, human dignity—are carefully considered while tailoring these technologies into practice, it is possible to capture the potential while mitigating the risks that go along with them.

## Ethical Challenges in AI and ML for Sports

While AI/ML seems to offer immense future prospects for sports, at the same time, it opens up a whole Pandora's box of ethical issues. One such major concern is algorithmic bias. The AI models are trained against large volumes of data that may contain, unabashedly, biases modeling the ones in society. These come in several ways, ranging from underrepresentation of an athlete population to justly predicting performance outcomes (Kapadiya et al., 2020).

Unchecked, biased algorithms are quite capable of perpetuating currently existing inequalities and acting against the very basic principles related to fair competition. Another critical issue revolves around privacy concerns. In many instances, sports analytics collects sensitive data about athletes, including biometric information, medical records, and performance metrics (Chang et al., 2023). Security of this data goes a long way in protecting the privacy of athletes and preventing unauthorized access or misuse of their data. This makes serious ethical questions considering the potential data breaches and use of personal information for commercial purposes. Transparency and explainability are at the core of building trust in AI and ML systems. A black-box model is one that generates an output without disclosing any logic through which such an output is generated. As such, it may turn out to be problematic in accountability, since errors or bias would be quite hard to find or rectify. This makes the transparency of AI algorithms essential, with clear explanations of their decisions necessary to retain public confidence and for ethical ends. Fairness and competitive advantage go hand-in-hand. Clearly, AI and ML can be utilized to gain performance and find talent; at the same time, however, there is the potential for an uneven playing field (Sampaio, 2024). Advanced technologies would be within reach of teams with more resources, rapidly creating an uneven playing field where talent would then gravitate to, holding dominance in the hands of very few. This raises questions over the long-term sustainability and fairness of the sport. Job displacement is yet another ethical consideration. The more sophisticated AI and ML systems become, the higher the potential for automating tasks, usually performed by humans, leading to the loss of certain jobs in the sports industry. Such developments should be carefully thought out in advance with plans in place to accommodate the workers that will be displaced through various retraining and upskilling programs. The ethical issues related to AI and ML in sport are multifaceted and multilayered. Any form of solution to the issues at hand calls for a multi-stakeholder platform that brings together athletes, coaches, teams, fans, policymakers, and ethicists. Only through a multi-stakeholder approach can problems associated with AI and ML be identified and consequently curbed at an early stage while their positive benefits are harnessed.

## Case Studies and Examples:

The latte is a crucial element in driving the point home of ethical complexity within sports analytics. Through case studies on real-world occurrences, researchers can help unveil practical implications for ethical dilemmas and provide insight into possible solutions

The most important area to worry about would be the field of player evaluation and recruitment tools that have alleged to let the algorithms be prejudiced against certain racial or ethnic groups (Abidin, 2021). For instance, in a case in which the historical data is filled with athletes from one specific background, the AI model might inadvertently develop a liking for players of that characteristic and miss talented athletes from a minority group.

There have been several high-profile privacy breaches in the sports world. Unauthorized revelation of such sensitive information about the health data of the athletes or their performance (Oytun et al., 2020) indicators may lead to the loss of reputation and career of the concerned persons. Hacking of the databases of teams or exploitation of data by some miscreants definitely dictates a requirement for great and strong safeguards on the protection of data.

In cases where AI-driven decisions had a huge impact on an athlete's career, issues related to transparency and explainability become very relevant. For example, if an AI system recommends early retirement for a player based on a forecasted performance decline, bases of the factors considered for making such a decision should be explained. In the absence of transparency, athletes may feel that they are being treated unfairly and that opportunities were being snatched from them.

When using AI to enhance player performance, there might also be ethical considerations around debates about the extent of one's allowable technological intervention, with dramatic cases involving athletes gaining an unfair advantage through the use of wearable devices or other technologies. It becomes a difficult balancing act among safeguarding fair means of competition, encouraging innovation, and preventing unethical behaviors (Olenich et al., 2020).

Moreover, the influence of AI over the sports workforce cannot be neglected either. There is a gradual increase in the number of displacements in jobs because of automation. To illustrate, AI video analysis tools might reduce the need for human scouts, thereby causing displacement. Investigating the effects of AI on the employment patterns in the sports industry and developing ways to counteract the negative impacts assume great significance.

## Case Study 1: Player Privacy and Data Security with Artificial Intelligence in the NFL

Following a humiliating defeat early in the 2021 season, the New England Patriots were determined to enhance their performance analytics by creating an avant-garde artificial intelligence and machine learning system that utilizes player GPS, biometric information, and fine-tuned performance measurements. Although the idea was to use this data to enhance the performance of the players and strategy planning, it opened up several major ethical issues concerning player privacy and security (Yang, 2024)

Of course, such massive data collection did ring the alarm bells in the minds of the players regarding their privacy. The most common fear of the players was the volume of data being collected and how it could be used apart from enhancing performance. Such concerns were sometimes even enhanced by fears of the data's use against them in contract negotiations, or even its public revelation, including that it could be shared with other people controlling it without the player's consent. This case highlighted the essential meaning and the essence of informed consent—players had to know exactly what kind of data will be collected and for what purposes that collected data would be used. First, there were consent forms in place, but the consent forms were full of legalese whereby the players could not understand them, then leading to the mix-ups and high wariness (Sangarsu, 2022)

The question of data security shot into prominence when the team suffered a breach in their data. Players' sensitive biometric data, including star quarterback Mac Jones and defensive lineman Matthew Judon, was exposed as part of a significant breach of trust. This incident reemphasized the need for stringent data security provisions so that the data collected was still secure from unauthorized access and its misuse. The breach not only outraged the involvement of potential legal liabilities but also aimed to spoil the relationship between the players and the management, thus calling for the importance of stringent security measures.

In light of all the aforementioned issues, the New England Patriots undertook a number of corrective actions. They updated their consent forms for clarity and transparency, and for being more easily understood and accessible by players. This was a key way to re-instill trust so that the players felt more secure and knowledgeable in the data collection processes. In the same breath, the team enhanced the protocols around data security with advanced encryption methods, very regular security audits, and hired third-party security experts for even more audits. These were efforts geared toward ensuring that such an incident did not recur and to protect the private data of the players.

The case study raises a shade on some of the ethical considerations that the use of AI and ML on sports analytics would have regarding players' privacy and data security. The experience of New England Patriots shows that clear communication, strong security measures, and deep commitment to transparency will be required in facing the ethical challenges. Indeed, it serves to be a reminder that technological advances, sometimes conveying massive boons to the performances found in sports, must all the same be counterbalanced by an equally increased measure of dedication to the preservation of players' rights and interests.

## Case Study 2: Bias in Talent Identification at FC Barcelona

FC Barcelona's famous youth academy, La Masia, was rolling out an AI-driven talent identification system to scout and develop young players in 2022. A system had been designed, designed to use a range of performance metrics ranging from physical attributes to game statistics and even to the biometric data of the individuals in predicting the future success of the young talents (Gour, 2024). Those prerequisites made the initiative one that was meant to be using cutting-edge technology to ensure that the legacy of the academy in churning out world-class footballers never faded. The implementation of this system lately exposed a myriad of ethical challenges, with the most important one being bias within the talent identification process.

In a matter of months, the AI system was already under concerns for being unfair and non-inclusive. Coaches and scouts started to realize that the AI system was being partial to the type of player with certain kinds of physical attributes and different categories of backgrounds. This bias reflected the training data on which the AI system was trained, biased to profiles of previously successful players at La Masia, such as Lionel Messi and Gerard Piqué. As such, it started to miss the top talents who belonged to less represented groups and those who were different from the conventional mold.

Algorithms being biased is the most ethical concern for the case. The bias of AI system to identify talents was facilitated by the historical and societal biases that were reflected in the data used for training the AI. This bias questioned the commitment of the academy to diversity and opportunity, as it threatened the opportunity for some of the world's most talented young players to develop and succeed. Fair and inclusive Artificial Intelligence systems are paramount; in this case, bias threatened to feed and build on previous inequalities in the sport.

The many ethical challenges brought about by this elicited a strong response from FC Barcelona. They pulled and diversified data for training, such as trying to balance the player profiles and performance metrics to build a more balanced and representative data set, which would eventually reduce the biases of the initial model. Noteworthy, the academy opted to combine the insights from AI with human judgment in a hybrid approach. Experienced scouts and coaches, including former players like Xavi Hernandez and Carles Puyol, were brought into the evaluation process to make sure of a holistic reach to young talents.

This case study underlines the importance of tackling bias in AI for fairness and inclusivity in sports analytics. The example of FC Barcelona's La Masia demonstrates that this involves continuous monitoring and updating of AI models to avoid making biased decisions or to correct them, even after the fact. Organizations can leverage the convergence of technology advancement and human experience to approximate a just and effective approach toward talent identification. This not only makes the system more accurate but also ensures that the ethical principles of fairness and equal opportunity are secured for all athletes who want to be on top of it.

## Case Study 3: Impact on Coaching and Decision-Making in the NBA

The Los Angeles Lakers, in 2023, integrated the AI system to assist in-game strategy and management of players. The system was developed in concurrence with one of the leading AI firms to give a recommendation for real-time analysis of the huge data pool about player performance, opponent tendencies, and game situation in match analysis to be proposed to coaches during the match (Pavitt et al., 2021). The goals involved enhancing decision-making and, therefore, enhancing game strategy. However, the implementation of the system raised serious ethical considerations in regards to the coaching and decision-making process.

Shortly after an AI was introduced, head coach Darvin Ham and his team first saw the conflicts between the judgment of the coach and recommendations made by the AI system. Many of the strategies or player rotations that the AI system suggested went against the instincts and the knowledge of the coaches. One foundational example is the AI would suggest benching LeBron during clutch times because it was "40 seconds to halftime Leone. This is where we have to get him out to rest him.". Consequently, such conflicts significantly lowered the feeling of agency by the coaching panel since they started feeling like the knowledge reserved to them is what the AI installed was ruling out.

What it became evident in this case is an ethical challenge in human-AI collaboration. While AI can add value with its insights, these should be balanced with human expertise. Many of these recommendations from the AI system were different from that of the coaches. It caused friction and low morale, where most of the time, the suggestions of the AI system were totally against the coaches' game plans. Non-transparency of the AI system in their recommendation process. The recommendation process of the AI system was not understood by the coaches and players, including top players like Anthony Davis and Russell Westbrook. Therefore, these recommendations were not trusted. Again, there was no understanding of how the AI system recommended the different recommendations it made; hence, accountability and transparency were an earlier issue.

Faced with these challenges, the Los Angeles Lakers have set the AI system to a rebrand from a lead actor to a supporting actor. In place were protocols that allowed for insight from AI to be just one among many inputs to arrive at a decision. This approach will allow Coach Ham and his staff to stay in the middle while getting the best data-driven recommendations from AI. The team also enhanced transparency by outlining how recommendations were being generated with the AI system; that helped bring understanding and better relations to trust between the coaching team and the players.

This is a case in point of ethics relating to the incorporation of AI into the sports analysis climate, more particularly in coaching and decision-making (DC, 2022). From what the Los Angeles Lakers encounters, with effective integration, there has to be great collaboration that potentially respects and enhances human judgment. What is more, it makes transparency and role clarity as institutional decisions for a greater positive and ethical work environment. A sports team could also perform at its best by using AI insights up to the point where it can equate to human judgment, or even better, as this shall enable them to preserve the trust and faith of the coaching staff and players towards the game.

## Case Study 4: Long-Term Health Implications in the English Premier League

In 2022, Manchester City—one of the top clubs in the English football Premier League—introduced an AI system that could track the physical condition of a player against an optimum training load to prevent injury (Claudino et al., 2019). It gave individual training recommendations, analyzing vast physiological and performance data, among other things like heart rate, muscle fatigue, and sleep. Whilst this was carried out with the aim of improving performance and attempting to prevent as many short-term injuries as could be, it did raise the ethical issues concerning the long-term health impacts if an individual were to follow AI-derived advice.

Players began to voice their misgivings over what the AI system's suggestions, usually driving them to the extreme physically. AI focused so much on short-term performance optimization that it frequently lost sight of the long-term players' welfare. For instance, the system would recommend extremely high-intensity training protocols that would be productive in the short run but rather increased the risk of developing chronic injuries or long-term health issues. This then raises some critical ethical questions pertaining to the trade-offs between short-term performances and the long-term health and safety of the athletes (Ayala, 2024).

Health and safety are major ethical considerations within sports analytics. The holistic health of the players was taken into serious consideration when making recommendations about the AI system. However, the overreliance on data-driven insights led to a situation whereby the players felt that health was secondary to the metrics portrayed in the performance. This situation brought out the realization for a broader perspective to take in both immediate performance and long-term health expectations.

For this, Manchester City consulted the medical professionals and sports scientists; this includes their lead physician, Dr. Max Sala, in order to balance AI recommendations against medical advice, effectively putting the players' health and safety first. In addition, it established follow-up for long-term health outcomes of the players trained as per the AI-guided regimens. This included ensuring that regular health check-ups were maintained and monitoring was done to check on symptoms of overstraining or being chronically fatigued.

Further, educating players on the AI system and its pilot status to players gets players informed and becomes key to better decision-making. With enabling the players to be fully informed on all possible risks and benefits, Manchester City is able to equip players through its duty so players are even more proactive in their health and performance.

This case epitomizes making the right long-term health and well-being decisions for the top athlete in sport analytics. The case of Manchester City epitomizes that critical decisions in ethical questions in sport analytics and medicine will require a collaborative, interdisciplinary approach with medical expertise integrated therein. With this balance, therefore, AI insights would be useful in the optimization of a certain performance without jeopardizing the health of the players within sports teams. This will not only enhance the ethical standards of sports analytics but foster a culture of trust and care within the team.

## Analysis of Ethical Considerations in Sports Analytics: Case Studies

Four case studies—concern for privacy and player data security, bias in talent identification, effect on coaching and decision-making, and long-term health consequences—point at critical ethical challenges that arise through the use of AI and ML in sports. The ethical concerns brought out in the case studies given above demonstrate how complex and multidimensional the use of such advanced technologies can be for sports analytics (Mountifield, 2023).

## Player Privacy- Data Security

Case of the New England Patriots: This is very critical in the best interest of player privacy and data security. Extended data collection, in this case—GPS and biometrics by players—raised a very critical player privacy concern. It was worsened when the data breach contained sensitive information, undermining the trust of the players. This presents a need for transparent communication and strong security mechanisms to protect the players' data. Informed consent, in this context, means that players should be given clear, simple-to-understand notices so that they can indeed understand the extent and the purposes of data collection. Besides, the use of more advanced security measures with regular auditing is an absolute requirement to prevent data breaches. In any case, constant vigilance needs to be applied to ensure that data is truly protected.

## Bias in Talent Identification

Indeed, the AI-based talent identification system used by FC Barcelona's La Masia academy epitomizes the ethical predicament that bias in AI models engenders. Relying on training data that was produced through unfair practice, it fosters preexisting inequalities since it had a partiality toward players of a certain size, physical ability, and background. This sets forth primacy in ensuring fairness and avoiding bias in the AI setting. This yields the two fundamental steps that can be taken to reducing bias: diversifying training data and implementing a hybrid approach of merging insights from AI with human judgment. One has to ensure that there are regular checks and updates in the models to avoid or correct biases and that talent identification processes are therefore principled under the banner of equality and diversity.

## Impact on Coaching and Decision-Making

The embedding of an AI system for game strategy and player management into the Los Angeles Lakers exposed the underlying ethical paradox of human-AI collaborations: Tensions between AI recommendations and the judgment of the coaches created an environment with a lesser sense of agency among the entire coaching staff. This case offers an illustration of why a more balanced approach that respects and enhances human expertise is called for. AI systems are meant to be supportive and not decision-making. There should be set protocols on how AI insights should be incorporated into the decision process. Transparency on the derivation of AI recommendations and ensuring accountability is key to sustaining the morale of the coaches and players.

## Long-Term Health Implications

The use of an AI system by Manchester City to optimize training loads in injury reduction speaks of the ethical consideration on the long-term health implications of the players. This means that the AI, in its pursuit of short-term gains in performance, may unwittingly sacrifice the long-term well-being of players. Of the main worry, there are skyrocketing cases of the player's chronic injury tagged to the program. Obviously, the lessons one can draw from such cases elevate the need to put health and safety at the top of the agenda in the field of sports analytics (Robel, 2023). More specifically, this should be carried out in a closely monitored multidisciplinary way that also involves medical professionals. Educating the players on what risks and benefits are possible with AI-driven regimens can prepare them to make an informed decision about their long-term health and safety. All the aforementioned case studies and examples indicate that there is an urgent need for serious ethical consideration when involving AI and ML technologies in the context of sport. Addressing such issues requires up-grouped strategies from collective stakeholders to ensure transparency, fairness, and above all the well-being of the athlete. Protecting player privacy and data safety through clear communication, effective security protocols, and continuous monitoring is paramount. Ensuring fairness and inclusivity within AI systems calls for the diversification of training data and integration of human judgment. AI insights must be balanced with human expertise and medical advice to maintain player trust and safeguard long-term player health. Abiding by these virtues of the organization, sports organizations should be able to use advanced technologies to better performance and at the same time, protect the rights and interests of the concerned stakeholders.

There have been many ethical concerns in sports analytics following the inclusion of artificial intelligence and machine learning, which should be handled carefully to ensure a positive net effect on the sector with the technology (Pashin, 2023). Part of that weight accepts ensuring the impact effectively benefits the players with safeguards in the athletes' rights and well-being. Analyzing cases of the New England Patriots, FC Barcelona's La Masia academy, Los Angeles Lakers, and Manchester City brings to light the key ethical challenges around privacy, bias, decision-making, and health implications.

The following case of the New England Patriots gives an example of how critical data security in player information is. The more in-depth data there is to be collected from athletes, such as the collection of biometric data and performance measures by sports agencies, the more it is possible to breach that information. This obviously requires stringent security measures and open communication to foster trust and protection of sensitive information about the players. This is one of the principles in upholding honesty in sports analytics: players should give informed consent so that they exactly know the data that should be collected and regulated.

The case with FC Barcelona represents one of the very basic ethical problems associated with bias in AI systems. The trained AI models, using the past data, might end up fortifying existing bias and end up treating groups underrepresented unfairly. This can deny many talented athletes opportunities because the data that go into training models for them are not properly diverse and predispositioned. The possible way to check and correct it is by increasing the amount and diversity of data used in training sports organizations and checking back on the AI status for any bias. The integration of human judgment with AI can create guardrails against these biases and help open up talent identification to the broad set of factors in terms of inclusivity.

The case of the Los Angeles Lakers exemplifies this best regarding the involvement of AI in the coaching process and real processes of decision-making. Even if AI could provide strategic input for the team, the balance between the recommendation power of AI and the human expertise in the field is important. Examples where such systems are believed to have the ultimate confirmation affect the authority and judgment of coaches. AI could support, but not replace, human decision-making to help foster a collaborative environment. Clear protocols and transparency in the means by which AI recommendations are generated would help underpin trust and morale in coaching staff and players.

Manchester City's AI application in optimizing training loads and preventing injuries surfaces an ethical consideration around long-term health implication. AI systems should be focused on short-term indicators of results in the athletic discipline, thus amplifying the possibility of chronic or other injuries and damage to health over the longer term. A holistic approach should be relevant to try and balance considerations of immediate performance along with well-being into the future. Health professionals should be included in the making of decisions, and players should be educated about the risks and benefits of AI-driven recommendations.

These represent multilevel ethical challenges that the use of artificial intelligence- and machine learning-supported technologies brings with it. Both a comprehensive strategy and the consequent actions are required. The bedrock principles on which the integration of these technologies must rest involve transparency, fairness, and concern for the well-being of the athletes. In case sports organizations uphold these ethical standards, then AI and ML may proceed to enhance performance and safeguard the rights and interests of athletes. Collaboration between and dialogue with each stakeholder are very important in an attempt to navigate the ethical quagmire that pervades the use of sports analytics (Giles et al., 2021).

## IMPLICATIONS

### Practical Implications

At this point, the integration of AI and ML in sports analytics shows several practical implications for the daily functioning of sports teams and organizations. In essence, these technologies have a great ability to enhance performance analysis, injury prevention, and strategic decision-making (Sampaio, 2024). For instance, AI-enabled systems can avail the real-time insights to the coaches during the games, thus allowing them to make informed decisions on the in-game players rotation and their strategies on the games. However, the practical adoption of those systems requires significant investments in technology and staffing training so as people are well equipped to interpret and apply the AI-generated data. Additionally, well-documented protocols on data collection, storage, and usage need to be followed strictly to develop confidence and trust in the respective players and stakeholders in the sports organizations.

## Ethical Considerations

The use of AI and ML in sports analytics carries deep and multifaceted significance (Paneru, 2024). Enhancing soccer pass receiver prediction in broadcast images through advanced deep learning techniques: a comprehensive study on model optimization and performance evaluation. Journal of Soft Computing Exploration, 5(2), 115-121. https://doi.org/10.52465/joscex.v5i2.301. The cases just discussed raise obvious concerns about the privacy and security of players, the long-term consequences of AI bias, and the effects on the health of athletes. This calls for ethical considerations, whereby sports organizations should, first and foremost, protect sensitive information about players through viable security measures that ensure transparent practices around data. Second, from a bias point of view, the AI systems have to be addressed to guarantee no discrimination during talent identification and development. It is of extreme importance to make sure that it guarantees the health and well-being of the athletes through the balancing of short-term performance gains with long-term health considerations. The ethical use of AI in sports analytics necessitates an ongoing vigilance and transparency, and commitment to fairness and respect to all athletes.

## Theoretical Implications

Integration of AI and ML in sports analytics presents several theoretical implications beyond application. The technologies force some level of re-evaluation on the traditional methodologies of performance analysis and decision-making. The use of AI requires a better understanding of how machine learning algorithms interact with human judgment and expertise (Chmait & Westerbeek, 2021). New theoretical frameworks are more likely to be developed that would unlock the understanding in proper terms and conceptualization of the nature and dynamics currently in place between AI systems and human judgment. Moreover, ethical considerations raised by AI in sports analytics can feed into larger debates on responsible technology use across fields and hence allow further development of more comprehensive ethical guidelines and standards.

## Managerial Implications

The proper implementation of AI and machine learning in sports analytics needs meticulous planning and strategic management from a managerial perspective. It is further the responsibility entrusted to the managers to see to it that AI should be "introduced in a way that is complementary to the coaches and other staff." This includes the facilitation of training and resources for staff toward the effective usage of AI tools (Chmait & Westerbeek, 2021). The setting of clear lines of accountability and transparency in making decisions is further a requisite to maintain trust and morale within the organization. What is more, managers are responsible for creating an ethical culture orientated at player well-being and fairness in the usage of AI regarding stated values and ethical standards.

## Societal Implications

The societal implications of AI and ML in sports analytics go beyond the immediate context of sports teams and organizations (Muniz & Flamand, 2022). How the tools are used will affect people's perceptions of fairness and inclusiveness in sports. An example is the issue of AI systems that may be fought through to change the existing perceptions and barriers among some groups in sports. An ethical use of AI in the analytics of sports now can actually set a precedent in the right way for other sectors; how can one responsibly use technology in the betterment of human performance? without compromising the rights of the individual. Using AI in sports more widely can help spur discussions on more ethical technology use across society, driving policy and practices that ultimately ensure the responsible use of technology, the fair treatment, and respect of all people (Liu et al., 2021).

## Limitations and Future Avenues of Research

But the one thing that should be obvious, really, is the quality and comprehensiveness of the data on which an AI system is trained. Incomplete or biased data will result in wrong predictions and further increase the existing inequalities, as in the case of the FC Barcelona talent identification system. Diverse and good-quality data are very important in developing reliable models. Furthermore, there is an issue of black-box challenge: for numerous AI algorithms, their functioning is quite opaque, so it could be problematic to understand or explain—if necessary—the basis for taken decisions. Such a lack of transparency undermines trust and accountability, calling for an approach that has a development process of more interpretable AI models (Salim et al., 2020).

Another limitation is the potential for over-reliance on AI at the expense of human expertise. While AI is helpful in giving insight, it is not infallible. In many cases, it can miss contextual factors that the human expert would notice. In the Los Angeles Lakers case, the resilience between AI recommendations and human judgment mirrors what has been called for: that of a balanced inspiration allowing for a role of AI insights alongside general knowledge built up through time spent in a profession. Also it is these ethical issues that can raise issues such as player privacy, data security, or long-term health impacts that call for persistent attention and a strict governing structure to assure the protection of the rights and well-being of the players (Houtmeyers et al., 2021).

One of the principal directions of future research in this area should be future clear. First, more in-depth studies of the evaluation and effectiveness and impact of AI systems in different sports contexts are needed. For example, it would be necessary to engage in longitudinal studies that investigate the long-lasting influence of the training regime powered by AI on the health and performance of the athlete (Sanjaykumar, 2024). Further research is called for ways to decrease bias in such AI models, whether in data sources or in algorithms built with the ability to consciously remove the prejudice in collected data.

Indeed, transparent and interpretable AI models are an important domain among others under research. Developments in XAI can help in making comprehensible the decision-making processes fostered by AI systems to coaches, players, and other stakeholders. Similarly, it should also consider looking at practices where AI insights can be integrated to result in better human judgments, their better understanding, and how this hybrid approach will influence it across different sports and organizational contexts.

Finally, ethical consideration must be paramount in ongoing research in this area. Studies should expound on the ethical implications of AI in sports analytics to a greater level, formulating a framework, and possibly guidelines that might aid organizations in moving through this complex ethical environment. It can be achieved by looking beyond immediate concerns on privacy and data security to the broader societal impact and the push for fairness and inclusivity in sports (Szymanski, 2020).

It is evident, from the discussion above, that, whilst AI and ML offer huge potential in augmenting sports analytics, the key to unlocking that potential and ensuring the right definition of use is going to be addressing their limitations and developing research in these critical areas. Finally, centered on data quality, transparency, bias mitigation, and ethical considerations of future work, it should enable the possible construction of AI systems that enhance performance without harm to the rights and well-being of athletes (Sanjaykumar, 2024)

## CONCLUSION

Artificial Intelligence and Machine Learning have, therefore, a place in sports analytics as a potentially very transformative development, to do with the potential result in performance and tactics within sports (Almarashi, 2024). As reflected in the case studies of the New England Patriots, FC Barcelona's La Masia academy, the Los Angeles Lakers, and Manchester City, the application of these technologies also raises a range of ethical considerations that must be carefully navigated. The issues involved range from player privacy (Liu, 2024), data security, bias in talent identification, the effect on coaching and decision making, to long-term health implications, which would otherwise warrant a balanced and responsible approach in AI and ML in sports. This poses an ethical question of how benefits can be reaped from AI in consideration of such issues that may encroach on ethics in AI application in sporting if sports were to be left entirely to machines (Constandt et al., 2020). Robust data governance, transparency, and infusion of human judgment with technological acumen in sports organizations is the solution that may help exploit benefits from AI and at the same time take note of issues that may raise questions of ethics when left entirely to machines. This will not just maximize system efficiency, but more importantly lead to fairness, inclusivity, and respect for the rights and well-being of the athletes. Beyond doubt, ongoing research and development should be followed so as not to take care of any backlogs in maintaining data quality and algorithmic bias, striving further in the domain of sports analytics in concurrence with the ethical standards demanded.

In conclusion, the future of sports analytics will increasingly rely on the responsible deployment of AI and ML. To balance the potential of the technologies against the need to maintain the integrity of the sport and the welfare of its participants, embracement of the salient ethical features of the technologies, and encouragement of collaboration between technology developers, sports professionals, and ethical advisors would be affected. Be that as it may, in such an evolving field, commitments must be made toward ethical practices and continuous improvements are invaluable to ensure that in evolving artificial intelligence and machine learning, they contribute to the positive advancement of sport and the enhancement of athlete performance (Musa et al., 2021).

## REFERENCES


Abidin, D. (2021). A case study on player selection and team formation in football with machine learning. *Turkish Journal of Electrical Engineering and Computer Sciences, 29*(3), 1672–1691. DOI: 10.3906/elk-2005-27

Almarashi, A., Daniyal, M., & Jamal, F. (2024). A novel comparative study of nnar approach with linear stochastic time series models in predicting tennis player's performance. *BMC Sports Science, Medicine and Rehabilitation, 16*(1), 28. Advance online publication. DOI: 10.1186/s13102-024-00815-7 PMID: 38273407

Ayala, R., Granados, D. P., Gutiérrez, C. A. G., Ruíz, M. A. O., Espinosa, N. R., & Heredia, E. C. (2024). Novel study for the early identification of injury risks in athletes using machine learning techniques. *Applied Sciences (Basel, Switzerland), 14*(2), 570. DOI: 10.3390/app14020570

Bin, L., & Xu, X. (2021). Application of artificial intelligence in basketball sport. *Journal of Education, Health and Sport, 11*(7), 54–67. DOI: 10.12775/JEHS.2021.11.07.005

Chang, K., Wang, W., & Peng, W. (2023). Where will players move next? dynamic graphs and hierarchical fusion for movement forecasting in badminton. *Proceedings of the AAAI Conference on Artificial Intelligence, 37*(6), 6998–7005. DOI: 10.1609/aaai.v37i6.25855

Chmait, N., & Westerbeek, H. (2021). Artificial intelligence and machine learning in sport research: An introduction for non-data scientists. *Frontiers in Sports and Active Living, 3*, 682287. Advance online publication. DOI: 10.3389/fspor.2021.682287 PMID: 34957395

Claudino, J., Capanema, D., Souza, T., Serrão, J., Pereira, A., & Nassis, G. (2019). Current approaches to the use of artificial intelligence for injury risk assessment and performance prediction in team sports: A systematic review. *Sports Medicine - Open, 5*(1), 28. Advance online publication. DOI: 10.1186/s40798-019-0202-3 PMID: 31270636

Constandt, B., Heres, L., Marlier, M., & Willem, A. (2020). A stakeholder perspective on ethical leadership in sport: Bridging the gap between the normative and descriptive lines of inquiry. *Psychologica Belgica, 60*(1), 381–395. DOI: 10.5334/pb.543 PMID: 33362936

Constandt, B., Heres, L., Marlier, M., & Willem, A. (2020). A stakeholder perspective on ethical leadership in sport: Bridging the gap between the normative and descriptive lines of inquiry. *Psychologica Belgica*, *60*(1), 381–395. DOI: 10.5334/pb.543 PMID: 33362936

Dc, S.DC. (2022). Artificial intelligence in sport: An ethical issue. *Unity Journal*, *3*(01), 27–39. DOI: 10.3126/unityj.v3i01.43313

Dyer, B. (2020). A pragmatic approach to resolving technological unfairness: The case of nike's vaporfly and alphafly running footwear. *Sports Medicine - Open*, *6*(1), 21. Advance online publication. DOI: 10.1186/s40798-020-00250-1 PMID: 32448974

Evans, R., McNamee, M., & Guy, O. (2016). Ethics, nanobiosensors and elite sport: The need for a new governance framework. *Science and Engineering Ethics*, *23*(6), 1487–1505. DOI: 10.1007/s11948-016-9855-1 PMID: 27995447

Giles, B., Peeling, P., Kovalchik, S., & Reid, M. (2021). Differentiating movement styles in professional tennis: A machine learning and hierarchical clustering approach. *European Journal of Sport Science*, *23*(1), 44–53. DOI: 10.1080/17461391.2021.2006800 PMID: 34781856

Glebova, E., Madsen, D. Ø., Mihaľová, P., Géczi, G., Mittelman, A., & Jorgič, B. (2024). Artificial intelligence development and dissemination impact on the sports industry labor market. *Frontiers in Sports and Active Living*, *6*, 1363892. Advance online publication. DOI: 10.3389/fspor.2024.1363892 PMID: 38606117

Gómez-Carmona, P., Fernández-Cuevas, I., Quintana, M., Arnaiz-Lastras, J., & Navandar, A. (2020). Infrared thermography protocol on reducing the incidence of soccer injuries. *Journal of Sport Rehabilitation*, *29*(8), 1222–1227. DOI: 10.1123/jsr.2019-0056 PMID: 32188790

Gour, P., & Khan, M. F. (2024). Utilizing machine learning for comprehensive analysis and predictive modelling of ipl-t20 cricket matches. *Indian Journal of Science and Technology*, *17*(7), 592–597. DOI: 10.17485/IJST/v17i7.2944

Houtmeyers, K., Jaspers, A., & Figueiredo, P. (2021). Managing the training process in elite sports: From descriptive to prescriptive data analytics. *International Journal of Sports Physiology and Performance*, *16*(11), 1719–1723. DOI: 10.1123/ijspp.2020-0958 PMID: 34686619

Kapadiya, C., Shah, A., Adhvaryu, K., Barot, P., & Principal, S. (2020). Intelligent cricket team selection by predicting individual players' performance using efficient machine learning technique. *International Journal of Engineering and Advanced Technology*, *9*(3), 3406–3409. DOI: 10.35940/ijeat.C6339.029320

Lan, H. (2024). Research on analytical model of participation and social influence of she sports activities based on multi-source data fusion. jes, 20(6s), 343-348. https://doi.org/DOI: 10.52783/jes.2652

Leeuw, A., Zwaard, S., Baar, R., & Knobbe, A. (2021). Personalized machine learning approach to injury monitoring in elite volleyball players. *European Journal of Sport Science*, *22*(4), 511–520. DOI: 10.1080/17461391.2021.1887369 PMID: 33568023

Leyva, A. (2020). Ethical aspects of organized contact sports for children as participants. *International Journal of Contemporary Pediatrics*, *7*(8), 1823. DOI: 10.18203/2349-3291.ijcp20203047

Liu, P., Li, X., Zang, B., & Diao, G. (2024). Privacy-preserving sports data fusion and prediction with smart devices in distributed environment. *Journal of Cloud Computing (Heidelberg, Germany)*, *13*(1), 106. Advance online publication. DOI: 10.1186/s13677-024-00671-3

Luccioni, A., & Bengio, Y. (2020). On the morality of artificial intelligence [commentary]. *IEEE Technology and Society Magazine*, *39*(1), 16–25. DOI: 10.1109/MTS.2020.2967486

Mountifield, C. (2023). Sport analytics: graduating from alchemy.. https://doi.org/DOI: 10.5772/intechopen.1002423

Muniz, M., & Flamand, T. (2022). Sports analytics for balanced team-building decisions. *The Journal of the Operational Research Society*, *74*(8), 1892–1909. DOI: 10.1080/01605682.2022.2118634

Musa, R., Majeed, A., Suhaimi, M., Abdullah, M., Razman, M., Deboucha, A., & Osman, N. (2021). Identification of high-performance volleyball players from anthropometric variables and psychological readiness: A machine-learning approach. *Proceedings of the Institution of Mechanical Engineers. Part P, Journal of Sports Engineering and Technology*, *237*(4), 317–324. DOI: 10.1177/17543371211045451

Olenich, T., Terarakelyants, V., Shestopalova, O., & Biryukov, I. (2020). Sport spirituality as an educational innovation (evidenced-based study). E3s Web of Conferences, 210, 17006. https://doi.org/DOI: 10.1051/e3sconf/202021017006

Ossa, L. (2024). Integrating ethics in ai development: A qualitative study. *BMC Medical Ethics*, *25*(1), 10. Advance online publication. DOI: 10.1186/s12910-023-01000-0 PMID: 38262986

Oytun, M., Tınazcı, C., Şekeroğlu, B., Açıkada, C., & Yavuz, H. (2020). Performance prediction and evaluation in female handball players using machine learning models. *IEEE Access : Practical Innovations, Open Solutions*, *8*, 116321–116335. DOI: 10.1109/ACCESS.2020.3004182

Paneru, B., Paneru, B., Poudyal, R., & Poudyal, K. (2024). Enhancing soccer pass receiver prediction in broadcast images through advanced deep learning techniques: A comprehensive study on model optimization and performance evaluation. *Journal of Soft Computing Exploration*, *5*(2), 115–121. DOI: 10.52465/joscex.v5i2.301

Pashin, N. (2023). Development of the mathematical model for calculating player ratings using soft calculations. E3s Web of Conferences, 419, 02023. https://doi.org/DOI: 10.1051/e3sconf/202341902023

Pavitt, J., Braines, D., & Tomsett, R. (2021). Cognitive analysis in sports: Supporting match analysis and scouting through artificial intelligence. *Applied AI Letters*, *2*(1), e21. Advance online publication. DOI: 10.1002/ail2.21

Robel, M. (2023). Cricket players selection for national team and franchise league using machine learning algorithms. Cloud Computing and Data Science, 108-139. https://doi.org/DOI: 10.37256/ccds.5120243741

Salim, F., Haider, F., Postma, D., Delden, R., Reidsma, D., Luz, S., & Beijnum, B. (2020). Towards automatic modeling of volleyball players' behavior for analysis, feedback, and hybrid training. *Journal for the Measurement of Physical Behaviour*, *3*(4), 323–330. DOI: 10.1123/jmpb.2020-0012

Sampaio, T., Oliveira, J. P., Marinho, D. A., Neiva, H. P., & Morais, J. E. (2024). Applications of machine learning to optimize tennis performance: A systematic review. *Applied Sciences (Basel, Switzerland)*, *14*(13), 5517. DOI: 10.3390/app14135517

Sampaio, T., Oliveira, J. P., Marinho, D. A., Neiva, H. P., & Morais, J. E. (2024). Applications of machine learning to optimize tennis performance: A systematic review. *Applied Sciences (Basel, Switzerland)*, *14*(13), 5517. DOI: 10.3390/app14135517

Sangarsu, R. (2022). Securing the organization's sensitive data in the ai era. *Design of Single Chip Microcomputer Control System for Stepping Motor*, *1-3*, 1–3. Advance online publication. DOI: 10.47363/JAICC/2022(1)175

Sanjaykumar, S., Udaichi, K., Rajendiran, G., Cretu, M., & Kozina, Z. (2024). Cricket performance predictions: A comparative analysis of machine learning models for predicting cricket player's performance in the one day international (odi) world cup 2023. *Health Sport Rehabilitation*, *10*(1), 6–19. DOI: 10.58962/HSR.2024.10.1.6-19

Szymanski, S. (2020). Sport analytics: Science or alchemy? *Kinesiology Review (Champaign, Ill.)*, *9*(1), 57–63. DOI: 10.1123/kr.2019-0066

Yang, L., Tian, M., Xin, D., Cheng, Q., & Zheng, J. (2024). Ai-driven anonymization: Protecting personal data privacy while leveraging machine learning. *Applied and Computational Engineering*, *71*(1), 7–13. DOI: 10.54254/2755-2721/71/2024MA0053

# Chapter 13
# Sports Analytics Case Studies

**Sandeep Kumar Singh**
https://orcid.org/0000-0002-1741-7254
*O.P. Jindal Global University, India*

**Geshwaree Huzooree**
https://orcid.org/0000-0001-8076-6636
*Edinburgh Napier University, UK*

## ABSTRACT

*This chapter examines the disruptive influence of sports analytics on the optimization of performance, game tactics, and fans' involvement in the game. Cases that varied in the book were as such player performance analysis, injury prevention, and game tactics. The chapter addresses data accuracy, stakeholder resistance, and the ethical considerations of using analytics that are bound into privacy concerns. It also covers future trends, including more advanced artificial intelligence, wearable technology, and immersive experiences, which will remain important dynamics moving into the future for teams seeking to tap into data as a source of competitive advantage.*

## INTRODUCTION TO SPORTS ANALYTICS

Sports analytics have today been regarded as the next revolution in modern sports, changing how teams, coaches, and athletes think about optimizing their performances and making strategic decisions. This used to be reliant almost single-handedly on intuition and experience but is now supplemented, and in many cases, entirely driven by data. Advanced analytics not only puts light on a broad range of metrics but also offers key evidence toward improving decision-making processes at all

DOI: 10.4018/979-8-3693-5385-1.ch013

levels of sports organizations- professional leagues and amateur teams. It enables them to gain a competitive edge through data-driven approaches while enhancing health or enriching the fan experience (Mondello & Kamke, 2014).

The roots of sports analytics are simple statistical tracking, but they have grown exponentially with the advancement of technology. From here, today data is accumulated from thousands of sources, including wearable devices, video analyses, social networks, and even biomechanical models. This amount of data impacts both sharp analysis at the microsecond as well as long-term player development in addition to influencing game tactics (Gorman, 2017). As more teams embrace these practices, predictive analytics, machine learning algorithms, and advanced statistical models have become just the norm, so it is possible to grade player potential and innate risks of injury, as well as games, much better and more accurately.

The talk about number-crunching with regards to sports analytics is not about crunching those numbers for the sake of counting but rather drawing insights and actionable data out from there. The real value, however, lies in interpreting the data through the incorporation of frameworks of decision-making. Sports analytics applied in multifaceted ways from scouting talents to optimizing game strategies, management of player health improvements, and also improved fan engagement can have wider implications. On the flip side, organizations that are successful in harnessing analytic power can not only improve their competitive standing but also revolutionize innovation within the broader sports ecosystem (Vinué & Epifanio, 2017).

## TYPES OF SPORTS ANALYTICS

Three primary types of sports analytics are: descriptive, predictive, and prescriptive analytics. Each kind of sports analytics serves a different kind of purpose. However, through all these three types, it presents an entire structure for understanding and further improving athletic performance, game strategies, and results in the world of business related to sports.

1. Descriptive Analytics

The basis of sports data analysis lies in descriptive analytics since it focuses more on the collection and interpretation of historical information. Such analysis helps summarise past events and gives insights into what has happened already in a game, in a season, or even the career of a player. Descriptive analytics includes common metrics such as player statistics, for instance, points scored, assists, rebounds; team performance in regard to possession percentages and turnovers (Kwartler, 2022), and the win-loss records. These types of metrics assist the coaches, analysts, and the decision-makers identify trends and patterns that inform decisions in strategic moves. Descriptive analytics sets the foundation for more complex analyses and is therefore very essential in finding benchmarks against which future performances can be measured.

2. Predictive Analytics

Predictive analytics is that analysis that goes beyond what already happened, giving a glimpse into what is likely to happen in the near future based on the available data. It involves historical data and advanced algorithms in forms such as machine learning models, regression analysis, neural networks, among others, to analyze and predict performance by players, chances of injury, or results in a game. Teams in professional sports use predictive analytics to evaluate the potential of their players, predict the chances of winning a game, and determine which strategy is more effective (Bouzarth et al., 2021). For example, predictive models can calculate a player's chances of getting injured during a match or season based on how much he has worked, his motion patterns, and his injury history. This helps the coach and the medical team to take proper decisions on resting and rehabilitating the player to avoid permanent damage.

3. Prescriptive Analytics

Prescriptive analytics is the most advanced and final type of sports data analysis. It does more than predicting outcomes; it recommends actions taken to achieve desired results. This implies that prescriptive analytics integrates a predictive model with optimization algorithms, which suggests strategies that may lead to best possible outcomes. For instance, through prescriptive analytics, the coaches will be able to identify what is the optimum set of in-game lineup combinations during a contest or when to bring in that critical substitution when to make key substitutions. Another example is to make an optimization of training schedules, nutritional plans, and game-day tactics. Prescriptive analytics enables organizations to make proactive data-informed decisions that will enhance team performance as well as operational efficiency (Alamar, 2024).

In conclusion, these three categories of sports analytics-descriptive, predictive, and prescriptive-appear to form the skeleton of a much larger, overarching framework of data-driven decision-making in sports. Be it the analysis of past performances or forecasting future outcomes or optimizing strategies, sports analytics continues to redefine how teams, players, and organizations approach competition (Bouzarth et al., 2021).

## CASE STUDIES

### Case Study 1: Player Performance Analysis

This is a major aspect of strategic decision-making in professional sports. A clear example of this is the Golden State Warriors, an NBA team from San Francisco, California. This team has been highly at the edge in applying analytics in assessing players' performances, leading to their success in multiple championship seasons. The strategy entails gathering data that covers player movement, shot accuracy, and even fatigue levels, followed by analysis of such data to decide on player development and game strategy (Hughes & Elkins, 2023).

The Warriors combine wearable technologies and advanced statistical models to monitor player performance in real-time. For example, during practice games and games, players are fitted with GPS trackers and accelerometers that give out the movement patterns of the player, the speed at which he is running, and the workload on his body. All these can then be analyzed with machine learning algorithms to identify inefficiencies in a player's technique, warn signs of fatigue, and optimize training regimens. Coaches can tailor individually framed training plans to maximum strengths and address weaknesses of any player by correlating movement data with outcomes such as shooting accuracy or defensive effectiveness. Actually, the Golden State Warriors used player performance analytics the summer before the 2017 season to manage star Stephen Curry's minutes. Advanced load management analytics applied by the coaching staff monitored Curry's physiological condition throughout the entire season. Patterns of fatigued conditions that could turn into injuries if not managed were identified; hence, strategic resting was applied for him during specific games. This proactive approach helped to diminish his risk of injury, while also keeping him in top performing form in the playoffs which consequently led to the championship (Miller, 2015).

Another example is in Major League Baseball, the Houston Astros of Houston, Texas. The Astros have utilized data analytics very heavily, judging the performance of players, mainly in batting techniques. Using high-speed cameras and motion-capture technology, Astros actually biomechanics swings of a player (Sch.oenfeld, 2023). The data acquired is continuously manipulated to make minute adjustments to a player's posture, swing trajectory, and timing. For example, from the analysis of swing data, coaches in the Astros helped players like Jose Altuve perfect their hitting mechanics, which greatly contributed to him having an MVP season in 2017.

It is well established that success for teams involved in teams actually translates to real on-field results when the insight gained through data-driven player performance analysis occurs. Advanced technologies like wearables, video analysis, and machine learning algorithms have swing the balance in favor of enabling teams to gain much more insight into ability and to optimize training programs accordingly. Continuous monitoring of performance data and changing approaches based on such data may continue to improve individual player development and overall team performance.

In conclusion, this case study of the Golden State Warriors and Houston Astros demonstrates the increasing significance of player performance analytics in professional sports. The teams are now able to use data-driven insights for improving player development, reducing injuries, and optimizing performance according to their advantage in ways that previously were impossible. If technology continues to evolve, player performance analytics will probably be much more integral to winning sports teams worldwide.

## Case Study 2: Injury Prevention and Management

One of the most basic applications of sports analytics lies in the prevention and management of injuries. Teams in any sport are now employing statistics to reduce the rate of injury, consequently lengthening the careers of players. A great example of this practice is in EPL football at Manchester City FC, Manchester, England. Manchester City has implemented the most advanced data analytic systems to track player health, provide early warnings on injury, and decide on player workload and periods of recovery (Chang et al., 2024).

Wearable technology, including GPS trackers and heart monitors, is used by Manchester City to obtain large amounts of data on all movements, efforts made, and physiological responses in training and matches. It feeds this data into machine learning models tracking key indicators of injury risk, such as sudden accelerations, decelerations, and overall workload. For example, their data analytics team has detected that player who exceeded a certain threshold of sprint distance per match had a higher likelihood of sustaining hamstring injuries. Based on these observations, training intensity was modified and recovery sessions with a target were incorporated to minimize injury (Argibay-González et al., 2022).

Among some positive applications of this approach was in the management of Kevin De Bruyne injury in rehabilitation of the season 2018-2019. After De Bruyne had injury to the knee ligaments, even his recovery was monitored by wearable devices measuring recovery of the muscles and movement patterns together with general physical stress. It is in this respect that through real-time data and his recovery, the medical personnel were in an excellent position to adjust his training load according to his improving condition, hence no strain to report back to full match intensity. In this regard, De Bruyne was able to return to the pitch without exacerbating the injury further and significantly aided the title-winning campaign for that season (Herberger & Litke, 2021).

More recently, US American football has also experienced pioneering clubs in the guise of the National Football League's (NFL) Seattle Seahawks, based in Seattle, Washington. The Seahawks collated sources of information on player bio-mechanics, sleep patterns, hydration levels, among other sources, for every player to compile individual player health profiles. One of the key focuses they have made is concussion prevention, an area that still haunts the NFL. Helmet sensors that track the force and angle of impacts on both practice and game days alert the Seahawks' medical staff to immediately obvious concussions and more subtle ones. Analyzing the impact data also helped change the Seahawks' tackling to minimize those risky, high-impact collisions (Ghasem et al., 2021).

In addition, the Seahawks applied predictive analytics to align training activities so that the workload of players would not be excessive and lead to non-contact injuries such as hamstring strains and muscle tears (Abbot, 2018). For example, they could take data from training sessions to choose when a player's workload exceeded his typical capacity, which was linked to injury likelihood. The Seahawks, basing their learnings, put each of the players into particular rest periods and recovery protocols that brought about an unprecedented 50% decline of the team's overall rate of injuries throughout the 2019 season (Del Prete, 2021).

These case studies demonstrate how advanced analytics changes the injury prevention and management approaches in sport. Aggregation and analysis of player movement, workload, and impact forces are thus deployed by teams in both proactive measures that reduce the probability of a range of injuries, while also raising the longevity of their players. Thus, it would therefore allow a sports organization to have a better view of what is happening to the health of the player, which would, in turn, lead to performance and competitiveness.

## Case Study 3: Game Strategy and Tactics

Game strategy and tactics have radically been influenced by the power of analytics, since teams now make use of data in order to optimally plan their approach to achieve an edge above the rest on the field. A very good example here is Major League Baseball, or MLB, and the Oakland Athletics, who play out of Oakland, California. This use of analytics was popularly coined as "Moneyball," which dramatically changed how the strategies for baseball are constructed. With General Manager Billy Beane, the Athletics, using advanced sabermetrics found low-cost players who successfully went unnoticed in respect to a less obvious but statistically significant area that was on-base percentage (Elitzur, 2020).

This changed the game strategy of Athletics, enabling the team to play against more affluent clubs with great success. Focusing more on the data and not to the traditional scouting, Athletics managed to build a team that was tactically efficient.

For example, placing high value on walks and getting players on base rather than focusing single-handedly on power hitting. This analytical analysis not only formed the directions of game tactics of individual games (Moorefield, 2021), like optimization of lineup and defensive positions but has also changed the way teams in the league assess talents in players as well as how they develop plans for their games

The next convincing example of analytics-based game strategy can be seen in basketball through Houston Rockets, a team in the National Basketball Association (NBA) based in Houston, Texas. Under General Manager Daryl Morey, the Rockets defined a data-driven approach to game strategy, in which they optimized shot selection in the context of advanced metrics. Morey and his cohorts were able to drive the argument that three-pointers and shots close to the hoop have, respectively, much higher efficiency rates than mid-range jumpers. As a result, the Rockets developed a game strategy emphasizing three-point shots and trips to the basket, thus transforming the team's mode of attacking significantly (Ford, 2018).

The 2017-2018 NBA season witnessed the Rockets attempt the most three-point shot attempts in the league-a testament to their analytically informed approach. In fact, the team's game plan-also colloquially known as "Moreyball"-is to try to score the most points per possession by shooting the most statistically valued field goal attempts. The data-driven approach led the Rockets to a franchise-record 65-win season and a deep playoff run, which narrowly excluded the Rockets from advancing into the NBA Finals. This not only helped them in scoring but also transformed how clubs prepare tactics for matches league wide as well (Davenport, 2014).

In soccer, FC Barcelona has been a leader in innovation regarding tactics for many years. In the past few years, they have embraced the use of data analytics in the popular possession-based "tiki-taka" style of play. For example, the coaching staff at Barcelona uses GPS technology and video analytics on player positioning and passing networks. They thus aim to optimize ball movement and spacing on the pitch in such a way that the ball is in the control of the players for longer periods. From data monitored and presented, Barcelona can alter its tactical arrangement, in real-time during the game, with factors like pass lanes, players' running patterns, and weaknesses of the opponent (Wisdom & Javed, 2023).

For example, in the 2018-19 La Liga season, there were many reports that Barcelona used data analytics to enhance its pressing game. The opposition's passing patterns and movement tendencies could be analyzed to establish the opportune moments to press and regain possession. This approach helped Barcelona dominate ball possession and contributed to their league title that year. The embedding of data in their game plan has since become a crucial enabler of their dominance both at the domestic and international level (Cacho-Elizondo & Álvarez, 2020).

These case studies thus illustrate how data analytics fundamentally changed game strategy and tactics in more than one sport-from Oakland Athletics' Moneyball to Houston Rockets' effective three-point shooting strategy, or to FC Barcelona's data-driven pressing tactics. Analytics enables teams to explore deeper insights into game dynamics. By optimizing strategies through the use of data and making informed tactical decisions, sports organizations are then bettered in their ability to outmanoeuvre opponents for consistent success.

## Case Study 4: Fan Engagement and Marketing

In recent years, sports organizations have become to increasingly make use of data analytics in the pursuit of fan engagement and driving marketing efforts. This yield teams a better understanding of fan behavior, tailors communications, and develops campaigns tailored toward increasing fan loyalty and revenue. Two examples include European football and cricket: teams and leagues there already utilize information in growing fans' attachment (Parganas & Anagnostopoulos, 2015).

One of the major cases of fan engagement through analytics comes from Liverpool FC in Liverpool, England. Of all teams in the English Premier League, Liverpool has taken huge investment in their digital strategy, making extensive use of fan data for engagement across platforms. The club collects its data through social media, the Liverpool FC mobile app, and ticketing systems, hence getting data from its global fan base. This data is then used to collect preference information from fans, including favourite players, what fans consume content-wise, and their buying behaviors (Rasooli et al., 2024).

It enables the club to personalize the content and offers for individual fans through a data-driven approach. For example, the club applies data analytics of fans to profile email marketing campaigns so that fans receive updates about merchandise, matchday experiences, or digital content that resonate well with their preferred tastes. So, this has resulted in increased product sales, particularly through targeted marketing at the right time, such as when kits are launched or during a good performance. And additionally, the matchday experience fan engagement strategy of Liverpool uses live data to further enhance the matchday experience as it offers individual mobile updates alongside unique content, therefore creating an interactive environment for spectators attending games.

Another great example of fan engagement and marketing through analytics is Cricket Australia, Australia's governing body of cricket, headquartered in Melbourne. Cricket Australia has developed a comprehensive fan engagement platform incorporating match attendance data, digital interactions, and fan clubs (Barve, 2023). The use of such data is making the organization connect with the fans more, which is beneficial for the delivery of content and focused marketing programs that drive fan engagement and lead to expanded participation in the sport.

One of the key analytics-based marketing strategies that Cricket Australia uses is the "MyCricket" application through which it enables the fan to track live scores, information regarding the player statistics, and special content. The app would, therefore, collect valuable data on the behavior of users such as which team's users follow, their viewing habits among other interaction with contents (Annamalai et al., 2022). Such data could then be analyzed in order to come up with customized content recommendations or personalized marketing messages. For instance, during the 2019 ICC Cricket World Cup, Cricket Australia effectively used fan data to send targeted updates on match scores and merchandise deals to fans about their favorite teams and players (Taylor, 2020). Apart from increasing fan engagement, this move also saw a massive surge in merchandise sales during the tournament.

Furthermore, La Liga is the top professional football division in Spain, located in Madrid, and has developed itself significantly within the analytics resources that enhance fan engagement. In its implementation of a wide-ranging digital transformation, La Liga simply used data to reach out to fans through different channels. The data it collects on fan preferences, match attendance, and content engagement are gathered through its mobile app and digital platforms. This information is then used to produce personalized digital experiences for instance privileged behind-the-scenes content and real-time match updates based on every fan's preference.

La Liga's data strategy was witnessed in operation during the COVID-19 pandemic when attendance at stadiums was barred. It utilized its digital platforms to stay the fans connected to the action through virtual experiences like immersive streams and interactive content. La Liga analyzed fan data to personalize digital campaigns, which sharply rose online engagement and social media interaction at a time when other common avenues of traditional fan engagement were out of bounds. This data-driven approach kept the interest of fans and at the same time made the league popular all around the world on the internet (Previati, 2020).

Using data analytics has not only acted as a facilitator for fan engagement and marketing in sports. Evidently, from the above illustration, whether it is about making use of personalized content at Liverpool FC or tailored marketing efforts for Cricket Australia (Mattesi, 2019), or digitizing La Liga, sports organizations increasingly rely on data to render more meaningful and engaging interactions with fans and get them further attached to a particular team or clubs. These cases prove that data-driven fan engagement fosters loyalty, increases revenue growth, and establishes a strong connection between teams and their followers.

## Case Study 5: Performance Analytics in Esports

Esports is a fast-evolving industry, and analytics are an integral part to the improvement of player performance and team strategy. As far as performance analytics in esports goes, its application would be in monitoring in-game player actions, keeping track of behaviors, and optimising strategies in real-time. Since their identity is digital, gathering data or information is easy, and teams can implement changes immediately. Two most notable cases where performance analytics has been adopted are those of the South Korean League of Legends esports scene and Danish teams that feature Counterstrike: Global Offensive.

As far as the extremely popular game League of Legends (LoL) is concerned, the most pioneering application of performance analytics for competitive advantage purposes could be seen in South Korea. These include the team T1, from Seoul, South Korea. This was the most victorious team in League of Legends history, with multiple world championships. Using advanced analytics, T1 monitors such in-game metrics as player positioning, reaction times, the efficiency of their decision-making under pressure, and how efficiently they carry out all the various game strategies. Through real-time data analysis, a team can assess the strength and weak points of each player regarding different champions (game characters), roles, and scenarios, according to Jayal et al., (2018).

For instance, according to Cho, T1 coaches use heatmaps to analyze movements on the game map, pointing out to areas as most vulnerable to enemy attacks or becoming inefficient in taking over the objective. By analysing these trends, the coaches will be able to train players so that they position themselves better in order to control key portions of the map, such as dragon pits and towers, holding the key to the game's success. This data-driven plan seemed to pay off during T1's run to the 2016 League of Legends World Championship as they dominated competitions through better control of the map and more decision-making capabilities (Novak et al., 2020).

There is the Danish Astralis in CS: Global Offensive (CS) from Copenhagen, Denmark. This team relies very much on performance analytics. Astralis has been one of the world's greatest CS teams, especially because of their groundbreaking analytics in optimizing team performance. It is a strategic first-person shooting game where team strategy and personal performance play a highly important role. The Danish team, Astralis (Kähärä, 2020), is increasingly using top-of-the-line data analytics to monitor in-game metrics such as reaction times for players, accuracy in shooting, grenade usage, and coordination with their team overall.

One area in which Astralis has excelled is in data utilization for fine-tuning the use of grenades, including smokes, flashes, and those that impede an opponent's vision or movement. Analyzing the in-game stats from game footage enabled Astralis to know the best possible positions and time for grenade smokes. They ensured to attain a position advantage over foes and extracted poor situations of the opponents. The extent of precision while executing strategies according to the performance analytics supported them in dominating the global CS landscape, winning four Major Championship titles between 2017 and 2019 (dos Santos, 2023).

Astralis makes use of biometric data to monitor player health and performance. This includes the integration of wearable devices data for analysis of players' heart rates and stress levels during practice sessions and competition to derive analyses relevant for sport psychologists to work with players for the management of stress while keeping concentration during the high-stakes matches. This integration of in-game analytics with performance-focused mental training has put Astralis atop the totem pole as one of the most consistent and successful teams in esports (Schöber et al., 2024).

Another example of performance analytics can be seen in Team Liquid, a North American esports organization based in Los Angeles, California. Competing in various titles such as Dota 2 and StarCraft II, Team Liquid has invested in using data to enhance player performance. For Dota 2, performance analytics is used for metrics like the gold per minute, experience per minute, and overall player efficiency in securing map objectives. From these analytics, the coaching staff of Team Liquid could find where the players were underperforming and make necessary adjustments in strategy (Orme, 2020).

Analytically, while running for The International 2017, the most notable annual Dota 2 tournament, Team Liquid could study, therefore, the draft phase in which teams pick and ban heroes. By doing so, through analyzing historical data on win rates, team compositions, and hero counters, the drafts from this team were optimized as it came out to be several times promising advantageous matchups that would give them strategic control even before the game has begun. This data-informed drafting strategy has so much to contribute toward their success in tournament.

In other words, the esports teams are making use of performance analytics to better their strategies during the games in order to make better decisions regarding their moves and heighten the overall prowess of the team. As demonstrated by teams such as T1, Astralis, and Team Liquid, analytics can be fitted to most esports' games, including League of Legends and CS

This team took it to Dota 2. From using data analytics, it is this key feature that teams employed in their attempt to keep on top in the competitive scene, demonstrating the increased reliance of performance analytics in the ever-fast-paced world of esports.

## CHALLENGES AND LIMITATIONS OF SPORTS ANALYTICS

Despite the powerful impact of sports analytics in terms of how teams and organizations actually work, there remain significant challenges and limitations affecting its full realization. Ranging from issues of data accuracy to more mundane problems resulting from resistance of coaches and players to an occasional worry over the privacy of the data itself, among many more, below are some of the key challenges faced in the sports analytics realm.

1. Data Quality and Accuracy

One of the greatest challenges in sports analytics is ensuring that data collected on any sport is of good quality and accurate. Misleading insights based on false information will likely have a negative impact on a team's strategies and player performance appraisals. Automated tracking systems and sensors may often be used in fast-paced sports, like soccer or basketball, to collect data. However, these systems are not immune to error-free conditions. These will sometime miss data points or wrongly track players. Wearable devices also create the possibility of factors such as interference from sources such as battery life, position of the device, or environmental conditions affecting the data gathered (Vinué & Epifanio, 2017).

Another issue apart from technical problems is inconsistency in data coming from different teams and leagues. For example, the tracking technologies or analytics platforms may vary between teams of a particular league; therefore, it will be challenging to establish standards while comparing players' performances or reach a general conclusion based on the collected data. This indeed adds a complexity layer to analysts and teams that need to make strategic decisions through data (Apostolou & Tjortjis, 2019).

2. Coaches' and Players' Push Back

Another challenging problem with the implementation of sport analytics is cultural resistance from coaching staffs, players, and other people involved. Long-term, experience-based, and intuitive-coaching staffs may view analytics as a threat to their power or as too technical. They would strongly resist the approach introduced through data-based methods. "Analytics cannot capture the intangible elements of sports: team chemistry, leadership, or clutch performances in crucial moments," they might argue (Sarlis & Tjortjis, 2020).

Players, too, may resent performance tracking and the continuous analysis of their actions. Some may feel that analytics trivializes their importance or makes their on-field decisions sound like counting. This is particularly true for older players or more experienced players who are less used to data gaining influence in sports decision-making. Stakeholders at all levels still find it difficult to be convinced by the merits of analytics (Miller, 2015).

3. Data Overload and Complexity

One of the critical dilemmas of today's big data era is the volume of data generated inside training sessions, matches, and tournaments. It can quickly overwhelm both teams and analysts as they are scrounging for actionable insights. Take, for example, the case of a premier league football team with terabytes of data from player tracking systems, performance metrics, and game footage generated during a season. It requires skills and tools that most teams do not have to sift through this data for meaningful patterns (Alamar, 2024).

Furthermore, even if the related data becomes accessible to it, it is pretty challenging for the data to become translated into proper coaching or game-day decisions. Relating advanced metrics or complicated statistical models may not be easy to comprehend for coaches and players. This simplification and communication of analytical insights in terms that stakeholders might understand is the biggest challenge in the expansive use of sports analytics.

4. Integration with Traditional Methods

Analytics is better to be used as a supplement to traditional forms of coaching rather than substituting them, and infusing analytics into the established framework of a sports team can be problematic. For instance, there could be conflict between the data-driven nature of choices made by analytics and the gut instincts that the veteran coaches would typically rely upon (Houtmeyers et al., 2021). Another concern would be that analytics does not supplant the emotional and mental exercises that encompass sports performance. A lot of attention to numbers might overpower the role played by motivation, teamwork, and confidence that are factors that can let them win the game in competitive sports.

A fine balancing act to achieve between human intuition and data-driven insights, such that not all teams have mastered it.

5. Data Privacy and Ethical Concerns

As sports analytics is increasingly working on gathering sensitive data, be it biometric information retrieved from wearable devices, concerns regarding data privacy and ethical considerations related to monitoring athletes are growing in number. The concerned biometric data include information about the athlete's heart rate, stress level, sleep pattern, and general physical health. Although useful for insight into performance optimization and injury prevention, these metrics also raise such questions as who owns this data, how it is being stored, and how it is used (Mondello & Kamke, 2014).

For instance, the players might find the level of tracking uncomfortable and fear that the information gathered will be used against them in contract renegotiation or career evaluation. Sensitive information leakage may lead to reputational damage or competitive disadvantages. As analytics become increasingly adopted, sports organizations will have to navigate through intricate data protection regulations and guidelines to ensure that the voices of the players are pronounced.

6. High Prices and Accessibility

The financial cost of implementing such advanced analytics systems is an important limitation, primarily to smaller teams or leagues with very few budgets. Advanced tracking systems, wearable devices, and experience data analysts require heavy investment. Teams in bigger leagues like the NFL or EPL can invest in these technologies, while smaller teams and organizations may find it hard to sustain the high demand for data-driven insights (Houtmeyers et al., 2021).

In addition, the inequality of access to analytics technology has created a performance gap between highly endowed teams that are able to provide advanced systems and poorly resourced teams that cannot. This can make the competitive gap even wider because less well endowed teams may take longer to compete with relatively data savvy organizations.

While sports analytics could revolutionize the sports world, however its applicability is strictly limited by a host of challenges and limitations. Problems associated with data quality, resistance by various stakeholders, or complications associated with the integration of analytics into the conventional methods of training have to be overcome. Other issues are data privacy concerns and higher analytics system costs. Yet, despite these challenges, the success stories in sport analytics keep the current trend of adoption in modern sports administration on course (Mondello & Kamke, 2014).

## FUTURE TRENDS IN SPORTS ANALYTICS

As sports analytics keeps growing, several emerging trends are expected to shape its future-which will, in turn, influence teams, athletes, and organizations in their performance optimization, engagement of fans, and strategic decision-making. Advances in AI and Machine Learning, personal health tracking, and immersive fan experiences promise a more data-driven, innovative tomorrow in the world of sports analytics.

1. Artificial Intelligence and Machine Learning

AI and machine learning will change the game entirely in sports analytics because it will allow the analysis of far more sophisticated data modeling and predictive approaches. With real-time processing of enormous amounts of data, teams can use algorithms from machine learning to identify patterns and trends that even the best human analysts might not have picked up. For instance, with AI, it is possible to predict a player's probability of fatigue (Vinué & Epifanio, 2017) and risk of injury and optimal strategy based on their previous game performance and other external conditions. Machine learning algorithms might also detect the opponent's tendencies and suggest changes during the game to use those vulnerabilities, giving them an edge in competition.

The implementation of AI in sports will not be restricted to the field-teams will thus be having better insights on their fan behavior and ticket sales and can better create marketing strategies. AI allows real-time analysis of the social media activities, purchasing patterns, and other digital interactions, hence helping organizations tailor their marketing efforts in such a way so that fans can be engaged in a much better way (Sarlis & Tjortjis, 2020).

2. Wearable Technology and Personalized Health Analytics

Wearable technology is already regarded nowadays as a basic structural component of modern sports; yet it is in future designs that the maximum extent to which personalized health analytics can be taken will be revealed. For instance, with increasingly sophisticated sensors, wearables will provide the athlete with information about his or her physical condition with all the precision needed-to the beat, in fact, relating to heart rate variability, muscle fatigue level, hydration level, and sleep quality. This shall lead to more customized specific training sessions and also fewer chances of injury, with athletes reaching the pinnacle of their performance, with minimized risks (Rubleske et al., 2020).

Wearables will become smaller, softer, and deeper integrated into clothing worn by the athlete. They'll talk in real-time to coaching staff and analytics, providing the athlete with immediate feedback about what they're actually doing. It would be a game-changer on how athletes should train, recover, and compete.

3. Advanced Video Analytics and Computer Vision

The other trend that is going to shape the future of sports analytics is increased development in advanced video analytics and computer vision technologies. Computer vision systems can recognize images quite efficiently with sophisticated image recognition algorithms, more accurately and in greater detail than ever before. These can track player movements, ball trajectories, and even body language, giving really valuable insights into performances and tactics (Alamar, 2024).

Computer vision technologies will, therefore, provide sports like soccer, basketball, and tennis with unprecedented insight into where the players are and how movement efficiency is or isn't enhanced, as well as decision-making under pressure. These insights would help coaches fine-tune their strategies and tactics in real-time. Video analytics would also aid performance analysis while promoting officiating with more accurate and unbiased decisions, reducing human error during critical moments.

4. Virtual and Augmented Reality for Training and Fan Engagement

Virtual reality and augmented reality are the next big thing in both training for a player and as an engaging tool for fans. Virtual reality and augmented reality would soon allow athletes to create scenarios of real-world games with all possible challenges without having the physical implications of actual games. In this regard, American football players can employ VR in modeling passing drills, as soccer players can use it in penalty kicks in virtual space (Bouzarth et al., 2021).

AR and VR, for fans, will revolutionize how people watch sports: totally immersive and interactive ways to view live sports. Fans will see through the eyes of a favorite player as if experiencing himself at a game or look in greater detail at stats overlays during a live game. This technology will make engagements deeper and sport interaction more personal.

5. Predictive Analytics and Data-Driven Decision Making

Predictive analytics is going to become much more important as teams look to forecast future performance, player development, and team dynamics. Analysis of historical data and leveraging machine learning models can predict outcomes such as games, player progression, and recovery of injuries with greater precision. Example: Predictive analytics could inform coaches to make decisions about which type of player is likely to excel in specific matchups or tactics to be used for the highest probabilities of success (Kwartler, 2022).

It will also make up the base of player scouting and recruitment. Teams will be able to uncover some of the best talents in performance metrics from every corner of the globe, bringing a competitive edge in the building of winning teams.

6. Blockchain Technology and Sports Data Security

The increasing concern in sports data collection and storage involves issues of data privacy and security. The blockchain technology is increasingly becoming an accepted solution to this problem since it can enable the decentralization and secure data storing and exchanging. Blockchain uptake by organizations in sports means that data that could be described as personal or sensitive, such as information on player metrics in terms of performance, biometric data, or even monetary transactions, will be encrypted and therefore cannot be accessed without permission (Miller, 2015).

In addition to safeguarding the data, it would, in that regard, give the sports persons the option to have the ownership of the performance data, making them, therefore, in control of who and to whom the data is accessed and shared. In a nutshell (Sarlis & Tjortjis, 2020), the contracts negotiation and assessment of the player would be more straightforward because both parties would have the precise numbers.

Advancements such as AI, wearable technology, video analytics, and immersive experiences will continue to define the future of sports analytics, besides making a much bigger deal out of data safety and security using blockchain. This will further continue to challenge the boundaries of what is possible in sports, bringing new avenues for teams, players, and organizations to gain a competitive advantage and engage fans. With more and more of it included in all aspects of sports, the scope for innovation is endless (Apostolou & Tjortjis, 2019).

## CONCLUSION

Sports analytics fundamentally changed the way an athlete, teams, and organizations would behave in terms of performance optimization, game strategy, and fan engagement. Data-backed insights help teams make better decisions in outcomes on the playing field as well as off-field activities. From analyzing player performance to injury prevention and game strategy optimization, sports analytics is rewriting the book on modern sports.

However, in diversified case studies, it has been observed that the mere implementation and adaptation of sports analytics carry inherent difficulties. Issues ranging from data accuracy to cultural resistance and ethical concerns like privacy and surveillance continue to pose setbacks. On the other hand, the technological advances by AI, wearable devices, and predictive analytics promise to solve most of these limitations and therefore more innovative solutions to be progressed in the future.

Beyond performance analysis, its application will extend to far broader areas for sports analytics as its functional role in the ongoing process continues to grow. Emerging trends include fan engagement, esports, and personalized health tracking where data-driven approaches will be applied more extensively. Besides, virtual reality and blockchain technology will let the future of sports analytics not only be more accurate but also more secure and immersive.

In the long run, sports analytics might be viewed as the dawn of a technological revolution in sports: the confluence of data, science, and technology bent on pushing the frontiers of human performance and business strategy. At such a rapid rate of change in the world of professional sports, embracing these innovations will be critical to staying competitive across teams and organizations.

## REFERENCES


Abbott, D. (2018). The transition of the college quarterback to the NFL: Why the hardest position in sports is getting easier.

Alamar, B. (2024). *Sports analytics: A guide for coaches, managers, and other decision makers*. Columbia University Press. DOI: 10.7312/alam20520

Alamar, B. (2024). *Sports analytics: A guide for coaches, managers, and other decision makers*. Columbia University Press. DOI: 10.7312/alam20520

Annamalai, B., ShabbirHusain, R. V., Chandrasekaran, S., & Varshney, S. (2022). Cultural differences in sports fan engagement on Facebook: A comparison of Australian and Indian cricket league. *International Journal of Sport Management and Marketing*, *22*(1-2), 120–141. DOI: 10.1504/IJSMM.2022.121251

Apostolou, K., & Tjortjis, C. (2019, July). Sports analytics algorithms for performance prediction. In *2019 10th International Conference on Information, Intelligence, Systems and Applications (IISA)* (pp. 1-4). IEEE. DOI: 10.1109/IISA.2019.8900754

Argibay-González, J. C., Vázquez-Estévez, C., Gutiérrez-Santiago, A., Paramés-González, A., Reguera-López-de-la-Osa, X., & Prieto-Lage, I. (2022). Analysis of injury patterns in men's football between the English league and the Spanish league. *International Journal of Environmental Research and Public Health*, *19*(18), 11296. DOI: 10.3390/ijerph191811296 PMID: 36141571

Barve, Y. D. (2023). Assessing the impacts of digital marketing and sponsorship on the football industry as a business and their implications on fan engagement (Doctoral dissertation, Dublin, National College of Ireland).

Bouzarth, E. L., Grannan, B. C., Harris, J. M., Hutson, K. R., & Keating, P. J. (2021). Storytelling with sports analytics. In *Tutorials in Operations Research: Emerging Optimization Methods and Modeling Techniques with Applications* (pp. 38-61). INFORMS. DOI: 10.1287/educ.2021.0230

Cacho-Elizondo, S., & Álvarez, J. D. L. (2020). Big data in the decision-making processes of football teams integrating a theoretical framework, applications and reach. *Journal of Strategic Innovation and Sustainability*, *15*(2), 21–44.

Chang, V., Sajeev, S., Xu, Q. A., Tan, M., & Wang, H. (2024). Football analytics: Assessing the correlation between workload, injury and performance of football players in the English Premier League. *Applied Sciences (Basel, Switzerland)*, *14*(16), 7217. DOI: 10.3390/app14167217

Davenport, T. H. (2014). What businesses can learn from sports analytics. *MIT Sloan Management Review*.

Del Prete, T. (2021). *The greatest teams never: Sports memories of near misses, total messes, and not-so-magical moments*. Gatekeeper Press.

dos Santos, M. (2023). The impact of Covid-19 on esports–Analysis of stock market and corporate governance.

Elitzur, R. (2020). Data analytics effects in major league baseball. *Omega, 90*, 102001. DOI: 10.1016/j.omega.2018.11.010

Ford, R. A. (2018). Trade secrets and information security in the age of sports analytics. In *The Oxford Handbook of American Sports Law*.

Ghasem, W., Valenzuela, J., & Saxon, L. A. (2021). Player tracking technology and data for injury prevention in the National Football League. *Current Sports Medicine Reports, 20*(9), 436–439. DOI: 10.1249/JSR.0000000000000873 PMID: 34524184

Gorman, D. (2017). Sports analytics: Analysis of the National Football League (Doctoral dissertation, Dublin, National College of Ireland).

Herberger, T. A., & Litke, C. (2021). The impact of big data and sports analytics on professional football: A systematic literature review. In *Digitalization, digital transformation and sustainability in the global economy: Risks and opportunities* (pp. 147-171). DOI: 10.1007/978-3-030-77340-3_12

Houtmeyers, K. C., Jaspers, A., & Figueiredo, P. (2021). Managing the training process in elite sports: From descriptive to prescriptive data analytics. *International Journal of Sports Physiology and Performance, 16*(11), 1719–1723. DOI: 10.1123/ijspp.2020-0958 PMID: 34686619

Hughes, K., & Elkins, E. (2023). Silicon Valley's team: The Golden State Warriors, datafied managerialism, and basketball's racialized geography. *American Quarterly, 75*(3), 471–499. DOI: 10.1353/aq.2023.a905860

Jayal, A., McRobert, A., Oatley, G., & O'Donoghue, P. (2018). *Sports analytics: Analysis, visualisation and decision making in sports performance*. Routledge. DOI: 10.4324/9781315222783

Kähärä, B. (2020). Analytical support in esports: Creating a new dimension using eye-tracking analysis.

Kwartler, T. (2022). *Sports analytics in practice with R*. John Wiley & Sons. DOI: 10.1002/9781119598084

Mattesi, R. (2019). Social-media as platform for football clubs to increase revenues and enhance brand value.

Miller, T. W. (2015). *Sports analytics and data science: Winning the game with methods and models*. FT Press.

Mondello, M., & Kamke, C. (2014). The introduction and application of sports analytics in professional sport organizations. *Journal of Applied Sport Management, 6*(2), 11. DOI: 10.7290/jasm06ldmv

Moorefield, J. (2021). The Oakland Athletics use of sabermetrics and the rise of big data analytics in business.

Novak, A. R., Bennett, K. J., Pluss, M. A., & Fransen, J. (2020). Performance analysis in esports: Modelling performance at the 2018 League of Legends World Championship. *International Journal of Sports Science & Coaching, 15*(5-6), 809–817. DOI: 10.1177/1747954120932853

Orme, S. (2020). Playing to win: The global esports industry and key issues. In *The Video Game Debate 2* (pp. 66–80). Routledge. DOI: 10.4324/9780429351815-6

Parganas, P., & Anagnostopoulos, C. (2015). Social media strategy in professional football: The case of Liverpool FC. *Choregia, 11*(2).

Previati, A. (2020). *The importance of fan engagement and fan management in sports*. St. John's University.

Rasooli, M., Mehri, S., & Aziziani, M. (2024). Analyzing Liverpool FC website through fan management perspective. *Sports Marketing Studies, 5*(2), 69–87.

Rubleske, J., Fletcher, T., & Westerfeld, B. (2020). E-sports analytics: A primer and resource for student research projects and lesson plans. *Journal of Instructional Pedagogies, 23*.

Sarlis, V., & Tjortjis, C. (2020). Sports analytics—Evaluation of basketball players and team performance. *Information Systems, 93*, 101562. DOI: 10.1016/j.is.2020.101562

Schöber, T., Stadtmann, G., Parshakov, P., & Tylkin, I. (2024). Survival of professional counter-strike: Global offensive teams: What matters? A research note. *Journal of Electronic Gaming and Esports, 2*(1). Advance online publication. DOI: 10.1123/jege.2022-0025

Schoenfeld, B. (2023). *Game of edges: The analytics revolution and the future of professional sports*. WW Norton & Company.

Vinué, G., & Epifanio, I. (2017). Archetypoid analysis for sports analytics. *Data Mining and Knowledge Discovery, 31*(6), 1643–1677. DOI: 10.1007/s10618-017-0514-1

Wisdom, C., & Javed, A. (2023). Machine learning for data analytics in football: Quantifying performance and enhancing strategic decision-making. *Available at SSRN* 4558733. DOI: 10.2139/ssrn.4558733

# Compilation of References

Abbott, D. (2018). The transition of the college quarterback to the NFL: Why the hardest position in sports is getting easier.

Abbott, A., Button, C., Pepping, G.-J., & Collins, D. (2005). Unnatural selection: Talent identification and development in sport. *Nonlinear Dynamics Psychology and Life Sciences*, *9*(1), 61–88. PMID: 15629068

Abidin, D. (2021). A case study on player selection and team formation in football with machine learning. *Turkish Journal of Electrical Engineering and Computer Sciences*, *29*(3), 1672–1691. DOI: 10.3906/elk-2005-27

Acar, G. (2023). The evolution of sports management: Through the lens of management science, trends, and future vision. *International Journal of Recreation and Sports Science*, *7*(1), 61–69. DOI: 10.46463/ijrss.1378131

Agarwal, S. (2023). Artificial intelligence in sports industry. In *Artificial intelligence for business* (pp. 250–269). Productivity Press. DOI: 10.4324/9781003358411-15

Ahmed, A., & Abdulkareem, A. M. (2023). Big data analytics in the entertainment Industry: Audience behavior analysis, content recommendation, and Revenue maximization. *Reviews of Contemporary Business Analytics*, *6*(1), 88–102.

Akhtar, R., Winsborough, D., Lovric, D., & Chamorro-Premuzic, T. (2019). Identifying and managing talent in the age of artificial intelligence. In *Workforce readiness and the future of work* (pp. 169–185). Routledge. DOI: 10.4324/9781351210485-10

Akyıldız, Z., Ocak, Y., Clemente, F., Birgonul, Y., Günay, M., & Nobari, H. (2022). Monitoring the post-match neuromuscular fatigue of young Turkish football players. *Scientific Reports*, *12*(1), 13835. Advance online publication. DOI: 10.1038/s41598-022-17831-7 PMID: 35974069

Alamar, B. (2024). *Sports analytics: A guide for coaches, managers, and other decision makers*. Columbia University Press. DOI: 10.7312/alam20520

Albert, E. T. (2019). AI in talent acquisition: A review of AI-applications used in recruitment and selection. *Strategic HR Review, 18*(5), 215–221. DOI: 10.1108/SHR-04-2019-0024

Alenezi, M. A., Alshehri, M. A., & Aldhafferi, F. H. (2022). Improving AI-based injury prediction models by addressing algorithmic biases. *Journal of Artificial Intelligence in Healthcare, 5*(1), 45–57.

Allal-Chérif, O., Aránega, A. Y., & Sánchez, R. C. (2021). Intelligent recruitment: How to identify, select, and retain talents from around the world using artificial intelligence. *Technological Forecasting and Social Change, 169*, 120822. DOI: 10.1016/j.techfore.2021.120822

Almarashi, A., Daniyal, M., & Jamal, F. (2024). A novel comparative study of nnar approach with linear stochastic time series models in predicting tennis player's performance. *BMC Sports Science, Medicine and Rehabilitation, 16*(1), 28. Advance online publication. DOI: 10.1186/s13102-024-00815-7 PMID: 38273407

Anik, A. I., Yeaser, S., Hossain, A. I., & Chakrabarty, A. (2018, September). Player's performance prediction in ODI cricket using machine learning algorithms. In 2018 4th international conference on electrical engineering and information & communication technology (iCEEiCT) (pp. 500-505). IEEE.

Annamalai, B., ShabbirHusain, R. V., Chandrasekaran, S., & Varshney, S. (2022). Cultural differences in sports fan engagement on Facebook: A comparison of Australian and Indian cricket league. *International Journal of Sport Management and Marketing, 22*(1-2), 120–141. DOI: 10.1504/IJSMM.2022.121251

Apostolou, K., & Tjortjis, C. (2019, July). Sports analytics algorithms for performance prediction. In *2019 10th International Conference on Information, Intelligence, Systems and Applications (IISA)* (pp. 1-4). IEEE. DOI: 10.1109/IISA.2019.8900754

Argibay-González, J. C., Vázquez-Estévez, C., Gutiérrez-Santiago, A., Paramés-González, A., Reguera-López-de-la-Osa, X., & Prieto-Lage, I. (2022). Analysis of injury patterns in men's football between the English league and the Spanish league. *International Journal of Environmental Research and Public Health, 19*(18), 11296. DOI: 10.3390/ijerph191811296 PMID: 36141571

Atlas, M., & Zhang, Y.-Q. (2004). Fuzzy neural agents for online NBA scouting. *IEEE/WIC/ACM International Conference on Web Intelligence (WI'04)*, 58–63. DOI: 10.1109/WI.2004.10047

Ayala, F., López-Valenciano, A., Martín, J. A. G., Croix, M. D. S., Vera-Garcia, F. J., del Pilar Garcia-Vaquero, M., & Myer, G. D. (2019). A preventive model for hamstring injuries in professional soccer: Learning algorithms. *International Journal of Sports Medicine*, *40*(05), 344–353. DOI: 10.1055/a-0826-1955 PMID: 30873572

Ayala, R., Granados, D. P., Gutiérrez, C. A. G., Ruíz, M. A. O., Espinosa, N. R., & Heredia, E. C. (2024). Novel study for the early identification of injury risks in athletes using machine learning techniques. *Applied Sciences (Basel, Switzerland)*, *14*(2), 570. DOI: 10.3390/app14020570

Baerg, A. (2016). Big data, sport, and the digital divide. *Journal of Sport and Social Issues*, *41*(1), 3–20. DOI: 10.1177/0193723516673409

Bahr, R., & Holme, I. (2003). Risk factors for sports injuries—A methodological approach. *British Journal of Sports Medicine*, *37*(5), 384–392. DOI: 10.1136/bjsm.37.5.384 PMID: 14514527

Bahr, R., & Krosshaug, T. (2005). Understanding injury mechanisms: A key component of preventing injuries in sport. *British Journal of Sports Medicine*, *39*(6), 324–329. DOI: 10.1136/bjsm.2005.018341 PMID: 15911600

Bairui, T., Cheng, C., Lubo, L., & Lishu, W. (2019). Analysis of Urban Talent Demand Model Based on Neural Network. *2019 11th International Conference on Measuring Technology and Mechatronics Automation (ICMTMA)*, 416–420.

Bajwa, S. S. (2024). Role of artificial intelligence (AI) in the promotion of sports. *Asian Journal of Research in Social Sciences and Humanities*, *14*(5), 1–7. DOI: 10.5958/2249-7315.2024.00012.X

Barron, D., Ball, G., Robins, M., & Sunderland, C. (2020). Identifying playing talent in professional football using artificial neural networks. *Journal of Sports Sciences*, *38*(11–12), 1211–1220. DOI: 10.1080/02640414.2019.1708036 PMID: 31941425

Bartlett, R. (2006). Artificial intelligence in sports biomechanics: New dawn or false hope? *Journal of Sports Science & Medicine*, *5*, 474–479. PMID: 24357939

Bartley, A., Hayden, J., & Scully, D. (2019). The application of AI for harm prediction and prevention: Ethical implications. *The Journal of Law, Medicine & Ethics*, *47*(3), 538–546.

Barve, Y. D. (2023). Assessing the impacts of digital marketing and sponsorship on the football industry as a business and their implications on fan engagement (Doctoral dissertation, Dublin, National College of Ireland).

Basit, A., Alvi, M. B., Jaskani, F. H., Alvi, M., Memon, K. H., & Shah, R. A. (2020, November). ICC T20 Cricket World Cup 2020 winner prediction using machine learning techniques. In 2020 IEEE 23rd International Multitopic Conference (INMIC) (pp. 1-6). IEEE.

Bayoumi, M. R., & Zaid, N. A. (2021). *Analytical study on the extent of the impact of modern technology on the management of sports institutions*. Modern Sport.

Beal, R., Norman, T. J., & Ramchurn, S. D. (2019). Artificial intelligence for team sports: A survey. *The Knowledge Engineering Review*, *34*, e28. DOI: 10.1017/S0269888919000225

Beck, P. J., Mohammadi-Aragh, M. J., Archibald, C., Jones, B. A., & Barton, A. (2018, October). Real-time metacognition feedback for introductory programming using machine learning. In *2018 IEEE Frontiers in Education Conference (FIE)* (pp. 1-5). IEEE. DOI: 10.1109/FIE.2018.8658973

Bergkamp, T. L. G., Frencken, W. G. P., Niessen, A. S. M., Meijer, R. R., & den Hartigh, R. J. R. (2022). How soccer scouts identify talented players. *European Journal of Sport Science*, *22*(7), 994–1004. DOI: 10.1080/17461391.2021.1916081 PMID: 33858300

Bergkamp, T. L. G., Niessen, A. S. M., den Hartigh, R. J. R., Frencken, W. G. P., & Meijer, R. R. (2019). Methodological issues in soccer talent identification research. *Sports Medicine (Auckland, N.Z.)*, *49*(9), 1317–1335. DOI: 10.1007/s40279-019-01113-w PMID: 31161402

Best, A., Sibson, R., & Morgan, A. (2024). Technology adoption and use in not-for-profit sport: A case study of an Australian state sporting association. *Managing Sport and Leisure*, *29*(2), 273–291. DOI: 10.1080/23750472.2021.2020678

Bilohur, V., Skrypchenko, I., & Nepsha, O. (2022). The concept of sports management as a factor of effective sports activities. *Humanities Studies*, (12), 60–70.

Bin, L., & Xu, X. (2021). Application of artificial intelligence in basketball sport. *Journal of Education, Health and Sport*, *11*(7), 54–67. DOI: 10.12775/JEHS.2021.11.07.005

Biró, A., Jánosi-Rancz, K. T., & Szilágyi, L. (2024, January). Real-time Artificial Intelligence Text Analysis for Identifying Burnout Syndromes in High-Performance Athletes. In *2024 IEEE 22nd World Symposium on Applied Machine Intelligence and Informatics (SAMI)* (pp. 000253-000258). IEEE. DOI: 10.1109/SAMI60510.2024.10432817

Biró, A., Cuesta-Vargas, A. I., & Szilágyi, L. (2023). AI-assisted fatigue and stamina control for performance sports on IMU-generated multivariate time series datasets. *Sensors (Basel), 24*(1), 132. DOI: 10.3390/s24010132 PMID: 38202992

Bittencourt, N. F., Meeuwisse, W. H., Mendonça, L. D., Nettel-Aguirre, A., Ocarino, J. M., & Fonseca, S. T. (2016). Complex systems approach for sports injuries: Moving from risk factor identification to injury pattern recognition—narrative review and new concept. *British Journal of Sports Medicine, 50*(21), 1309–1314. DOI: 10.1136/bjsports-2015-095850 PMID: 27445362

Bosch, B., & Mansell, H. (2015). Interprofessional collaboration in health care: Lessons to be learned from competitive sports. *Canadian Pharmacists Journal/ Revue des Pharmaciens du Canada, 148*(4), 176-179.

Bouzarth, E. L., Grannan, B. C., Harris, J. M., Hutson, K. R., & Keating, P. J. (2021). Storytelling with sports analytics. In *Tutorials in Operations Research: Emerging Optimization Methods and Modeling Techniques with Applications* (pp. 38-61). INFORMS. DOI: 10.1287/educ.2021.0230

Bruton, G., & Sheng, N. (2023). When monetary profit maximization does not rule: Historical analysis of english quakers and the role of religious institutional logic. *Journal of Management History, 29*(4), 502–517. DOI: 10.1108/JMH-07-2022-0027

Byeon, H. (2023). Advances in value-based, policy-based, and deep learning-based reinforcement learning. *International Journal of Advanced Computer Science and Applications, 14*(8). Advance online publication. DOI: 10.14569/IJACSA.2023.0140838

Cacho-Elizondo, S., & Álvarez, J. D. L. (2020). Big data in the decision-making processes of football teams integrating a theoretical framework, applications and reach. *Journal of Strategic Innovation and Sustainability, 15*(2), 21–44.

Callejo, M. B., & Forcadell, F. J. (2006). Real Madrid football club: A new model of business organization for sports clubs in Spain. *Global Business and Organizational Excellence, 26*(1), 51–64. DOI: 10.1002/joe.20121

Cao, L. (2022). Design and optimization of a decision support system for sports training based on data mining technology. *Scientific Programming, 2022*(1), 1846345. DOI: 10.1155/2022/1846345

Chamorro-Premuzic, T., Winsborough, D., Sherman, R. A., & Hogan, R. (2016). New talent signals: Shiny new objects or a brave new world? *Industrial and Organizational Psychology: Perspectives on Science and Practice, 9*(3), 621–640. DOI: 10.1017/iop.2016.6

Chang, C. (2013). Integrating action-based defect prediction to provide recommendations for defect action correction. *International Journal of Software Engineering and Knowledge Engineering*, *23*(02), 147–172. DOI: 10.1142/S0218194013500022

Chang, K., Wang, W., & Peng, W. (2023). Where will players move next? dynamic graphs and hierarchical fusion for movement forecasting in badminton. *Proceedings of the AAAI Conference on Artificial Intelligence*, *37*(6), 6998–7005. DOI: 10.1609/aaai.v37i6.25855

Chang, V., Sajeev, S., Xu, Q. A., Tan, M., & Wang, H. (2024). Football analytics: Assessing the correlation between workload, injury and performance of football players in the English Premier League. *Applied Sciences (Basel, Switzerland)*, *14*(16), 7217. DOI: 10.3390/app14167217

Cheng, G., Zhang, Z., Kyebambe, M., & Kimbugwe, N. (2016). Predicting the outcome of nba playoffs based on maximum entropy principle. DOI: 10.20944/preprints201609.0103.v1

Cheng, H. (2024). Study on talent cultivation management model of universities based on fuzzy neural network algorithm. *International Journal of Maritime Engineering*, *1*(1), 521–530. DOI: 10.1049/ijme.2024.05.024

Chen, W., Jhou, M., Lee, T., & Lu, C. (2021). Hybrid basketball game outcome prediction model by integrating data mining methods for the national basketball association. *Entropy (Basel, Switzerland)*, *23*(4), 477. DOI: 10.3390/e23040477 PMID: 33920720

Cheungsirakulvit, T., & Girdwichai, P. (2023). The development of Thailand's national sports development fund (NSDF) and the NSDF management strategy. *Unpublished manuscript.*

Chidambaram, S., Maheswaran, Y., Patel, K., Sounderajah, V., Hashimoto, D. A., Seastedt, K. P., McGregor, A. H., Markar, S. R., & Darzi, A. (2022). Using artificial intelligence-enhanced sensing and wearable technology in sports medicine and performance optimization. *Sensors (Basel)*, *22*(18), 6920. DOI: 10.3390/s22186920 PMID: 36146263

Chien, C.-F., & Chen, L.-F. (2008). Data mining to improve personnel selection and enhance human capital: A case study in high-technology industry. *Expert Systems with Applications*, *34*(1), 280–290. DOI: 10.1016/j.eswa.2006.09.003

Chmait, N., & Westerbeek, H. (2021). Artificial intelligence and machine learning in sport research: An introduction for non-data scientists. *Frontiers in Sports and Active Living, 3*, 682287. Advance online publication. DOI: 10.3389/fspor.2021.682287 PMID: 34957395

Ciechanowski, L., Przegalinska, A., Magnuski, M., & Gloor, P. (2019). In the shades of the uncanny valley: An experimental study of human–chatbot interaction. *Future Generation Computer Systems, 92*, 539–548. DOI: 10.1016/j.future.2018.01.055

Clark, D. (2020). *Artificial intelligence for learning: How to use AI to support employee development.* Kogan Page Publishers.

Claudino, J., Capanema, D., Souza, T., Serrão, J., Pereira, A., & Nassis, G. (2019). Current approaches to the use of artificial intelligence for injury risk assessment and performance prediction in team sports: A systematic review. *Sports Medicine - Open, 5*(1), 28. Advance online publication. DOI: 10.1186/s40798-019-0202-3 PMID: 31270636

Clemente, F., Silva, R., Chen, Y., Aquino, R., Praça, G., Castellano, J., Nobari, H., Mendes, B., Rosemann, T., & Knechtle, B. (2021). Accelerometry-workload indices concerning different levels of participation during congested fixture periods in professional soccer: A pilot study conducted over a full season. *International Journal of Environmental Research and Public Health, 18*(3), 1137. DOI: 10.3390/ijerph18031137 PMID: 33525533

Constandt, B., Heres, L., Marlier, M., & Willem, A. (2020). A stakeholder perspective on ethical leadership in sport: Bridging the gap between the normative and descriptive lines of inquiry. *Psychologica Belgica, 60*(1), 381–395. DOI: 10.5334/pb.543 PMID: 33362936

Costa, M., Oliveira, D., Pinto, S., & Tavares, A. (2019). Detecting driver's fatigue, distraction, and activity using a non-intrusive AI-based monitoring system. *Journal of Artificial Intelligence and Soft Computing Research, 9*(4), 247–266. DOI: 10.2478/jaiscr-2019-0007

Coutinho, D., Gonçalves, B., Wong, D., Travassos, B., Coutts, A., & Sampaio, J. (2018). Exploring the effects of mental and muscular fatigue in soccer players' performance. *Human Movement Science, 58*, 287–296. DOI: 10.1016/j.humov.2018.03.004 PMID: 29549745

Cust, E. E., Sweeting, A. J., Ball, K., & Robertson, S. (2019). Machine and deep learning for sport-specific movement recognition: A systematic review of model development and performance. *Journal of Sports Sciences, 37*(5), 568–600. DOI: 10.1080/02640414.2018.1521769 PMID: 30307362

Daga, B., Checker, J., Rajan, A., & Deo, S. (2020). Computer science career recommendation system using artificial neural network. *International Journal of Computer Trends and Technology*, *68*(3), 84–88. DOI: 10.14445/22312803/IJCTT-V68I3P117

Daly, E., Pearce, A., Esser, P., & Ryan, L. (2022). Evaluating the relationship between neurological function, neuromuscular fatigue, and subjective performance measures in professional rugby union players. *Frontiers in Sports and Active Living*, *4*, 1058326. Advance online publication. DOI: 10.3389/fspor.2022.1058326 PMID: 36439623

Darian, J. C., & Coopersmith, L. (2001). Integrated marketing and operations team projects: Learning the importance of cross-functional cooperation. *Journal of Marketing Education*, *23*(2), 128–135. DOI: 10.1177/0273475301232006

Davenport, T. H. (2014). What businesses can learn from sports analytics. *MIT Sloan Management Review*.

Davis, J., Bransen, L., Devos, L., Jaspers, A., Meert, W., Robberechts, P., Van Haaren, J., & Van Roy, M. (2024). Methodology and evaluation in sports analytics: Challenges, approaches, and lessons learned. *Machine Learning*, *113*(9), 6977–7010. DOI: 10.1007/s10994-024-06585-0

Dc, S.DC. (2022). Artificial intelligence in sport: An ethical issue. *Unity Journal*, *3*(01), 27–39. DOI: 10.3126/unityj.v3i01.43313

Deb, K., Pratap, A., Agarwal, S., & Meyarivan, T. (2002, August). A fast and elitist multiobjective genetic algorithm: NSGA-II. *IEEE Transactions on Evolutionary Computation*, *6*(2), 182–197. DOI: 10.1109/4235.996017

Del Prete, T. (2021). *The greatest teams never: Sports memories of near misses, total messes, and not-so-magical moments*. Gatekeeper Press.

Delecroix, B., McCall, A., Dawson, B., Berthoin, S., & Dupont, G. (2018). Workload and non-contact injury incidence in elite football players competing in European leagues. *European Journal of Sport Science*, *18*(9), 1280–1287. DOI: 10.1080/17461391.2018.1477994 PMID: 29860935

Dergaa, I., & Chamari, K. (2024). Big data in sports medicine and exercise science: Integrating theory and practice for future innovations. *TJSSM*, *2*(1), 1–13. DOI: 10.61838/kman.tjssm.2.1.1

Donath, L., Schmidt, M., & Knaflitz, M. (2021). Opportunities and challenges for AI-driven sports injury prediction. *European Journal of Sport Science*, *21*(4), 560–571.

dos Santos, M. (2023). The impact of Covid-19 on esports–Analysis of stock market and corporate governance.

Dyer, B. (2020). A pragmatic approach to resolving technological unfairness: The case of nike's vaporfly and alphafly running footwear. *Sports Medicine - Open*, *6*(1), 21. Advance online publication. DOI: 10.1186/s40798-020-00250-1 PMID: 32448974

Eid, A. I. A., Miled, A. B., Fatnassi, A., Nawaz, M. A., Mahmoud, A. F., Abdalla, F. A., Jabnoun, C., Dhibi, A., Allan, F. M., Elhossiny, M. A., Belhaj, S., & Mohamed, I. B. (2024). Sports prediction model through cloud computing and big data based on artificial intelligence method. *Journal of Intelligent Learning Systems and Applications*, *16*(2), 53–79. DOI: 10.4236/jilsa.2024.162005

Ekegren, C. L., Gabbe, B. J., & Finch, C. F. (2016). Sports injury surveillance systems: A review of methods and data quality. *Sports Medicine (Auckland, N.Z.)*, *46*(1), 49–65. DOI: 10.1007/s40279-015-0410-z PMID: 26423419

Elitzur, R. (2020). Data analytics effects in major league baseball. *Omega*, *90*, 102001. DOI: 10.1016/j.omega.2018.11.010

El-Maghrabi, Y., & Sharif, M. (2022). Game Changers or Game Predictors? Big Data Analytics in Sports for Performance Enhancement and Fan Engagement. *Journal of Contemporary Healthcare Analytics*, *6*(6), 19–39.

Evans, R., McNamee, M., & Guy, O. (2016). Ethics, nanobiosensors and elite sport: The need for a new governance framework. *Science and Engineering Ethics*, *23*(6), 1487–1505. DOI: 10.1007/s11948-016-9855-1 PMID: 27995447

Fenil, E., Manogaran, G., Vivekananda, G. N., Thanjaivadivel, T., Jeeva, S., & Ahilan, A. (2019). Real-time violence detection framework for football stadium comprising of big data analysis and deep learning through bidirectional LSTM. *Computer Networks*, *151*, 191–200. DOI: 10.1016/j.comnet.2019.01.028

Finch, C. (2006). A new framework for research leading to sports injury prevention. *Journal of Science and Medicine in Sport*, *9*(1-2), 3–9. DOI: 10.1016/j.jsams.2006.02.009 PMID: 16616614

Flores-Hernández, I., Bonilla-Huerta, E., Quintero-Flores, P. M., Ponce, O. A., & Hernández-Hernández, J. C. (2019). Applying intelligent techniques for talent recruitment. *Applied Computer Science*, *15*(2), 63–72. DOI: 10.35784/acs-2019-14

Ford, R. A. (2018). Trade secrets and information security in the age of sports analytics. In *The Oxford Handbook of American Sports Law*.

Ford, P. R., Bordonau, J. L. D., Bonanno, D., Tavares, J., Groenendijk, C., Fink, C., Gualtieri, D., Gregson, W., Varley, M. C., Weston, M., Lolli, L., Platt, D., & Di Salvo, V. (2020). A survey of talent identification and development processes in the youth academies of professional soccer clubs from around the world. *Journal of Sports Sciences, 38*(11–12), 1269–1278. DOI: 10.1080/02640414.2020.1752440 PMID: 32378447

Fotache, M., Cojocariu, I. C., & Bertea, A. (2021, June). High-level machine learning framework for sports events ticket sales prediction. In *Proceedings of the 22nd International Conference on Computer Systems and Technologies* (pp. 55-60). DOI: 10.1145/3472410.3472426

Gaál, L., Szolgay, J., Kohnová, S., Hlavčová, K., & Viglione, A. (2010). Inclusion of historical information in flood frequency analysis using a bayesian mcmc technique: A case study for the power dam orlík, czech republic. *Contributions to Geophysics and Geodesy, 40*(2). Advance online publication. DOI: 10.2478/v10126-010-0005-5

Gee, C. J., Marshall, J. C., & King, J. F. (2010). Should coaches use personality assessments in the talent identification process? A 15 year predictive study on professional hockey players. *International Journal of Coaching Science, 4*(1).

Gerrard, B. (2017). The role of analytics in assessing playing talent. In *Routledge handbook of talent identification and development in sport* (pp. 422–431). Routledge. DOI: 10.4324/9781315668017-30

Ghasem, W., Valenzuela, J., & Saxon, L. A. (2021). Player tracking technology and data for injury prevention in the National Football League. *Current Sports Medicine Reports, 20*(9), 436–439. DOI: 10.1249/JSR.0000000000000873 PMID: 34524184

Giles, B., Peeling, P., Kovalchik, S., & Reid, M. (2021). Differentiating movement styles in professional tennis: A machine learning and hierarchical clustering approach. *European Journal of Sport Science, 23*(1), 44–53. DOI: 10.1080/17461391.2021.2006800 PMID: 34781856

Giorgi, A., Ronca, V., Vozzi, A., Aricò, P., Borghini, G., Capotorto, R., Tamborra, L., Simonetti, I., Sportiello, S., Petrelli, M., Polidori, C., Varga, R., van Gasteren, M., Barua, A., Ahmed, M. U., Babiloni, F., & Di Flumeri, G. (2023). Neurophysiological mental fatigue assessment for developing user-centered Artificial Intelligence as a solution for autonomous driving. *Frontiers in Neurorobotics, 17*, 1240933. DOI: 10.3389/fnbot.2023.1240933 PMID: 38107403

Glebova, E., Madsen, D. Ø., Mihaľová, P., Géczi, G., Mittelman, A., & Jorgič, B. (2024). Artificial intelligence development and dissemination impact on the sports industry labor market. *Frontiers in Sports and Active Living*, *6*, 1363892. Advance online publication. DOI: 10.3389/fspor.2024.1363892 PMID: 38606117

Goebert, C. (2020). Augmented reality in sport marketing: Uses and directions. *Sports Innovation Journal*, *1*, 134–151. DOI: 10.18060/24227

Goes, F., Meerhoff, L., Bueno, M., Rodrigues, D., Moura, F., Brink, M., Elferink-Gemser, M. T., Knobbe, A. J., Cunha, S. A., Torres, R. S., & Lemmink, K. (2020). Unlocking the potential of big data to support tactical performance analysis in professional soccer: A systematic review. *European Journal of Sport Science*, *21*(4), 481–496. DOI: 10.1080/17461391.2020.1747552 PMID: 32297547

Golchi, S. (2020). Use of historical individual patient data in analysis of clinical trials. https://doi.org//arxiv.2002.09910DOI: 10.48550

Gómez-Carmona, P., Fernández-Cuevas, I., Quintana, M., Arnaiz-Lastras, J., & Navandar, A. (2020). Infrared thermography protocol on reducing the incidence of soccer injuries. *Journal of Sport Rehabilitation*, *29*(8), 1222–1227. DOI: 10.1123/jsr.2019-0056 PMID: 32188790

Gorman, D. (2017). Sports analytics: Analysis of the National Football League (Doctoral dissertation, Dublin, National College of Ireland).

Gour, P., & Khan, M. F. (2024). Utilizing machine learning for comprehensive analysis and predictive modelling of ipl-t20 cricket matches. *Indian Journal of Science and Technology*, *17*(7), 592–597. DOI: 10.17485/IJST/v17i7.2944

Grant, M. J., & Booth, A. (2009). An examination of 14 review kinds and related techniques to create a taxonomy of reviews. *Journal of Health Information & Libraries*, *26*(2), 91–108. DOI: 10.1111/j.1471-1842.2009.00848.x

Guelmami, N., Fekih-Romdhane, F., Mechraoui, O., & Bragazzi, N. L. (2023). Injury Prevention, Optimized Training and Rehabilitation: How Is AI Reshaping the Field of Sports Medicine. *New Asian Journal of Medicine*, *1*(1), 30–34. DOI: 10.61186/najm.1.1.30

Guenter, R. W., Dunn, J. G. H., & Holt, N. L. (2019). Talent identification in youth ice hockey: Exploring “intangible” player characteristics. *The Sport Psychologist*, *33*(4), 323–333. DOI: 10.1123/tsp.2018-0155

Guillén, F., & Martínez-Alvarado, J. R. (2014). The sport engagement scale: An adaptation of the Utrecht Work Engagement Scale (UWES) for the sports environment. *Universitas Psychologica*, *13*(3), 975–984.

Hakes, J. K., and Sauer, R. D. (2016). An economic evaluation of the Moneyball hypothesis. J. Econ. Perspect. 20, 173–186. doi: . 3.173DOI: 10.1257/jep.20

Halilaj, E., Rajagopal, A., Fiterau, M., Hicks, J. L., Hastie, T. J., & Delp, S. L. (2018). Machine learning in human movement biomechanics: Best practices, common pitfalls, and new opportunities. *Journal of Biomechanics, 81*, 1–11. DOI: 10.1016/j.jbiomech.2018.09.009 PMID: 30279002

Harris, J. G., Craig, E., & Light, D. A. (2011). Talent and analytics: New approaches, higher ROI. *The Journal of Business Strategy, 32*(6), 4–13. DOI: 10.1108/02756661111180087

Hasanika, D., Dilhara, R., Liyanage, D., Bandaranayake, A., & Deegalla, S. (2021, December). Data mining system for predicting a winning cricket team. In 2021 IEEE 16th International Conference on Industrial and Information Systems (ICIIS) (pp. 92-97). IEEE.

Hassan, Y., Pandey, J., Varkkey, B., Sethi, D., & Scullion, H. (2022). Understanding talent management for sports organizations: Evidence from an emerging country. *International Journal of Human Resource Management, 33*(11), 2192–2225. DOI: 10.1080/09585192.2021.1971736

Herberger, T. A., & Litke, C. (2021). The impact of big data and sports analytics on professional football: A systematic literature review. In *Digitalization, digital transformation and sustainability in the global economy: Risks and opportunities* (pp. 147-171). DOI: 10.1007/978-3-030-77340-3_12

Hoch, M. C., McKeon, P. O., Ross, S. E., & Calmbach, W. L. (2020). Physical therapists' roles in preventing injuries and helping athletes return to the field. *. *International Journal of Sports Physical Therapy, 15*(2), 179–194.

Hong, W. (2023). Research and application of talent training evaluation model based on deep learning. *Sixth International Conference on Intelligent Computing, Communication, and Devices (ICCD 2023), 12703*, 247–252.

Houtmeyers, K., Jaspers, A., & Figueiredo, P. (2021). Managing the training process in elite sports: From descriptive to prescriptive data analytics. *International Journal of Sports Physiology and Performance, 16*(11), 1719–1723. DOI: 10.1123/ijspp.2020-0958 PMID: 34686619

Howard, M. C. (2017). A meta-analysis and systematic literature review of virtual reality rehabilitation programs. *Computers in Human Behavior, 70*, 317–327. DOI: 10.1016/j.chb.2017.01.013

Huang, L.-C., Huang, K.-S., Huang, H.-P., & Jaw, B.-S. (2004). Applying fuzzy neural network in human resource selection system. *IEEE Annual Meeting of the Fuzzy Information, 2004. Processing NAFIPS'04., 1*, 169–174.

Huang, X. (2023). Business Talent Demand Prediction Model Based On Neural Network in Integration of Industry and Education in Greater Bay Area. *2023 IEEE 5th Eurasia Conference on IOT, Communication and Engineering (ECICE)*, 382–385.

Huang, M. H., & Rust, R. T. (2021). A strategic framework for artificial intelligence in marketing. *Journal of the Academy of Marketing Science, 49*(1), 30–50. DOI: 10.1007/s11747-020-00749-9

Huda, N. U., Jensen, K., Gade, R., & Moeslund, T. B. (2018). Estimating the number of soccer players using simulation-based occlusion handling. *2018 IEEE/CVF Conference on Computer Vision and Pattern Recognition Workshops (CVPRW)*. DOI: 10.1109/CVPRW.2018.00236

Hughes, K., & Elkins, E. (2023). Silicon Valley's team: The Golden State Warriors, datafied managerialism, and basketball's racialized geography. *American Quarterly, 75*(3), 471–499. DOI: 10.1353/aq.2023.a905860

Humphreys, K., Vernon, H., & Kroeling, P. (2019). A systematic analysis of the prevention of musculoskeletal injuries with chiropractic care was published in the. *Journal of Manipulative and Physiological Therapeutics, 42*(9), 675–684.

Ibsen, B., & Levinsen, K. (2019). Collaboration between sports clubs and public institutions. *EJSS European Journal for Sport and Society, 16*(2), 187–204. DOI: 10.1080/16138171.2019.1610619

Jaffar, Z., Noor, W., & Kanwal, Z. (2019). Predictive human resource analytics using data mining classification techniques. *Int. J. Comput, 32*(1), 9–20.

Jantan, H., Hamdan, A. R., & Othman, Z. A. (2011). Talent knowledge acquisition using data mining classification techniques. *2011 3rd Conference on Data Mining and Optimization (DMO)*, 32–37.

Jantan, H., Hamdan, A. R., & Othman, Z. A. (2012). Human talent forecasting using data mining classification techniques. In *Human Resources Management: Concepts, Methodologies, Tools, and Applications* (pp. 486–499). IGI Global.

Jantan, H., Hamdan, A. R., & Othman, Z. A. (2010). Classification and prediction of academic talent using data mining techniques. *International Conference on Knowledge-Based and Intelligent Information and Engineering Systems*, 491–500. DOI: 10.1007/978-3-642-15387-7_53

Jasni, N. H., Mustapha, A., Tenah, S. S., Mostafa, S. A., & Razali, N. (2022). Prediction of player position for talent identification in association netball: A regression-based approach. *International Journal of Advances in Intelligent Informatics*, *8*(1), 84. Advance online publication. DOI: 10.26555/ijain.v8i1.707

Jauhiainen, S., Äyrämö, S., Forsman, H., & Kauppi, J. P. (2019). Talent identification in soccer using a one-class support vector machine. *International Journal of Computer Science in Sport*, *18*(3), 125–136. DOI: 10.2478/ijcss-2019-0021

Jayal, A., McRobert, A., Oatley, G., & O'Donoghue, P. (2018). *Sports analytics: Analysis, visualisation and decision making in sports performance*. Routledge. DOI: 10.4324/9781315222783

Jenkins, S., & Evans, N. (2020, April). Cybersecurity impact of the growth of data in sports. In *Cyber Sensing 2020* (Vol. 11417, pp. 84–100). SPIE. DOI: 10.1117/12.2557898

Jha, A., Dichwalkar, A., Shaikh, A., & Pawar, G. (n.d.). *Talent Explorer using Data Mining*.

Jin, X., Zhao, S., and Jiang, H. (2022). AI-driven injury prediction and prevention: ethical considerations. 22(1), 68–81; "Ethics in Science and Environmental Politics".

Kadiri, P., Anusha, P., Prabhu, M., Asuncion, R., Pavan, V. S., & Suman, J. V. (2024, July). Morphed Picture Recognition using Machine Learning Algorithms. In *2024 Second International Conference on Advances in Information Technology (ICAIT)* (Vol. 1, pp. 1-6). IEEE.

Kähärä, B. (2020). Analytical support in esports: Creating a new dimension using eye-tracking analysis.

Kalaivani, V., & Elamparithi, M. M. (2014). An efficient classification algorithms for employee performance prediction. *International Journal of Research in Advent Technology*, *2*(9), 27–32.

Kalinina, O., Suschenko, V., Shchegolev, V., & Barykin, S. (2018). Logistic development and use of personnel motivation system based on the chosen strategy of sports organization. In *MATEC Web of Conferences* (Vol. 193, p. 05063). EDP Sciences. DOI: 10.1051/matecconf/201819305063

Kaluarachchi, A., & Aparna, S. V. (2010, December). CricAI: A classification based tool to predict the outcome in ODI cricket. In *2010 Fifth International Conference on Information and Automation for Sustainability* (pp. 250-255). IEEE.

Kapadiya, C., Shah, A., Adhvaryu, K., Barot, P., & Principal, S. (2020). Intelligent cricket team selection by predicting individual players' performance using efficient machine learning technique. *International Journal of Engineering and Advanced Technology*, *9*(3), 3406–3409. DOI: 10.35940/ijeat.C6339.029320

Kaur, A., Kaur, R., & Jagdev, G. (2021). Analyzing and exploring the impact of big data analytics in sports sector. *SN Computer Science*, *2*(3), 184. Advance online publication. DOI: 10.1007/s42979-021-00575-y

Khadartsev, A. A., Nesmeyanov, A. A., Eskov, V. M., Filatov, M. A., & Pan, W. (2017). Fundamentals of chaos and self-organization theory in sports. *Integrative Medicine International*, *4*(1-2), 57–65. DOI: 10.1159/000458153

Khan, N. J., Ahamad, G., Naseem, M., & Sohail, S. S. (2023). Computational efficiency in sports talent identification-a systematic review. *International Journal of Applied Decision Sciences*, *16*(3), 358–384. DOI: 10.1504/IJADS.2023.130600

Khan, S. M., & Shah, M. (2005, November). Detecting group activities using rigidity of formation. In *Proceedings of the 13th annual ACM international conference on Multimedia* (pp. 403-406).

Khurana, R., Yadav, M., Quttainah, M., Srivastava, A. P., Baludi, A., & Singh, P. K. (2023). Neural Networks in Recruitment: Trends and Future Directions. *2023 International Conference on Ambient Intelligence, Knowledge Informatics and Industrial Electronics (AIKIIE)*, 1–5. DOI: 10.1109/AIKIIE60097.2023.10390017

Kim, H. S., & Kim, M. (2020). Viewing sports online together? Psychological consequences on social live streaming service usage. *Sport Management Review*, *23*(5), 869–882. DOI: 10.1016/j.smr.2019.12.007

King, M., Brown, M., Cox, J., McLellan, R., Towlson, C., & Barrett, S. (2024). Talent identification in soccer: The influence of technical, physical and maturity-related characteristics on a national selection process. *PLoS One*, *19*(3), e0298359. DOI: 10.1371/journal.pone.0298359 PMID: 38478494

Kirola, M., Memoria, M., & Dumka, A. (2023). Optimized U-Net convolutional neural network based breast cancer prediction for accuracy increment in big data. *Concurrency and Computation*, *35*(9), e7652. Advance online publication. DOI: 10.1002/cpe.7652

Kjeldsen, T., Macdonald, N., Lang, M., Mediero, L., Albuquerque, T., Bogdanowicz, E., Brázdil, R., Castellarin, A., David, V., Fleig, A., Gül, G. O., Kriauciuniene, J., Kohnová, S., Merz, B., Nicholson, O., Roald, L. A., Salinas, J. L., Sarauskiene, D., Šraj, M., & Wilson, D. (2014). Documentary evidence of past floods in europe and their utility in flood frequency estimation. *Journal of Hydrology (Amsterdam), 517*, 963–973. DOI: 10.1016/j.jhydrol.2014.06.038

Komskienė-Žukauskienė, D., Švagždienė, B., & Benetytė, M. (2009). Development of loyalty of employees in contemporary sports organization. *Socialiniai Tyrimai*, (2), 32–41.

Kononenko, I. (2001). Machine learning for medical diagnosis: History, state of the art and perspective. *Artificial Intelligence in Medicine, 23*(1), 89–109. DOI: 10.1016/S0933-3657(01)00077-X PMID: 11470218

Kumar, A., Labshetwar, A., Kawale, A., & Aland, P. (2024). INDPLAY: A software solution for uncovering India's sporting talent. *International Journal of Innovative Research in Computer Science & Technology, 12*(3), 23–27. DOI: 10.55524/ijircst.2024.12.3.5

Kwartler, T. (2022). *Sports analytics in practice with R*. John Wiley & Sons. DOI: 10.1002/9781119598084

Lahat, D., Adali, T., & Jutten, C. (2015). Multimodal data fusion: An overview of methods, challenges, and prospects. *Proceedings of the IEEE, 103*(9), 1449–1477. DOI: 10.1109/JPROC.2015.2460697

Lam, M. H., Hong, Y., & Fong, D. T. (2020). A comprehensive evaluation was conducted to predict football-related sports injuries. The. *Journal of Science and Medicine in Sport, 23*(1), 52–57. PMID: 32928654

Lampis, T., Ntzoufras, I., Vasilios, V., & Stavrianna, D. (2023). Predictions of european basketball match results with machine learning algorithms. *Journal of Sports Analytics, 9*(2), 171–190. DOI: 10.3233/JSA-220639

Lan, H. (2024). Research on analytical model of participation and social influence of she sports activities based on multi-source data fusion. jes, 20(6s), 343-348. https://doi.org/DOI: 10.52783/jes.2652

Lapham, A. C., & Bartlett, R. M. (1995). The use of artificial intelligence in the analysis of sports performance: A review of applications in human gait analysis and future directions for sports biomechanics. *Journal of Sports Sciences, 13*(3), 229–237. DOI: 10.1080/02640419508732232 PMID: 7563290

Larkin, P., & Reeves, M. J. (2018). Junior-elite football: Time to re-position talent identification? *Soccer and Society*, *19*(8), 1183–1192. DOI: 10.1080/14660970.2018.1432389

Lee, K. F., & Qiufan, C. (2021). [*Ten visions for our future*. Crown Currency.]. *AI*, •••, 2041.

Lee, K., Feibus, K. B., & Lo, M. C. (2020). AI-driven injury prediction and prevention: Ethical implications. *Ethics, Medicine, and Public Health*, *15*, 100571.

Leeuw, A., Zwaard, S., Baar, R., & Knobbe, A. (2021). Personalized machine learning approach to injury monitoring in elite volleyball players. *European Journal of Sport Science*, *22*(4), 511–520. DOI: 10.1080/17461391.2021.1887369 PMID: 33568023

Lehtonen, K. (2017). Building of the legitimacy of a sports organization in a hybridized operating environment: Case Finland. *EJSS European Journal for Sport and Society*, *14*(2), 166–181. DOI: 10.1080/16138171.2017.1318199

Leo, F. M., García-Calvo, T., González-Ponce, I., Pulido, J. J., & Fransen, K. (2019). How many leaders does it take to lead a sports team? The relationship between the number of leaders and the effectiveness of professional sports teams. *PLoS One*, *14*(6), e0218167. DOI: 10.1371/journal.pone.0218167 PMID: 31181130

Leo, M., Mosca, N., Spagnolo, P., Mazzeo, P. L., D'Orazio, T., & Distante, A. (2008, July). Real-time multiview analysis of soccer matches for understanding interactions between ball and players. In *Proceedings of the 2008 international conference on Content-based image and video retrieval* (pp. 525-534).

Lewis, M. (2014). *Moneyball: The Art of Winning an Unfair Game*. WW Norton and Company.

Lewis, M., & Yoon, Y. (2016). An empirical examination of the development and impact of star power in Major League Baseball. *Journal of Sports Economics*, *19*(2), 155–187. DOI: 10.1177/1527002515626220

Leyva, A. (2020). Ethical aspects of organized contact sports for children as participants. *International Journal of Contemporary Pediatrics*, *7*(8), 1823. DOI: 10.18203/2349-3291.ijcp20203047

Liberati, A., Tetzlaff, J., Altman, D. G., & Moher, D. (2015). For systematic reviews and meta-analyses, the preferred reporting item is the PRISMA statement. *Journal of Clinical Epidemiology*, *62*(10), 1006–1012.

Li, J., Liu, S., Wang, Z., & Guo, J. (2020). Neutrosophy theory based visualization report of sports news data. *International Journal of Electrical Engineering Education*, •••, 0020720920940581.

Li, J., Li, X., & Dong, B. (2021). The [presents a systematic overview of artificial intelligence in public health.]. *Journal of Medical Artificial Intelligence*, *3*(1), e2007.

Li, S., Chen, S., & Li, Y. (2021). [Application of machine learning in sports injury prediction: A systematic review.]. *Journal of Sports Sciences*, *39*(3), 255–266.

Liu, P., Li, X., Zang, B., & Diao, G. (2024). Privacy-preserving sports data fusion and prediction with smart devices in distributed environment. *Journal of Cloud Computing (Heidelberg, Germany)*, *13*(1), 106. Advance online publication. DOI: 10.1186/s13677-024-00671-3

Liu, Z., & Zhang, X. (2024). Construction and optimization of sports athlete selection and talent cultivation system based on data analysis. *Journal of Electrical Systems*, *20*(6s), 2070–2081. DOI: 10.52783/jes.3122

Looser, C. E., Guntupalli, J. S., & Wheatley, T. (2013). Multivoxel patterns in face-sensitive temporal regions reveal an encoding schema based on detecting life in a face. *Social Cognitive and Affective Neuroscience*, *8*(7), 799–805.

Lowman, G. H. (2016). Moving beyond identification: Using gamification to attract and retain talent. *Industrial and Organizational Psychology: Perspectives on Science and Practice*, *9*(3), 677–682. DOI: 10.1017/iop.2016.70

Lubis, A. E., Raharjo, F. M., & Nugroho, A. (2020). A Model of Basic Skill Test for Talent Scouting Soccer Athlete Candidates. *1st Unimed International Conference on Sport Science (UnICoSS 2019)*, 79–86. DOI: 10.2991/ahsr.k.200305.025

Luccioni, A., & Bengio, Y. (2020). On the morality of artificial intelligence [commentary]. *IEEE Technology and Society Magazine*, *39*(1), 16–25. DOI: 10.1109/MTS.2020.2967486

Lüdin, D., Donath, L., & Romann, M. (2023). Disagreement between talent scouts: Implications for improved talent assessment in youth football. *Journal of Sports Sciences*, *41*(8), 758–765. DOI: 10.1080/02640414.2023.2239614 PMID: 37490515

Ma, H., & Ding, A. (2022). Construction and implementation of a college talent cultivation system under deep learning and data mining algorithms. *The Journal of Supercomputing*, *78*(4), 5681–5696. DOI: 10.1007/s11227-021-04036-4

Mandil, W., Nazari, K., & Ghalamzan, A. (2022). Action conditioned tactile prediction: case study on slip prediction.. DOI: 10.15607/RSS.2022.XVIII.070

Mandorino, M., Tessitore, A., Leduc, C., Persichetti, V., Morabito, M., & Lacome, M. (2023). A new approach to quantify soccer players' readiness through machine learning techniques. *Applied Sciences (Basel, Switzerland), 13*(15), 8808. DOI: 10.3390/app13158808

Mann, D. L., Dehghansai, N., & Baker, J. (2017). Searching for the elusive gift: Advances in talent identification in sport. *Current Opinion in Psychology, 16*, 128–133. DOI: 10.1016/j.copsyc.2017.04.016 PMID: 28813336

Marcu, V., & Buhaş, S. D. (2014). Sports organizations–management and science. *Procedia: Social and Behavioral Sciences, 117*, 678–682. DOI: 10.1016/j.sbspro.2014.02.281

Marlapudi, K., & Lenka, U. (2024). Unlocking the potential: Redefining talent and competency mapping for Industry 4.0. *Management Research Review, 47*(11), 1805–1832. Advance online publication. DOI: 10.1108/MRR-07-2023-0496

Martinho, D., Rebelo, A., Field, A., Ribeiro, A. S., Pereira, F., Bizarro, B., Ribeiro, J., Len, S. M., Gouveia, É. R., & Sarmento, H. (2024). The quantification of physical performance and internal training load in youth male soccer players during preseason. *International Journal of Sports Physiology and Performance, 19*(5), 480–486. DOI: 10.1123/ijspp.2023-0312 PMID: 38437841

Mason, C. (2019). Adapting sports for young children. In *The physical development needs ofyoung children* (pp. 144–156). Routledge. DOI: 10.4324/9780429469831-12

Mastromartino, B., Ross, W. J., Wear, H., & Naraine, M. L. (2020). Thinking outside the 'box': A discussion of sports fans, teams, and the environment in the context of COVID-19. *Sport in Society, 23*(11), 1707–1723. DOI: 10.1080/17430437.2020.1804108

Mat-Rasid, S. M., Abdullah, M. R., Juahir, H., Maliki, A. B., Kosni, N. A., Musa, R. M., Hashim, M. R., Alnamat, A. S. F., Alias, N., & Najmi, N. (2019). Applied multidimensional analysis for assessing youth performance in sports talent identification program. *Int J Recent Technol Eng*Https://Doi. Org/10.35940/Ijrte. *B, 1051*, 0782S719.

Mat-Rasid, S. M., Abdullah, M. R., Juahir, H., Maliki, A., Musa, R. M., Kosni, N. A., Hashim, M. R., Eswaramoorthi, V., & Najmi, N. (2019). Determining youth profile using principle component analysis for identifying talent in sports. *International Journal of Recent Technology and Engineering, 8*(2), 212–215.

Mattesi, R. (2019). Social-media as platform for football clubs to increase revenues and enhance brand value.

McAuley, A. B., Baker, J., Johnston, K., & Kelly, A. L. (2024). Artificial intelligence in talent identification and development in sport. In *Artificial intelligence in sports, movement, and health* (pp. 255–270). Springer Nature Switzerland., DOI: 10.1007/978-3-031-67256-9_15

McCall, A., Dupont, G., & Ekstrand, J. (2016). Injury prevention strategies, coach compliance and player adherence of 33 of the UEFA Elite Club Injury Study teams: A survey of teams' head medical officers. *British Journal of Sports Medicine*, *50*(12), 725–730. DOI: 10.1136/bjsports-2015-095259 PMID: 26795611

McCullagh, J. (2010). Data mining in sport: A neural network approach. *International Journal of Sports Science and Engineering*, *4*(3), 131–138.

Mgaya, G. B., Liu, H., & Zhang, B. (2021). A survey on applications of modern deep learning techniques in team sports analytics. In *Proceedings of the 12th International Conference on Soft Computing and Pattern Recognition (SoCPaR 2020)* 12 (pp. 434-443). Springer International Publishing. DOI: 10.1007/978-3-030-73689-7_42

Miah, A., Fenton, A., & Chadwick, S. (2020). Virtual reality and sports: The rise of mixed, augmented, immersive, and esports experiences. *21st century sports: How technologies will change sports in the digital age*, 249-262.

Mielke, J., Schmidli, H., & Jones, B. (2018). Incorporating historical information in biosimilar trials: Challenges and a hybrid bayesian-frequentist approach. *Biometrical Journal. Biometrische Zeitschrift*, *60*(3), 564–582. DOI: 10.1002/bimj.201700152 PMID: 29532950

Miller, T. W. (2015). *Sports analytics and data science: Winning the game with methods and models*. FT Press.

Mishra, R., Rodriguez, R., & Portillo, V. (2020). An ai based talent acquisition and benchmarking for job. *ArXiv Preprint ArXiv:2009.09088.*

Mishra, N., Habal, B. G. M., Garcia, P. S., & Garcia, M. B. (2024, June). Harnessing an AI-Driven Analytics Model to Optimize Training and Treatment in Physical Education for Sports Injury Prevention. In *Proceedings of the 2024 8th International Conference on Education and Multimedia Technology* (pp. 309-315). DOI: 10.1145/3678726.3678740

Mondello, M., & Kamke, C. (2014). The introduction and application of sports analytics in professional sport organizations. *Journal of Applied Sport Management*, *6*(2), 11. DOI: 10.7290/jasm06ldmv

Moorefield, J. (2021). The Oakland Athletics use of sabermetrics and the rise of big data analytics in business.

Mosley, R. (2014). *Employer brand management: Practical lessons from the world's leading employers*. John Wiley & Sons.

Mountifield, C. (2023). Sport analytics: graduating from alchemy.. https://doi.org/ DOI: 10.5772/intechopen.1002423

Muniz, M., & Flamand, T. (2023). Sports analytics for balanced team-building decisions. *The Journal of the Operational Research Society*, *74*(8), 1892–1909. DOI: 10.1080/01605682.2022.2118634

Munoz-Macho, A. A., Domínguez-Morales, M. J., & Sevillano-Ramos, J. L. (2024). Performance and healthcare analysis in elite sports teams using artificial intelligence: A scoping review. *Frontiers in Sports and Active Living*, *6*, 1383723. DOI: 10.3389/fspor.2024.1383723 PMID: 38699628

Musa, R., Majeed, A., Suhaimi, M., Abdullah, M., Razman, M., Deboucha, A., & Osman, N. (2021). Identification of high-performance volleyball players from anthropometric variables and psychological readiness: A machine-learning approach. *Proceedings of the Institution of Mechanical Engineers. Part P, Journal of Sports Engineering and Technology*, *237*(4), 317–324. DOI: 10.1177/17543371211045451

Mustafa, B., & Branch, J. (2024). Innovations in the Metaverse: Merging Augmented Reality and Artificial Intelligence for Immersive User Experiences. *Innovations*, •••, 110.

Mwaro, P. N., Ogada, K., & Cheruiyot, W. (2021). Neural network model for talent recruitment and management for employee development and retention. *2021 IEEE AFRICON*, 1–6.

Myrén, A., & Neto, P. S. (2017). *Evaluation of Machine Learning Algorithms in Recommender Systems: Candidate Recommender Systems in the Staffing Industry*.

Nagai, T. (2017). Predicting herbicide mixture effects on multiple algal species using mixture toxicity models. *Environmental Toxicology and Chemistry*, *36*(10), 2624–2630. DOI: 10.1002/etc.3800 PMID: 28316094

Nahavandi, D., Alizadehsani, R., Khosravi, A., & Acharya, U. R. (2022). Application of artificial intelligence in wearable devices: Opportunities and challenges. *Computer Methods and Programs in Biomedicine*, *213*, 106541. DOI: 10.1016/j.cmpb.2021.106541 PMID: 34837860

Naik, B. T., Hashmi, M. F., & Bokde, N. D. (2022). A comprehensive review of computer vision in sports: Open issues, future trends and research directions. *Applied Sciences (Basel, Switzerland)*, *12*(9), 4429. DOI: 10.3390/app12094429

Najjar, M. C. (2023). Legal and Ethical Issues Arising from the Application of Data Analytics and Artificial Intelligence to Traditional Sports. *Alb. LJ Sci. & Tech.*, *33*, 51.

Nobari, H., Gorouhi, A., Mallo, J., Lozano, D., Prieto-González, P., & Mainer-Pardos, E. (2023). Variations in cumulative workload and anaerobic power in adolescent elite male football players: Associations with biological maturation. *BMC Sports Science, Medicine and Rehabilitation*, *15*(1), 11. Advance online publication. DOI: 10.1186/s13102-023-00623-5 PMID: 36721183

Novak, A. R., Bennett, K. J., Pluss, M. A., & Fransen, J. (2020). Performance analysis in esports: Modelling performance at the 2018 League of Legends World Championship. *International Journal of Sports Science & Coaching*, *15*(5-6), 809–817. DOI: 10.1177/1747954120932853

Nunes Rodrigues, A. C., Santos Pereira, A., Sousa Mendes, R. M., Araújo, A. G., Santos Couceiro, M., & Figueiredo, A. J. (2020). Using artificial intelligence for pattern recognition in a sports context. *Sensors (Basel)*, *20*(11), 3040. DOI: 10.3390/s20113040 PMID: 32471189

Olenich, T., Terarakelyants, V., Shestopalova, O., & Biryukov, I. (2020). Sport spirituality as an educational innovation (evidenced-based study). E3s Web of Conferences, 210, 17006. https://doi.org/DOI: 10.1051/e3sconf/202021017006

Oliva, A., & Olcina, J. (2023). Historical floods and territorial planning: Lessons learned and opportunities lost after the santa teresa flood (1879) in the segura basin (spain). *Land (Basel)*, *13*(1), 28. DOI: 10.3390/land13010028

Orme, S. (2020). Playing to win: The global esports industry and key issues. In *The Video Game Debate 2* (pp. 66–80). Routledge. DOI: 10.4324/9780429351815-6

Ossa, L. (2024). Integrating ethics in ai development: A qualitative study. *BMC Medical Ethics*, *25*(1), 10. Advance online publication. DOI: 10.1186/s12910-023-01000-0 PMID: 38262986

Oytun, M., Tınazcı, C., Şekeroğlu, B., Açıkada, C., & Yavuz, H. (2020). Performance prediction and evaluation in female handball players using machine learning models. *IEEE Access : Practical Innovations, Open Solutions*, *8*, 116321–116335. DOI: 10.1109/ACCESS.2020.3004182

Ozcaglar, C., Geyik, S., Schmitz, B., Sharma, P., Shelkovnykov, A., Ma, Y., & Buchanan, E. (2019). Entity personalized talent search models with tree interaction features. *The World Wide Web Conference*, 3116–3122. DOI: 10.1145/3308558.3313672

Panaccio, A., Mayo, N. E., and Pucher, K. (2019). Journal of Sport Rehabilitation, 28(2), 190-199. A comprehensive study of the relationship between physical fitness and the risk of musculoskeletal injuries: Part 2-Muscular strength and endurance.

Paneru, B., Paneru, B., Poudyal, R., & Poudyal, K. (2024). Enhancing soccer pass receiver prediction in broadcast images through advanced deep learning techniques: A comprehensive study on model optimization and performance evaluation. *Journal of Soft Computing Exploration*, *5*(2), 115–121. DOI: 10.52465/joscex.v5i2.301

Parganas, P., & Anagnostopoulos, C. (2015). Social media strategy in professional football: The case of Liverpool FC. *Choregia, 11*(2).

Parra-Martinez, F. A., & Wai, J. (2023). Talent identification research: A bibliometric study from multidisciplinary and global perspectives. *Frontiers in Psychology*, *14*, 1141159. DOI: 10.3389/fpsyg.2023.1141159 PMID: 37303914

Pashin, N. (2023). Development of the mathematical model for calculating player ratings using soft calculations. E3s Web of Conferences, 419, 02023. https://doi.org/DOI: 10.1051/e3sconf/202341902023

Pavitt, J., Braines, D., & Tomsett, R. (2022). Cognitive analysis in sports: Supporting match analysis and scouting through artificial intelligence. *Applied AI Letters*, *2*(1), e22.

Perumal, V. (2022). The future of US data privacy: Lessons from the GDPR and State Legislation. *Notre Dame J. Int'l Comp. L.*, *12*, 99.

Pinheiro, P., & Cavique, L. (2020). A bi-objective procedure to deliver actionable knowledge in sport services. *Expert Systems: International Journal of Knowledge Engineering and Neural Networks*, *37*(6), e12617. Advance online publication. DOI: 10.1111/exsy.12617

Previati, A. (2020). *The importance of fan engagement and fan management in sports*. St. John's University.

Pruna, R., Miñarro Tribaldos, L., & Bahdur, K. (2018). Player talent identification and development in football. *Apunts Sports Medicine*, *53*(198), 43–46. DOI: 10.1016/j.apunts.2018.02.002

Qin, C., Zhang, L., Zha, R., Shen, D., Zhang, Q., Sun, Y., Zhu, C., Zhu, H., & Xiong, H. (2023). A comprehensive survey of artificial intelligence techniques for talent analytics. *ArXiv Preprint ArXiv:2307.03195.*

Radicchi, E., & Mozzachiodi, M. (2016a). Social talent scouting: A new opportunity for the identification of football players? *Physical Culture and Sport Studies and Research*, *70*(1), 28–43. DOI: 10.1515/pcssr-2016-0012

Rafiq, M., Rafiq, G., Agyeman, R., Choi, G. S., & Jin, S. I. (2023). Scene classification for sports video summarization using transfer learning. *Sensors (Basel)*, *20*(6), 1702. DOI: 10.3390/s20061702 PMID: 32197502

Rasooli, M., Mehri, S., & Aziziani, M. (2024). Analyzing Liverpool FC website through fan management perspective. *Sports Marketing Studies*, *5*(2), 69–87.

Ráthonyi, G., Müller, A., & Rathonyi-Odor, K. (2018). How digital technologies are changing sport? *Apstract, Applied Studies in Agribusiness and Commerce*, *12*(3-4), 89–96. DOI: 10.19041/APSTRACT/2018/3-4/10

Ratno, P., Suprayitno, S., Hasibuan, R., & Fadli, Z. (2019). The Development of Karate Talent Scouting Identification Instrument. *Proceedings of The 5th Annual International Seminar on Trends in Science and Science Education, AISTSSE 2018,* 18-19 October 2018, Medan, Indonesia. DOI: 10.4108/eai.18-10-2018.2287433

Razali, N., Mustapha, A., Yatim, F. A., & Ab Aziz, R. (2017). Predicting player position for talent identification in association football. *IOP Conference Series. Materials Science and Engineering*, *226*(1), 012087. DOI: 10.1088/1757-899X/226/1/012087

Reeves, M. J., McRobert, A. P., Lewis, C. J., & Roberts, S. J. (2019). A case study of the use of verbal reports for talent identification purposes in soccer: A Messi affair! *PLoS One*, *14*(11), e0225033. DOI: 10.1371/journal.pone.0225033 PMID: 31714943

Reilly, T., Williams, A. M., & Richardson, D. (2003). Identifying talented players. In *Science and soccer* (pp. 315–334). Routledge. DOI: 10.4324/9780203417553

Rein, I., Shields, B., & Grossman, A. (2015). *The sports strategist: Developing leaders for a high-performance industry*. Oxford University Press.

Reyaz, N., Ahamad, G., Khan, N. J., & Naseem, M. (2022). Machine Learning in Sports Talent Identification: A Systematic Review. *2022 2nd International Conference on Emerging Frontiers in Electrical and Electronic Technologies (ICEFEET)*, 1–6.

Reyaz, N., Ahamad, G., Khan, N. J., Naseem, M., & Ali, J. (2024). SVMCTI: Support vector machine based cricket talent identification model. *International Journal of Information Technology : an Official Journal of Bharati Vidyapeeth's Institute of Computer Applications and Management*, *16*(3), 1931–1944. DOI: 10.1007/s41870-023-01686-w

Reynoso-Sanchez, L. F. (2023). Tech-driven talent identification in sports: Advancements and implications. *Health Nexus, 1*(3), 77–82. DOI: 10.61838/kman.hn.1.3.11

Rija, T. H., Mohammed, T. K., & Kadhlm, R. A. (2023). The role of organizational development in improving the reality of the work of the administrative bodies to manage active sports clubs in Baghdad. *Revista Iberoamericana de Psicología del Ejercicio y el Deporte, 18*(3), 298–304.

Robel, M. (2023). Cricket players selection for national team and franchise league using machine learning algorithms. Cloud Computing and Data Science, 108-139. https://doi.org/DOI: 10.37256/ccds.5120243741

Rossi, A., Pappalardo, L., Cintia, P., Iaia, F. M., Fernández, J., & Medina, D. (2018). Effective injury forecasting in soccer with GPS training data and machine learning. *PLoS One, 13*(7), e0201264. DOI: 10.1371/journal.pone.0201264 PMID: 30044858

Roychoudhury, S., & Neuenschwander, B. (2020). Bayesian leveraging of historical control data for a clinical trial with time-to-event endpoint. *Statistics in Medicine, 39*(7), 984–995. DOI: 10.1002/sim.8456 PMID: 31985077

Rubleske, J., Fletcher, T., & Westerfeld, B. (2020). E-sports analytics: A primer and resource for student research projects and lesson plans. *Journal of Instructional Pedagogies, 23*.

Ryan, C. W. (2014). In Runyan, C. W. (Ed.), *Overview of preventing injuries. *Handbook of Injury and Violence Prevention* (pp. 3–20). Springer.

Sajadi, S. M., Baghaie, S., & Rezaei, R. (2024). Optimizing sports development: Identifying and prioritizing key indicators for professional and competitive sports. *World Development, 180*, 106651. DOI: 10.1016/j.worlddev.2024.106651

Salim, F., Haider, F., Postma, D., Delden, R., Reidsma, D., Luz, S., & Beijnum, B. (2020). Towards automatic modeling of volleyball players' behavior for analysis, feedback, and hybrid training. *Journal for the Measurement of Physical Behaviour, 3*(4), 323–330. DOI: 10.1123/jmpb.2020-0012

Sampaio, T., Oliveira, J. P., Marinho, D. A., Neiva, H. P., & Morais, J. E. (2024). Applications of machine learning to optimize tennis performance: A systematic review. *Applied Sciences (Basel, Switzerland), 14*(13), 5517. DOI: 10.3390/app14135517

Sandamal, K., Arachchi, S., Erkudov, V. O., Rozumbetov, K. U., & Rathnayake, U. (2024). Explainable artificial intelligence for fitness prediction of young athletes living in unfavorable environmental conditions. *Results in Engineering, 23*, 102592. DOI: 10.1016/j.rineng.2024.102592

Sangarsu, R. (2022). Securing the organization's sensitive data in the ai era. *Design of Single Chip Microcomputer Control System for Stepping Motor, 1-3*, 1–3. Advance online publication. DOI: 10.47363/JAICC/2022(1)175

Sanjaykumar, S., Udaichi, K., Rajendiran, G., Cretu, M., & Kozina, Z. (2024). Cricket performance predictions: A comparative analysis of machine learning models for predicting cricket player's performance in the one day international (odi) world cup 2023. *Health Sport Rehabilitation, 10*(1), 6–19. DOI: 10.58962/HSR.2024.10.1.6-19

Sarkar, P., & Ghosh, M. M. (2023, December). Virtual reality in sports–Redefining audience engagement and expectations. In *AIP Conference Proceedings* (Vol. 2914, No. 1). AIP Publishing. DOI: 10.1063/5.0175846

Sarlis, V., & Tjortjis, C. (2020). Sports analytics—Evaluation of basketball players and team performance. *Information Systems, 93*, 101562. DOI: 10.1016/j.is.2020.101562

Sarmento, H., Anguera, M. T., Pereira, A., & Araújo, D. (2018). Talent identification and development in male football: A systematic review. *Sports Medicine (Auckland, N.Z.), 48*(4), 907–931. DOI: 10.1007/s40279-017-0851-7 PMID: 29299878

Savić, Z., Ranđelović, N., Stojanović, N., Stanković, V., & Šiljak, V. (2018). The sports industry and achieving top sports results. *Facta Universitatis. Series: Physical Education and Sport, 15*(3), 513–522. DOI: 10.22190/FUPES1703513S

Sayal, A., Jha, J., Chaithra, N., Gupta, V., Gupta, A., Gupta, O., & Memoria, M. (2023). Neural Networks And Machine Learning. *2023 IEEE 5th International Conference on Cybernetics, Cognition and Machine Learning Applications (IC-CCMLA)*, 58–63.

Schöber, T., Stadtmann, G., Parshakov, P., & Tylkin, I. (2024). Survival of professional counter-strike: Global offensive teams: What matters? A research note. *Journal of Electronic Gaming and Esports, 2*(1). Advance online publication. DOI: 10.1123/jege.2022-0025

Schoenfeld, B. (2023). *Game of edges: The analytics revolution and the future of professional sports*. WW Norton & Company.

Selmi, O., Ouergui, I., Muscella, A., My, G., Marsigliante, S., Nobari, H., Suzuki, K., & Bouassida, A. (2022). Monitoring psychometric states of recovery to improve performance in soccer players: A brief review. *International Journal of Environmental Research and Public Health, 19*(15), 9385. DOI: 10.3390/ijerph19159385 PMID: 35954741

Seng, K. P., Ang, L. M., Peter, E., & Mmonyi, A. (2023). Machine learning and AI technologies for smart wearables. *Electronics (Basel)*, *12*(7), 1509. DOI: 10.3390/electronics12071509

Serôdio, A., Claudino, R., Santos-Rocha, R., & Sobreiro, P. (2018). Approach to management by processes in a sports department of a local government organization. *Motricidade*, *14*(2-3), 79–94. DOI: 10.6063/motricidade.13760

Seshadri, D. R., Li, R. T., Voos, J. E., Rowbottom, J. R., Alfes, C. M., Zorman, C. A., & Drummond, C. K. (2019). Wearable sensors for monitoring the internal and external workload of the athlete. *NPJ Digital Medicine*, *2*(1), 71. DOI: 10.1038/s41746-019-0149-2 PMID: 31372506

Shapiro, N. I., Miller, S. C., & Brown, T. M. (2020). Using machine learning to predict physiological deterioration within 72 hours. *Journal of Hospital Medicine*, *15*(12), 714–720.

Sikorska, I., Serban, I., Mihaela, T., & Sorin, C. (2014, May). Sports as a protective factor in adaptation to disability. In *The Second World Congress on Resilience: From Person to Society* (pp. 1209-1212).

Silacci, A., Taiar, R., & Caon, M. (2020). Towards an AI-based tailored training planning for road cyclists: A case study. *Applied Sciences (Basel, Switzerland)*, *11*(1), 313. DOI: 10.3390/app11010313

Singh, A., Nath, C., & Kumari, P. (2020). * [Artificial intelligence and machine learning algorithms: Understanding the applications in healthcare industry.]. *Journal of Clinical and Diagnostic Research : JCDR*, *14*(5), ZE10–ZE14.

Skora, L., Seth, A., & Scott, R. (2020). Sensorimotor predictions shape reported conscious visual experience in a breaking continuous flash suppression task. DOI: 10.31234/osf.io/hwkdj

Smith, A., & Westerbeek, H. (2004). *The sport business future*. Bound in Great Britain. DOI: 10.1057/9780230513693

Son, N. T., Van Thanh, L., Duong, T. B., & Anh, B. N. (2018, August). A decision support tool for cross-functional team selection: Case study in ACM-ICPC team selection. In *Proceedings of the 1st International Conference on Information Management and Management Science* (pp. 133-138). DOI: 10.1145/3277139.3277149

Spaaij, R., & Thiel, A. (2017). Big data: Critical questions for sport and society. *European Journal of Sport Science*, *14*(1), 1–4. DOI: 10.1080/16138171.2017.1288374 PMID: 27800713

Sridevi, G. M., & Kamala Suganthi, S. (2021). Artificial intelligence-based job applicant profile quality assessment and relevance ranking using clusters in talent acquisition process. *Applications of Artificial Intelligence in Engineering: Proceedings of First Global Conference on Artificial Intelligence and Applications (GCAIA 2020)*, 461–472.

Starling, L., Nellemann, S., Parkes, A., & Lambert, M. (2019). The fatigue and fitness test for teams (FFITT): A practical option for monitoring athletes in a team as individuals. *European Journal of Sport Science, 20*(1), 106–114. DOI: 10.1080/17461391.2019.1612951 PMID: 31109238

Starling, L., Nellemann, S., Parkes, A., & Lambert, M. (2020). The sensitivity of the fatigue and fitness test for teams (FFITT) to measure the demands of a rugby match. *European Journal of Sport Science, 21*(6), 803–810. DOI: 10.1080/17461391.2020.1780327 PMID: 32511079

Subha, T., Ranjana, R., Aarthi, B., Pavithra, S., & Srinidhi, M. S. (2022). Skill Analysis and Scouting Platform Using Machine Learning. *2022 International Conference on Communication, Computing and Internet of Things (IC3IoT)*, 1–6. DOI: 10.1109/IC3IOT53935.2022.9767872

Sullivan, P. J., & Callow, N. (2005). A cross-cultural examination of the factor structure of the scale for effective communication in team sports. *Group Dynamics, 9*(2), 87–92. DOI: 10.1037/1089-2699.9.2.87

Sümer, S. I., & Parilti, N. (Eds.). (2023). *Social Media Analytics in Predicting Consumer Behavior*. CRC Press. DOI: 10.1201/9781003200154

Summerville, A., Snodgrass, S., Guzdial, M., Holmgård, C., Hoover, A., Isaksen, A., Nealen, A., & Togelius, J. (2018). Procedural content generation via machine learning (pcgml). *IEEE Transactions on Games, 10*(3), 257–270. DOI: 10.1109/TG.2018.2846639

Suresh Babu, C. V., Akshayah, N. S., & Maclin Vinola, P. (2024). Artificial Intelligence in Healthcare: Assessing Impacts, Challenges, and Recommendations for Achieving Healthcare Independence. In Geada, N., & Jamil, G. (Eds.), *Perspectives on Artificial Intelligence in Times of Turbulence: Theoretical Background to Applications* (pp. 61–80). IGI Global., DOI: 10.4018/978-1-6684-9814-9.ch005

Suresh Babu, C. V., & Praveen, S. (2023). Swarm Intelligence and Evolutionary Machine Learning Algorithms for COVID-19: Pandemic and Epidemic Review. In Suresh Kumar, A., Kose, U., Sharma, S., & Jerald Nirmal Kumar, S. (Eds.), *Dynamics of Swarm Intelligence Health Analysis for the Next Generation* (pp. 83–103). IGI Global., DOI: 10.4018/978-1-6684-6894-4.ch005

Szymanski, S. (2020). Sport analytics: Science or alchemy? *Kinesiology Review (Champaign, Ill.)*, *9*(1), 57–63. DOI: 10.1123/kr.2019-0066

Tan, X. (2023). Enhanced sports predictions: A comprehensive analysis of the role and performance of predictive analytics in the sports sector. *Wireless Personal Communications*, *132*(3), 1613–1636. DOI: 10.1007/s11277-023-10585-z

Tekade, P., Markad, K., Amage, A., & Natekar, B. (2020). Cricket match outcome prediction using machine learning. *International Journal of Advance Scientific Research and Engineering Trends*, *5*(7).

Thomas, G., Gade, R., Moeslund, T. B., Carr, P., & Hilton, A. (2017). Computer vision for sports: Current applications and research topics. *Computer Vision and Image Understanding*, *159*, 3–18. DOI: 10.1016/j.cviu.2017.04.011

Thorne, K., & Pellant, A. (2007). *The essential guide to managing talent: How top companies recruit, train, & retain the best employees*. Kogan Page Publishers.

Till, K., & Baker, J. (2020). Challenges and [possible] solutions to optimizing talent identification and development in sport. *Frontiers in Psychology*, *11*, 664. DOI: 10.3389/fpsyg.2020.00664 PMID: 32351427

Uddin, M. F., & Lee, J. (2017). Predicting Educational Relevance For an Efficient Classification of Talent. *2017 ASEE Northeast Section Conference*.

Utamayasa, I. G. D. (2021). Talent Identification of Future Sportsmen Using Sport Search Application. *Budapest International Research and Critics Institute-Journal (BIRCI-Journal)*, *4*(1), 690–695.

Vasiljevas, M., Damaševičius, R., & Maskeliūnas, R. (2023). A human-adaptive model for user performance and fatigue evaluation during gaze-tracking tasks. *Electronics (Basel)*, *12*(5), 1130. DOI: 10.3390/electronics12051130

Vennila, G., Mounica, P., Prasanna, P. L., Kumar, P. P., & Sirisha, R. (2024, May). Enhancing Speech Emotion Recognition using Deep Learning Networks on Live Calls. In 2024 5th International Conference for Emerging Technology (INCET) (pp. 1-8). IEEE.

Vilela, T., Portela, F., & Santos, M. F. (2018). Towards a Pervasive Intelligent System on Football Scouting-A Data Mining Study Case. *Trends and Advances in Information Systems and Technologies*, *3*(6), 341–351. DOI: 10.1007/978-3-319-77700-9_34

Vinué, G., & Epifanio, I. (2017). Archetypoid analysis for sports analytics. *Data Mining and Knowledge Discovery*, *31*(6), 1643–1677. DOI: 10.1007/s10618-017-0514-1

Waheed, S., Zaim, A. H., Zaim, H., Sertbas, A., & Akyokus, S. (2014). Application of neural networks in talent management. *2013 International Conference on Electrical Information and Communication Technology (EICT)*, 1–4. DOI: 10.1109/EICT.2014.6777833

Wang, J., Liu, S., & Li, S. (2021).. . *Journal of Business Ethics*, *169*(4), 603–615. DOI: 10.1007/s10551-020-04549-7

Wang, Z., & Gao, Z. (2021). Analysis of real-time heartbeat monitoring using wearable device Internet of Things system in sports environment. *Computational Intelligence*, *37*(3), 1080–1097. DOI: 10.1111/coin.12337

Wertheim-Heck, S., & Spaargaren, G. (2015). Shifting configurations of shopping practices and food safety dynamics in hanoi, vietnam: A historical analysis. *Agriculture and Human Values*, *33*(3), 655–671. DOI: 10.1007/s10460-015-9645-4

WHO. (2020). *Injuries and violence: The facts*. World Health Organization.

Williams, A. M., Ford, P. R., & Drust, B. (2020). Talent identification and development in soccer since the millennium. *Journal of Sports Sciences*, *38*(11–12), 1199–1210. DOI: 10.1080/02640414.2020.1766647 PMID: 32568000

Williams, A. M., & Reilly, T. (2000). Talent identification and development in soccer. *Journal of Sports Sciences*, *18*(9), 657–667. DOI: 10.1080/02640410050120041 PMID: 11043892

Wisdom, C., & Javed, A. (2023). Machine learning for data analytics in football: Quantifying performance and enhancing strategic decision-making. *Available atSSRN* 4558733. DOI: 10.2139/ssrn.4558733

Wishart, D. S., & Cruz, J. A. (2020). Machine learning applications in environmental sciences and human health. *. *Briefings in Bioinformatics*, *21*(4), 1239–1251.

Woods, C. T., Joyce, C., & Robertson, S. (2016). What are talent scouts actually identifying? Investigating the physical and technical skill match activity profiles of drafted and non-drafted U18 Australian footballers. *Journal of Science and Medicine in Sport*, *19*(5), 419–423. DOI: 10.1016/j.jsams.2015.04.013 PMID: 25963663

Wrang, C. M., Rossing, N. N., Agergaard, S., & Martin, L. J. (2022). The missing children: A systematic scoping review on talent identification and selection in football (soccer). *EJSS European Journal for Sport and Society*, *19*(2), 135–150. DOI: 10.1080/16138171.2021.1916224

Wu, C. W., Shieh, M. D., Lien, J. J. J., Yang, J. F., Chu, W. T., Huang, T. H., Hsieh, H.-C., Chiu, H.-T., Tu, K.-C., Chen, Y.-T., Lin, S.-Y., Hu, J.-J., Lin, C.-H., & Jheng, C. S. (2022). Enhancing fan engagement in a 5G stadium with AI-based technologies and live streaming. *IEEE Systems Journal, 16*(4), 6590–6601. DOI: 10.1109/JSYST.2022.3169553

Xiao, Q., Zhong, X., & Zhong, C. (2020). Application research of KNN algorithm based on clustering in big data talent demand information classification. *International Journal of Pattern Recognition and Artificial Intelligence, 34*(06), 2050015. DOI: 10.1142/S0218001420500159

Xu, H., Yu, Z., Yang, J., Xiong, H., & Zhu, H. (2016). Talent circle detection in job transition networks. *Proceedings of the 22nd ACM SIGKDD International Conference on Knowledge Discovery and Data Mining*, 655–664. DOI: 10.1145/2939672.2939732

Yan, C. (2022). The impact of artificial intelligence on sports. International Journal of Sports, Yoga and Physical Activity, ISSN, 3005-5083.

Yang, L., Tian, M., Xin, D., Cheng, Q., & Zheng, J. (2024). Ai-driven anonymization: Protecting personal data privacy while leveraging machine learning. *Applied and Computational Engineering, 71*(1), 7–13. DOI: 10.54254/2755-2721/71/2024MA0053

Ye, J., Hu, H., & Chai, C. (2009). A talent classification method based on SVM. *2009 International Symposium on Intelligent Ubiquitous Computing and Education*, 160–163. DOI: 10.1109/IUCE.2009.63

Yi, F., Yu, Z., Xu, H., & Guo, B. (2019). Talents recommendation with multi-aspect preference learning. *Green, Pervasive, and Cloud Computing:13th International Conference, GPC 2018,Hangzhou, China,May 11-13, 2018, Revised Selected Papers 13*, 409–423.

Youping, L., & Jiangang, S. (2022). Talent Recruitment Platform for Large-Scale Group Enterprises Based on Deep Learning. *2022 7th International Conference on Cloud Computing and Big Data Analytics (ICCCBDA)*, 172–176.

Zhou, H., & Xiong, Z. (2024). Navigating the Digital Frontier: Inherent Mechanisms, Challenges, and Strategies for Sports Consumption Upgrade in the Digital Economy. *Journal of the Knowledge Economy*, •••, 1–40. DOI: 10.1007/s13132-024-02005-9

Zilio, F., Prates, M., & Lamb, L. (2018). Neural networks models for analyzing magic: the gathering cards., 227-239. DOI: 10.1007/978-3-030-04179-3_20

# About The Contributors

**Tanupriya Choudhury** completed his undergraduate studies in Computer Science and Engineering at the West Bengal University of Technology in Kolkata (2004-2008), India, followed by a Master's Degree in the same field from Dr. M.G.R University in Chennai, India (2008-2010). In 2016, he successfully obtained his PhD degree from Jagannath University, Jaipur. With a total of 16 years of experience in both teaching and research, Dr. Choudhury holds the position of Visiting Professor at Daffodil International University Bangladesh. Currently, he is working as a Professor at UPES Dehradun India, prior to this role he had worked as Associate Dean of Research at Graphic Era Deemed to be University, Dehradun, India. Prior to this role, he served Symbiosis International Deemed University Pune, Graphic Era Hill University Dehradun (Research Professor), UPES Dehradun (Professor and Research Head Informatics), Amity University Noida (Assistant Professor Grade 3 and International Dept. Head), and other prestigious academic institutions (Dronacharya College of Engineering Gurgaon, Lingaya's University Faridabad, Babu Banarsi Das Institute of Technology Ghaziabad, Syscon Solutions Pvt. Ltd. Kolkata etc.). Recently recognized for his outstanding contributions to education with the Global Outreach Education Award for Excellence in Best Young Researcher Award at GOECA 2018. His areas of expertise encompass Human Computing, Soft Computing, Cloud Computing, Data Mining among others. Notably accomplished within his field thus far is filing 25 patents and securing copyrights for 16 software programs from MHRD (Ministry of Human Resource Development). He has actively participated as an attendee or speaker at numerous National and International conferences across India and abroad. With more than 150 research papers (Scopus) authored to date on record; Dr. Choudhury has also been invited as a guest lecturer or keynote speaker at esteemed institutions such as Jamia Millia Islamia University, Maharaja Agersen College (Delhi University), Duy Tan University Vietnam etc.He has also contributed significantly to various conferences throughout India serving roles like TPC member and session chairperson. As an active professional within the technical community; Dr.Choudhury holds lifetime membership with IETA (International Engineering & Technology Association) along with being affiliated with IEEE (Institute of Electrical and Electronics Engineers), IET(UK) (Institution of Engineering & Technology UK),and other reputable technical societies.Additionally, he is associated with corporate entities and serves as a Technical Adviser for Deetya Soft Pvt. Ltd., Noida, IVRGURU, and Mydigital360.He is also serving a Editor's in reputed Journals. He currently serves as the Honorary Secretary in IETA (Indian Engineering Teacher's Association-India), alongside his role as the Senior Advisor Position in INDO-UK Confederation of Science, Technology and Research Ltd., London, UK and International Association of Professional and Fellow Engineers-Delaware-USA.

***

**Priyanka Bharti**, received B.E., M. Tech and PhD Degree in Computer Science & Engg. from Visveswaraya Technological University, Belagavi. She is currently working as an Associate Professor at REVA University, Bengaluru, INDIA. She has experience of around 15 years in teaching and research. She is involved in research in areas of Cloud and HPC applications.

**Ajay Chandel** is working as an Associate Professor at Mittal School of Business, Lovely Professional University, Punjab. He has 14 years of teaching and research experience. He has published papers in SCOPUS, WOS, and UGC listed Journals in areas like Social Media Marketing, E-Commerce, and Consumer Behaviour. He has published cases on SMEs and Social Entrepreneurship in The Case Centre, UK. He also reviews The Case Journal, Emerald Group Publishing, and International Journal of Business and Globalisation, Inderscience. He has authored and developed MOOCs on Tourism and Hospitality Marketing under Epg-Pathshala- A gateway to all postgraduate courses (a UGC-MHRD project under its National Mission on Education Through ICT (NME-ICT).

**Suman Devi** is currently working as Assistant Professor in School of Computing Science & Engineering. She has total experience of more than 11 years of teaching and has been associated with Galgotias University since 2017. Along with she is a research scholar in the Department of CSE at Galgotias University, India. She is firm Believer of productivity and efficiency in work. She exhibits an honest work ethic with the ability to excel in fast-paced, time-sensitive environment. Being a passionate teacher, she believes that teaching is not merely restricted to making the students understand the underlying concepts of a course but also to develop critical thinking and evaluate alternate approaches for problem solving. He always put his efforts towards the overall developments of her students. Her research interest area is Wireless sensor networks, Security. She has published several papers in peer reviewed journal and international conferences. She also organized and attended several workshops.

**Toufique Ahammad Gazi** is pursuing a PhD from UEM in Kolkata. He earned his MTech from Supreme Knowledge Foundation Group of Institutions West Bengal, India, in 2017 and his BTech from Kalyani Government Engineering College, India, in 2010. He currently works as an Assistant Professor in the Department of Computer Science and Engineering at Techno International New Town in India. He has around 11 years of teaching experience. His research interests include network security, machine learning for recommendation systems, mobile robot navigation planning with soft computing, and digital image processing.

**Geshwaree Huzooree** serves as the Programme Leader for BA Business Management and lecturer specialising in Strategy and Project Management within the MBA Programme at Edinburgh Napier University. Before joining the faculty at Edinburgh Napier, she held the position of Senior Lecturer at Curtin Mauritius for a commendable eight years. Driven by her passion for the field, she brings seven years of valuable experience in the IT industry, focusing on software application development and project management. Her academic achievements include a Ph.D. in Computer Science (2020), an MSc in Software Engineering Projects and Management (2014), and a BSc in Computer Science and Engineering (2007), all earned from the esteemed University of Mauritius. Dr. Geshwaree's professional reach extends globally, fostering close collaborations with various universities and institutions. Her research pursuits encompass diverse areas such as project management, remote working, the future workforce, health informatics, and digital technologies. She is dedicated to conducting innovative research that addresses national challenges, contributing to a better future.

**Preet Kanwal** completed her Post-Doctoral Fellowship at the ESG, University of Quebec in Montreal, Quebec, Canada, furthering research expertise in her field. During her Post Doctoral Fellowship, she worked on exploring demographic sensitivity and its impact on discrimination in HEIs while considering insights from Canada and India. Dr. Kanwal is an academician and researcher with over 22 years of experience in Human Resource Management. She holds a PhD in Human Resource Management from I.K. Gujral Punjab Technical University, Punjab, India, where she conducted an empirical study on the quality of work life in the textile industry of Punjab, India. She also has international experience teaching MBA students from Victoria University (Online), Australia, and Sunway University (Online),

Malaysia. Dr. Kanwal's research interests revolve around the quality of work-life, work-life balance, industrial relations, labour laws, social security and labour welfare, organizational stress, and behaviour, particularly in the context of the textile industry. She has presented her research at numerous national and international conferences and published her work in Scopus-indexed and UGC-listed Journals. Additionally, she has authored more than 25 book chapters and research papers on related topics, underscoring her commitment to advancing knowledge in her field. Her contributions extend beyond teaching and research; she has been actively involved in organizing and leading training sessions, workshops, and conferences, both as a participant and as a session chair. Currently, she is working on a funded project titled, "Empowering Women Artisans for Vision Viksit Bharat@2047: Financial Inclusion, Market Access, and Skill Development in Selected States of India". She has organised an ICSSR-sponsored International Conference, "Empowering Women Artisans for Vision Viksit Bharat@2047: Financial Inclusion, Market Access, and Skill Development" at Mittal School of Business, Lovely Professional University.

**Tarun Kumar** is currently working as Assistant Professor in School of Computer Science & Engineering. He has total experience of more than 18 years of teaching and has been associated with Galgotias University since 2017. Along with he is a research scholar in the Department of CSE at the National Institute of Technology Patna, Bihar, India. He is firm Believer of productivity and efficiency in work. He exhibits an honest work ethic with the ability to excel in fast-paced, time-sensitive environment. Being a passionate teacher, he believes that teaching is not merely restricted to making the students understand the underlying concepts of a course but also to develop critical thinking and evaluate alternate approaches for problem solving. He always put his efforts towards the overall developments of his students. His research interest area is Cloud Computing, DNA Computing. He has published several papers in peer reviewed journal and international conferences. He also organized and attended several workshops and conferences.

**Minakshi** is an accomplished academician with 18+ years of experience in computer science and engineering domains. Currently an Assistant Professor at King Khalid University, she has taught at esteemed institutions like Uttaranchal University and Tula's Institute. A prolific researcher with 80 Scopus publications, 18 patents, and 3 software copyrights, she has received accolades like Outstanding Section Volunteer Award (IEEE UP Section), Research Excellence Award, and HOD of the Year Award. Adept at curriculum development, research guidance, project management, and team leadership, Dr. Minakshi brings a holistic approach to education, fostering student success through quality instruction and innovative pedagogical methods.

**Thi Minh Ngoc Luu** is currently the Head of the Department of Economics and Management at the International School, Vietnam National University, Hanoi. She has over 17 years of experience in teaching and researching human resource management, management control, corporate governance, individual and organizational behavior, leadership, and sustainable development.

**Shashank Mittal** has done his FPM in Organizational behavior and Human Resource from Indian Institute of Management Raipur. He holds B. Tech from I.E.T. Lucknow. His post FPM work experience includes almost five years of industry and academics exposures in multiple roles. Prior to joining FPM, he has over two years of industrial experience and three years of teaching experience in various organizations. He has published multiple papers in ABDC ranked and SSCI indexed journals of international repute such as Journal of Knowledge Management, Journal of Behavioral and Experimental Finance, International Journal of Conflict Management, Journal of Management and Organization and Current Psychology. His current research interest includes Social identity, Knowledge exchanges, Status, Proactive helping, Employer branding, Organizational justice, and Humanitarian relief management. He enjoys badminton and cycling during leisure time.

**Anusha Palagati** is an Assistant Professor in the Department of Computer Science and Engineering at Guru Nanak Institute of Technology, Hyderabad. She has a diverse educational background, having completed her B.Tech in IT from JB Women's Engineering College, Tirupati, in 2012, and her M.Tech in CSE with Distinction from Geethanjali Institute of Technology, Nellore, in 2015. Currently, she is pursuing a Ph.D. at Anna University, Chennai. She holds 9 years of experience in the teaching field. She has made significant contributions to her field, having published 2 books and 2 book chapter, 16 articles in reputed journals, and 14 patent publications. Additionally, she has attended 10 conferences at both national and international levels.

**Kaushik Paul**, After H.S. he has completed B.Sc.(Mathematics) in 2003 from Barasat Govt. College(C.U.), then he has completed M.C.A. from Techno India(W.B.U.T.) in 2006 and after that he has completed M.Tech(IT) from RCCIIT(MAKAUT) in 2017. From 2007 he worked as a full time faculty in DOEACC computer centre, then worked in Kingston Engineering college from 2010 and after that he worked in Regent Education and Research Foundation from 2012 to January, 2023 as a Assistant Professor in CSE Department, then from 2023,february he worked at Elitte Engineering College as a Assistant Professor in CST Department and he is working now at Brainware University from November, 2023 as a Assistant Professor in CSE Department. In between he worked as visiting faculty at Techno

India, Camellia Institute of Technology, Torsa Management Institute side by side doing permanent job.

**Rohit** is a Research Associate at Thumbay College of Management and AI in Healthcare, Gulf Medical University, UAE. He is MBA from Kurukshetra University Kurukshetra (A state government public university), India. He has published research papers in international journals and participated in various international conferences, workshops, and seminars. He worked as a management trainee and intern in the Thumbay Hospital, United Arab Emirates (UAE); Decathlon, Zirakpur, India; and Bajaj Allianz General Insurance, India. He completed various MOOCs from Copenhagen Business School, University of New Mexico, University of California, Irvine, University of London, and many other. His areas of interest are Entrepreneurship, consumer behavior, marketing strategies and strategic management. He is inspired with thought leadership and a regular contributor to educational magazines, debates, and cultural activities. He can be reached at rohit27.sr@gmail.com

**Gopal Krishna Shyam**, received B.E., M. Tech and PhD Degree in Computer Science & Engg. from Visveswaraya Technological University, Belagavi. He is currently working as a Professor and HoD in School of Computer Engineering, Presidency University, Bengaluru, INDIA. He has experience of around 17 years in teaching and research. He is involved in research in areas of Cloud/Grid computing, E-commerce, Protocol engineering, and Artificial intelligence applications. As per google scholar, he has around 1500 citations. Some of his publications on Resource Management in Cloud Computing are among top down loaded articles in Elsevier Journals of Network and Computer Applications. He is reviewer of several international/national Journals published by Elsevier, IEEE, ACM, Springer, etc. He has been technical program committee member of more than 5 National/International Conferences. He has guided 32 B.E/ MTech Candidates, 2 PhD candidates and is currently guiding 4 PhD Scholars. He has given 5 invited talks at various engineering colleges.

**Sandeep Kumar Singh** is a faculty in the area of Information Systems and Analytics at Jindal Global Business School, O.P. Jindal Global University, Sonipat. Prior to joining Jindal Global Business School, he worked as an Assistant Professor at JKLU Jaipur for two years. He has earned his Ph.D. in computational physics from Antwerpen University, Belgium. His PhD work focused on mathematical modeling and simulation of two-dimensional materials. Post to his PhD, he worked as a research scientist in Sweden for four years in energy storage systems, bioelectronics. He also did MTech in industrial mathematics and scientific computing from IIT

Madras, Chennai. His current research interests are to apply complex mathematical modeling in the business and financial world.

**C.V. Suresh Babu** is a pioneer in content development. A true entrepreneur, he founded Anniyappa Publications, a company that is highly active in publishing books related to Computer Science and Management. Dr. C.V. Suresh Babu has also ventured into SB Institute, a center for knowledge transfer. He holds a Ph.D. in Engineering Education from the National Institute of Technical Teachers Training & Research in Chennai, along with seven master's degrees in various disciplines such as Engineering, Computer Applications, Management, Commerce, Economics, Psychology, Law, and Education. Additionally, he has UGC-NET/SET qualifications in the fields of Computer Science, Management, Commerce, and Education. Currently, Dr. C.V. Suresh Babu is a Professor in the Department of Information Technology at the School of Computing Science, Hindustan Institute of Technology and Science (Hindustan University) in Padur, Chennai, Tamil Nadu, India.

**Huy Hung Ta**, Lecture in Economics and Management, International School, Vietnam National University Hanoi, former of Vice Director International Program cooperate between Toulon University and Academy of Finance

**Mohit Yadav** is an Associate Professor in the area of Human Resource Management at Jindal Global Business School (JGBS). He has a rich blend of work experience from both Academics as well as Industry. Prof. Mohit holds a Ph.D. from Department of Management Studies, Indian Institute of Technology Roorkee (IIT Roorkee) and has completed Master of Human Resource and Organizational Development (MHROD) from prestigious Delhi School of Economics, University of Delhi. He also holds a B.Com (Hons.) degree from University of Delhi and UGC-JRF scholarship. He has published various research papers and book chapters with reputed publishers like Springer, Sage, Emerald, Elsevier, Inderscience etc. and presented research papers in national and International conferences both in India and abroad. He has many best paper awards on his credit too. He is reviewer of various international journals like Computers in Human Behavior, Policing etc. His areas of interest are Organizational Behavior, HRM, Recruitment and Selection, Organizational Citizenship Behavior, Quality of work life and role.

**Shubhankar Yadav**, Currently, he is pursuing B.Tech in Cybersecurity. He loves learning new things, networking with like minded people and sharing his experience, thought and ideas. In regards to future career, he has a wish of learning and understanding the complete existing working of the industry and then get himself into the same with a team of his who matches the same enthusiasm.

# Index

## A



## B



## C



## D



## E

## F



## G



## H



## I



## M



## P



## R

## S



## T



## V



## W

www.ingramcontent.com/pod-product-compliance
Lightning Source LLC
LaVergne TN
LVHW061548290926
849162LV00004B/948